**The Eye in Clinical Practice**

# The Eye in Clinical Practice

## Peggy Frith
Consultant Ophthalmic Physician
The Eye Hospital
Oxford

## Roger Gray
Consultant Ophthalmologist
Taunton and Somerset
NHS Trust

## Sally MacLennan
Clinical Assistant
The Eye Hospital
Oxford

## Phillip Ambler
General Practitioner, Wantage
and Clinical Assistant in Ophthalmology
The Eye Hospital
Oxford

SECOND EDITION

*b*

**Blackwell
Science**

© 1994, 2001 by
Blackwell Science Ltd
Editorial Offices:
Osney Mead, Oxford OX2 0EL
25 John Street, London WC1N 2BS
23 Ainslie Place, Edinburgh EH3 6AJ
350 Main Street, Malden
   MA 02148-5018, USA
54 University Street, Carlton
   Victoria 3053, Australia
10, rue Casimir Delavigne
   75006 Paris, France

Other Editorial Offices:
Blackwell Wissenschafts-Verlag GmbH
Kurfürstendamm 57
10707 Berlin, Germany

Blackwell Science KK
MG Kodenmacho Building
7–10 Kodenmacho Nihombashi
Chuo-ku, Tokyo 104, Japan

Iowa State University Press
A Blackwell Science Company
2121 S. State Avenue
Ames, Iowa 50014-8300, USA

First published 1994
Second edition 2001

Set by Best-set Typesetter Ltd., Hong Kong
Printed and bound by Imprimerie Pollina SA, Luçon

The Blackwell Science logo is a
trade mark of Blackwell Science Ltd,
registered at the United Kingdom
Trade Marks Registry

DISTRIBUTORS
Marston Book Services Ltd
PO Box 269
Abingdon, Oxon OX14 4YN
(*Orders*: Tel: 01235 465500
          Fax: 01235 465555)

USA
Blackwell Science, Inc.
Commerce Place
350 Main Street
Malden, MA 02148-5018
(*Orders*: Tel: 800 759 6102
                781 388 8250
          Fax: 781 388 8255)

Canada
Login Brothers Book Company
324 Saulteaux Crescent
Winnipeg, Manitoba R3J 3T2
(*Orders*: Tel: 204 837 2987)

Australia
Blackwell Science Pty Ltd
54 University Street
Carlton, Victoria 3053
(*Orders*: Tel: 3 9347 0300
          Fax: 3 9347 5001)

A catalogue record for this title
is available from the British Library

ISBN 0-632-05895-1

Library of Congress
Cataloging-in-publication Data

The eye in clinical practice / Peggy Frith . . . [*et al.*]. —2nd ed.
     p.   ;   cm.
   Includes index.
   ISBN 0-632-05895-1
     1. Eye—Diseases.   2. Family medicine.   I. Frith, Peggy.
   [DNLM: 1. Eye Diseases—diagnosis.   2. Eye Diseases—
   therapy.
   WW 140 E966 2001]
   RE46 .E94   2001
   617.7—dc21                                    00-060808

For further information on
Blackwell Science, visit our website:
www.blackwell-science.com

# Contents

# Preface

Eye problems are common and may cause much concern to their owners as well as to the non-specialist confronted by them, who may find difficulty in confident management. This is partly due to the size of the eye and the barrier of getting to grips with the magnifying tools sometimes needed to see in detail, partly to the crowded medical student curriculum with little time to spend on the specialty, and perhaps partly to an unspoken feeling that the eye is so complicated, sensitive and delicate that it is best left 'untouched'.

We have written this book for the doctor with little or no specialized eye training (apart from very basic anatomy and physiology) who wants to approach problems with the eye and vision to decide whether he or she can cope, in a few cases what risks there may be in doing so, and when and how urgently to refer for a specialist opinion. We have tried to avoid both too formal a style and the jargon which often obscures the subject, though we have included a glossary in case any has crept in or appears in specialist correspondence about patients.

We have adopted a practical approach, explaining how to elucidate symptoms and signs without necessarily using anything more sophisticated than a vision-testing chart and an ophthalmoscope, though the extra information visible with a slit-lamp has been included when of value. Management has been suggested, with some of the common pitfalls and cautions, and a formulary deals with common eye medications, both topical and systemic. While every effort has been made to ensure that the doses mentioned are correct, the reader is advised to check dosages, adverse effects and contraindications in the current *British National Formulary* (or *Drug Information* in the USA).

We believe this book will appeal particularly to doctors in general practice who are confronted directly by eye problems, but hope that medical students may find the practical aspects of interest and value, even though they may feel less immediate appeal in common but uncomfortable conditions such as blepharitis, dry eye and allergic conjunctivitis. The book may interest others involved in eye care such as optometrists and specialist ophthalmic nurses.

We hope we have shown that eyes are intriguing, approachable, understandable and rewarding to treat, often without needing specialist referral.

## Acknowledgements

We wish to thank all those who have contributed to the text or to the photographs. These include Paul Parker and the Department of Medical Illustration at the John Radcliffe Hospital in Oxford, Adrien Shun-Shin, the Optometry Department at the Oxford Eye Hospital, and Bill Stanton, Vanessa Venning, Paul Wordsworth and Eleanor Clough from the Department of Social Work. Lizzie Ambler contributed several of the diagrams. Mr John Salmon kindly updated the section on glaucoma. Mr David Taylor kindly gave permission to use some of the illustrations from *Pediatric Ophthalmology*, published by Blackwell Science.

We are most grateful to the staff of Blackwell Science for their help and enthusiasm in preparing the book. We owe a great debt of thanks to our spouses and children for giving us the time to write.

# Chapter 1  **Introduction**

For too many doctors, ophthalmology is a subject at the margin of their familiar territory. The word itself is difficult to pronounce and to spell. It conjures up an image of a mysterious interpretation of findings with the ophthalmoscope which many medical students in honesty are unable to see for themselves (Fig. 1.1). All this is done in the obscurity of a darkened room and compounded by incomprehensible medical jargon.

Undergraduate training in 'eyes' seems to leave the student with vivid memories of the dire consequences of mistakes, and too little knowledge or skill to feel confident in the management of many of the simpler conditions. This is a great pity, since eye problems are common, and present frequently in general practice and in other medical areas.

We stated in the introduction to the first edition of *The Eye in Clinical Practice* that the book is written for generalists who would like to gain confidence in practical ophthalmology. Recognizing that the specialty is often described in unfamiliar jargon and surrounded with an unnecessary mystique, we sought to bring some clarity to the subject. It was our hope that this would enable GPs and other general clinicians to give better explanations and treatments to their patients, and when necessary to make an informed referral. The writing of this second edition is based on the apparent success of that approach.

The current language of health care talks of 'journeys, pathways and interfaces' and, though it is jargon we ourselves seek to avoid, an important principle is relevant to this book as most patients still first seek medical help through their GP. It is estimated that eye problems account for 2–3% of GP consultations and without a basic level of skill, the doctor may either fail to treat effectively, or may place an undue burden on the local eye unit by inappropriate referral. Neither works to the benefit of the patient or doctor. With an increasing emphasis on Specialists within Primary Care providing a point of referral for other GPs in their locality, it is important that all family doctors have sufficient understanding of the subject to know how this system might work for them. We have therefore retained a systematic approach to the diagnosis and treatment of eye conditions as they are likely to be encountered in general practice.

On the other hand it may be reassuring to know that a study of treatment and referral patterns (Sheldrick *et al. British Medical Journal* 1992; **304**: 1096) showed that most cases of misdiagnosis had no serious consequences for the patient. The most common confusion is between infective and allergic conjunctivitis, and the most common mistakes in diagnosis are in not recognizing blepharitis and dry eyes, which both have specific treatments.

## Primary eye care in general practice

This usually means the GP, but under the chapters on screening and refractive problems the roles of health visitors, school nurses, child health clinics, orthoptists and optometrists (opticians) will be shown as part of a team. Nurse practitioners are also establishing their role in Primary Health Care Teams, with 'Walk-in' and 'Out of Hours' Centres.

In Chapter 2, we explain how to examine the patient with an eye problem, using only the time and the equipment which would normally be available in general practice. The subsequent chapters then consider the variety of symptoms which might be met, giving advice on their management. Practical procedures and surgery are explained, either for GPs to do themselves, or to help

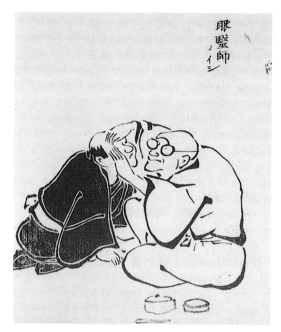

**Fig. 1.1** The ophthalmologist at work, using only spectacles. Japanese woodcut, circa 1740.

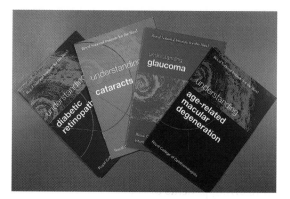

**Fig. 1.2** Royal National Institute for the Blind (RNIB) leaflets on a range of important subjects.

**Table 1.1** Professionals involved in eye care

| |
|---|
| GP |
| Hospital eye specialist |
|   Casualty |
|   Outpatient |
| Orthoptist |
| Optometrist (optician) |
| Community hospital |
| Child health clinic |
| School health service |
| Health visitor |

them and their patients understand what the ophthalmologist may do on referral to hospital.

Ophthalmology currently forms a significant component of all three parts of the membership examination for the Royal College of General Practitioners. In addition to specific questions on eye diseases, other questions concern the implications of systemic illnesses or treatments for the eye. The integration of eye problems with other diseases and with social factors is emphasized in this book, allowing ophthalmology to take its place in overall care provided for patients.

GPs might consider providing for their patients some of the booklets produced by agencies such as the RNIB (see Appendix 2). These include cataract, glaucoma, macular degeneration and diabetic eye disorders (Fig. 1.2). The leaflets can also have a role in encouraging screening and in advertising charity services. There are also HMSO leaflets about sight tests.

## Secondary care by other eye professionals (Table 1.1)

Whilst usually meaning a hospital eye unit, this could mean a 'high street' optometrist or community orthoptist. Under each subject, an attempt has been made to advise what should be referred for specialist help, to whom, and with what degree of urgency. Much will depend upon the local arrangements for eye care, and the skill, confidence and equipment of the referring doctor. GPs themselves may be a point of referral from optometrists or health visitors.

An eye casualty will provide immediate care for those patients who need 'same day' referral, whilst outpatients is the usual channel for most conditions. Even here, a good history and examination by the referring doctor will help the ophthalmologist assess the likely urgency of the problem, and whether other investigations, such as a refraction or visual field test will be needed before the patient is seen. Often the patient is frightened of blindness, and an informed

GP may be able to allay those fears while the patient waits for an appointment. Equally, fear of what the specialist might do is common: tales of eyeballs dangling on the cheek are believed by otherwise sensible people, and the GP may be someone they trust enough to discuss these fears. So, it is important that the doctor is accurately informed. This is what this book is hopefully all about.

### Referral letter and GOS 2 form

In referring patients to hospital eye services it is important to include enough information for prioritization of cases. Include in the referral letter information about speed of onset of symptoms, which eye(s) are involved and a measure of visual acuity as well as any other eye findings. It is helpful to state a possible diagnosis. Also give information about past eye history, current health and medication both general and given for the eyes. If available, always include the optometrist's form (GOS 2), filling in the relevant section of additional information asked from the GP. Some optometrists are approved to refer patients with cataracts directly to the hospital outpatient clinic, which can work well provided the GP is also involved, with an understanding of how the cataract relates to the patient's medical and social background.

### Training

We have assumed that the reader has had only an undergraduate training in ophthalmology which is to be reinforced, updated and expanded with the addition of a few simple practical procedures. We hope that this will encourage some readers to seek further training. Whilst postgraduate courses may help, it is really by experience and practice that confidence and skills are gained. This can best be done by linking with local ophthalmologists or the casualty or orthoptic departments, perhaps with the GP attending a session on a regular basis for a period of a few weeks at first. Time and payment are always scarce, but will be repaid if more of the provision of eye care can take place in the community as a result. This may also lead to a GP specialist role and could be facilitated by formation of Primary Care Trusts.

### Basic equipment (Fig. 1.3)

Firstly, the doctor needs dilating drops, and a good ophthalmoscope. A suitable torch (in North American, a flashlight!), preferably with a cobalt blue filter as an option, will be needed to look at the eye surface, to display corneal abrasions and to test pupil reactions. Fluorescein stain is invaluable and so are topical anaesthetic drops for removing foreign bodies from the cornea. A Snellen chart, pin hole, reading type and Ishihara colour vision testing book form the basic extras for the examination. Some sort of vision test for young children (Stycar or Sheridan Gardiner) is needed, and a patch. All of these are readily available and relatively inexpensive (see Appendix 2).

#### Slit-lamp

As the GP does more, so interest and skill will grow. At some stage it may be worth investing in a slit-lamp and in training in its use in an eye department. The lamp not only gives a magnified and properly illuminated view of the lids, linings and cornea, but also allows the diagnosis of iritis, assessment of cataracts, measurement of intra-ocular pressure and, with additional lenses and practice, gives a stable stereoscopic view of the retina. Elsewhere in this book the words 'should only be done under slit-lamp supervision' implies that the GP in a position to use a slit-lamp should not hold back if his or her skills are secure.

New, a good lamp (and it is never worth getting a bad one) may cost several thousands of pounds and is unlikely to be considered unless it can serve a group of doctors in a large practice or health centre, particularly if the services of a visiting ophthalmologist are also available. If care increasingly devolves to the Primary Care Group or Trust, this may be worthwhile. As the Health Service undergoes further changes it is a good time for GPs to re-evaluate their provision of eye care. We hope that this book will allow them to make informed decisions.

### Some old wives' tales in ophthalmology

It is perhaps worth trying to dispel some misconceptions about eyes which are surprisingly common.

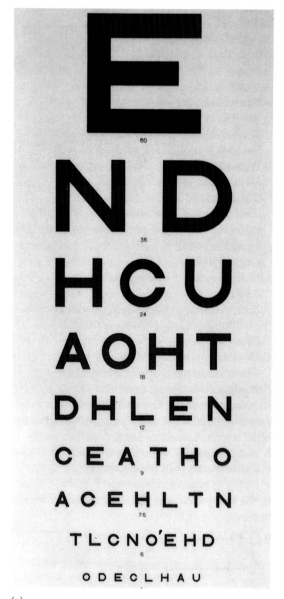

(a)

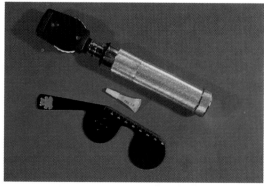

(b)

**Fig. 1.3** Basic equipment to examine eyes includes: (a) a Snellen's chart for testing vision at 6 metres' distance; (b) a pin hole device, dilating drops and an ophthalmoscope.

- Normal eyes are not damaged by:
  Reading in bright or poor light
  Reading too close or too far away
  Sunglasses
  Wearing the wrong glasses
  Not wearing glasses
  Using one eye alone
  'Crossing eyes'—voluntarily converging them
  Watching television (which only risks damaging the brain!)
  Using a VDU.
- Normal eyes are not helped by:
  Bathing with lotions
  Exercises, even when focus for near is worse with age
  Eating carrots.

- Headache is not caused by:
Glaucoma of the common chronic type
Reading with normal eyes.
- A cataract is not a film over the eye but opacification of the lens internally, so it cannot be 'peeled off'.
- The eyes are not removed from their socket for full examination, nor for eye surgery.

- Difficulty reading in later years is due to changes in the lens protein and not to weakness of the eye muscles.
- Contact lenses cannot get lost behind or inside the eye.

# Chapter 2 **A practical approach to the eye and visual problems**

Eye problems have always seemed daunting to the non-specialist. The eye is small and is usually thought to be delicate, although it is actually surprisingly resilient. Some doctors are reluctant to admit that they feel squeamish about eyes. Special equipment is needed to get a really good view of the outside and the inside, and it needs experience and practice to master these. Testing visual acuity and visual fields seems unreliable and not often important.

Despite these problems all doctors need to be able to assess what they can and can't deal with and to feel confident of giving the right treatment initially. This chapter suggests that a doctor with a good ophthalmoscope, to examine both the surface and inside the eye, can tackle the eye and become more confident in knowing what is found. The difficulty in a busy clinical setting is to know what to look for and how to look without wasting time on irrelevancies. It should be possible to assess the eye patient adequately in the allotted time if the procedures are sensibly selected, clearly understood and occasionally practiced. The precautions needed with giving dilating drops are discussed, as in practice this adds a great deal in selected patients with little 'wasted' time.

Most patients will have a problem either with the eyes' appearance, how the eyes feel or how the eyes see. The chapters which follow outline these symptoms and discuss the commoner causes. This chapter deals with the practical approach to looking for the physical signs.

## Equipment (Fig. 2.1)

### Magnifying aids
A hand-held magnifying lens (loupe) may help give confidence in diagnosis, particularly with corneal lesions. It is obviously difficult to do any-

thing practical such as removing foreign bodies with a hand-held lens and magnifying spectacles may help. Wear reading spectacles if you normally would for close tasks.

### Slit-lamp examination
The GP who has some training in ophthalmology will be familiar with the slit-lamp and with the benefits of looking at a stationary patient with bright illumination and magnification. One partner in a practice may opt to become skilled in its use and anyone with a training knows that a lamp is invaluable, allowing signs to be clearly seen, located and quantified (Fig. 2.2). Cells in the front or back chambers are visible. Ocular pressure can be accurately measured. The optic disc and retinal lesions can be examined in detail with an accessory lens.

## Abnormal eye appearance
Look carefully with a bright light shone from both front and side. A good ophthalmoscope, using the largest spot and on the brightest setting, often has a better light than a pen-torch. Look for discharge, swelling or redness of the lids or conjunctivae, or of the eyeball itself. Look carefully at the cornea, particularly if the eye is painful.

To examine the eyeball, pull down the lower eyelid with the patient looking up and pull up the upper lid with the patient looking down (Fig. 2.3). Ask the patient to look to either side as well. Decide if all the conjunctiva is inflamed or just part of it. If the eye is red but painless, suspect conjunctivitis (which is usually sticky) or episcleritis (which is often sectorial). If itching is prominent suspect an allergic reaction, especially if there is also swelling of the conjunctiva. Examine both eyes to compare them and decide if the problem affects one or both eyes.

If redness is mostly around the limbus or in a particular sector of the eyeball, look carefully at the cornea for a scratch, foreign body or ulcer. Red eye with pain rather than discomfort also suggests a more serious problem either of the cornea (when tearing is common) or of iritis (when photophobia is characteristic). Corneal abrasions can occur without a clear history of injury, especially in children. Beware also of the patient who has acquired a rust foreign body whilst working under the car, or the welder with 'arc eye' and of the contact lens wearer.

## Anaesthetic drops to examine a painful eye

If the eye is very painful it may be necessary to give local anaesthetic drops, perhaps 'minims' of benoxinate, to examine. Be particularly wary of painful red eyes in contact lens wearers, especially soft lenses. Anaesthetic drops should be used with caution if a contact lens is in place, and soft lenses will be temporarily stained by fluorescein (which can be bleached out with dilute hydrogen perox-

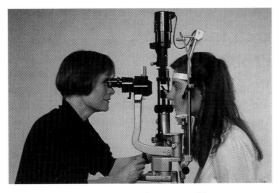

**Fig. 2.2** The slit-lamp in use. This gives stable magnification of the eye surface and interior.

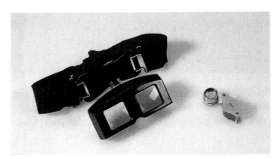

**Fig. 2.1** Magnifying aids, e.g. a hand-held single loupe or a binocular magnifier with headband.

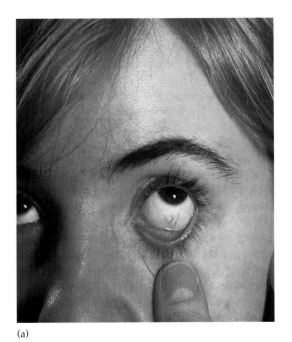

(a)

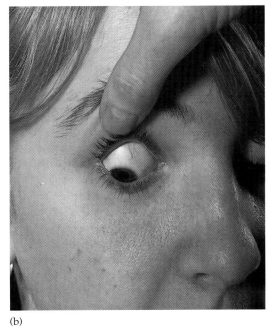

(b)

**Fig. 2.3** Examine all the eye surface by pulling the lower lid down and the upper lid up while the patient looks in the opposite direction.

ide). The lens should not be worn again until the pain and redness have subsided. If a child is reluctant to open the eyes for drops, try lying the child down and put a drop at the inner canthus. Prevent the child from wiping the drop away and as soon as the child opens the eye to see what is going on, the drop will run in without problem (though the child may feel a bit cheated) (Fig. 2.4).

Basic equipment needed:
• Snellen's chart
• pin hole device
• ophthalmoscope
• torch and Anglepoise light
• dilating drops
• local anaesthetic drops
• fluorescein strips
• a good book on eyes

A GP should be able to:
• measure vision and use a pin hole
• assess afferent pupil responses
• evert the upper eyelid
• use fluorescein
• use drops to dilate the pupil
• use the ophthalmoscope

To examine the eye surface:
• a bright light is essential
• a magnifying aid is useful

To give eye drops or ointment to a child try with them lying flat with the eye closed and put at the inner corner

## Fluorescein staining the cornea: to indicate loss of surface cells

If there is a possible corneal problem (particularly with pain, tearing or photophobia) stain with fluorescein. This comes as drops in 'minims' form, but a more convenient amount is dispensed from a moistened filter paper strip impregnated with fluorescein. This can be wetted with tears or tapwater, neither of which is sterile, though sterile saline is recommended (Fig. 2.5). The fluorescein film can be looked at with a bright white light, although a bright blue light is best. Some-

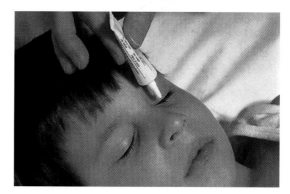

Fig. 2.4 Giving ointment to the inner corner of a closed eye in a child reluctant to open his or her eyes, with the child lying down (drops can be given in a similar way).

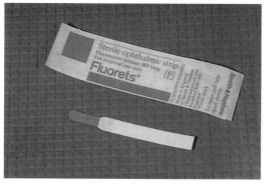

(a)

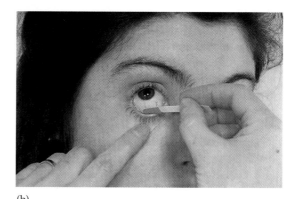

(b)

Fig. 2.5 (a) Fluorets (Smith and Nephew Pharmaceuticals, Romford, UK) are paper strips impregnated with fluorescein for staining the cornea. (b) The strip is wetted and touched to the inside of the eyelid.

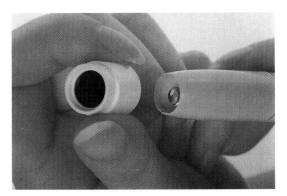

**Fig. 2.6** A pen-torch may be fitted with a cobalt blue filter for use with fluorescein stain.

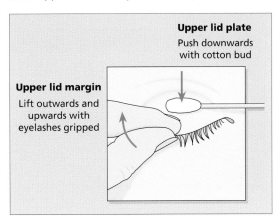

**Fig. 2.8** Eversion of the upper eyelid.

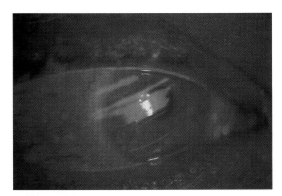

**Fig. 2.7** A corneal abrasion with the area of lost epithelium stained green with fluorescein and blue light. (Courtesy of Mr A. Shun-Shin.)

times pharmaceutical companies provide cobalt blue filters to attach to a pocket-torch (Fig. 2.6), and some ophthalmoscope manufacturers will fit a blue filter in the 'scope', but these are rarely standard. If the cornea is scratched or ulcerated, fluorescein stains the lesion which shows bright yellow in white light or lime green in blue light (Fig. 2.7).

## Upper eyelid eversion: an essential simple skill

If the eye is acutely red and uncomfortable with a foreign body feeling and a corneal foreign body is not seen, examine the everted upper lid for a subtarsal foreign body. Upper lid eversion can be managed in most patients with a bit of practice, though it is best to rehearse this at leisure on a will-ing colleague before tackling patients. It is a useful trick also in contact lens wearers if they 'lose' the lens under the upper lid. Ask the patient to look down. Grip the lashes of the upper lid, and pull downwards and away from the eye surface. With surface tension broken, the plate of cartilage within the lid flips over if pushed down with a cotton bud (or extended paper clip) as the lashes are lifted up (Figs 2.8 and 2.9b). Tell the patient that it feels uncomfortable but is not painful, and is a harmless procedure. The foreign body or lens is usually obvious with a good light, the former stuck to the lid and the latter often stuck to the eyeball. The patient will be very grateful when the foreign body has been wiped off with the cotton bud. The lid will flip itself back particularly if the lashes are pulled forwards again. It is rarely necessary to give local anaesthetic drops to achieve this unless the eye is very painful. It may be difficult to evert a swollen lid. The lower lid can be everted as shown in Fig. 2.9a. It is surprising how often patients believe that it may be necessary to remove the eyeball from its socket to examine properly, so re-assure the occasional patient about this if they seem reluctant to let you touch them.

## The red painful eye

If the eye is red and painful but no corneal or subtarsal problem is found, consider iritis or, less likely, acute glaucoma. Haziness of the cornea or anterior chamber is always significant (Fig. 2.10), and should be referred up to eye casualty.

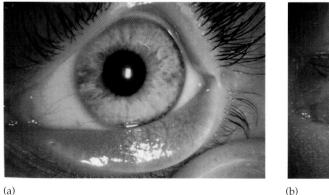

(a)

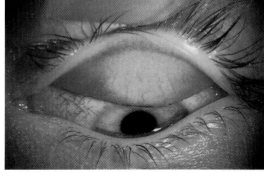

(b)

**Fig. 2.9** Learn to evert the lower lid by pressing it up and over your fingers (a). The upper lid is everted as shown in (b).

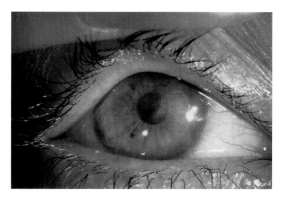

**Fig. 2.10** Corneal haze visible as an opacity using torch light—this was an indolent ulcer in a contact lens wearer.

Reduced vision or photophobia are common in the more serious 'front of eye' problems. In acute glaucoma with an overinflated eye the eyeball feels like a cricket ball to touch through closed lids, rather than the usual squash ball feel to finger pressure.

If there is a history of eye injury it is important to get a clear story and to examine the eye itself carefully as well as checking the vision (medicolegal implications perhaps). In this setting, irregularity, dilatation or sluggish response of the pupil is particularly important as it may signify a penetrating injury or iris trauma. Always ask specifically about hammer and chisel use (see Chapter 10) otherwise there may be a medicolegal sequel if there is a tiny high-velocity iron foreign body within the eye. Subconjunctival haemorrhage is quite common with relatively minor trauma, but

warrants an assessment of vision and a good look at the cornea and iris. Spontaneous subconjunctival haemorrhage, on the other hand, warrants measurement of blood pressure, enquiry to exclude a bleeding disorder (very rare cause) and reassurance. Bleeding within the eye will produce hazy media—hazy cornea from blood in the front chamber and hazy retinal view in the back chamber.

Most cases with sticky discharge are simple conjunctivitis, but beware if the problem is painful (there might be an underlying corneal problem or foreign body) or particularly itchy (the cause might be an allergy). Be careful also in contact lens wearers and in the very young or very old in whom the organism might be atypical. The sticky eye in neonates is discussed elsewhere. Recurrent stickiness with watering is likely to be due to poor tear drainage. Consider if there is also chronic blepharitis with redness and scaling of the lids.

Swelling may affect the lids or conjunctiva, or both, and may arise from an underlying surface problem such as a foreign body, so have a good look at the eye surface. It may be difficult to prize the lids apart, particularly if they are painful or slippery with tears or ointment, so use a gauze pad (Fig. 2.11). If there is swelling or asymmetry around the eyes, an important extra sign, often missed but not necessarily difficult to detect, is proptosis. This implies that the eye is pushed forwards by something behind in the orbit. It may be seen best if the patient puts chin to chest and the doctor sights down the brows and nose. Another

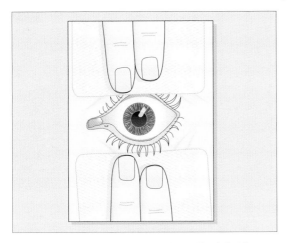

**Fig. 2.11** Examination of an eye with swollen lids. The eyelids are separated with two gauze swabs and gentle pressure.

cause of swelling is an enlarged lacrimal gland. This can be felt through the upper lid at the outer corner, and is often just visible if the upper lid is pulled up in this area with the patient looking down and in towards the nose (see Fig. 5.54).

### Schirmer testing for dryness (Fig. 2.12)

If there are symptoms suggesting dryness it may be helpful to test tear production. This is done within a few minutes using small standardized Schirmer filter paper strips. These are folded and placed (without using anaesthetic drops) hooking over the outer part of the lower eyelids for a timed 5-minute period. The patient may be most comfortable if the eyes are closed. Reassure them that the strips feel uncomfortable but are harmless. Wetting down the strip length is measured in millimetres from the fold. Anything less than 10 mm is suggestive of dryness; under 5 mm is diagnostic.

### Cover test for the squinting eye (Fig. 2.13)

Childhood squint is discussed in Chapters 7 and 9. It is worth being able to do a simple cover test to detect squint. This is best learned by visiting an orthoptic department to see and practice under supervision. If there is double vision, look at the range of horizontal and vertical following eye movements and get the patient to decide where the doubleness is most pronounced as this will help to define the likely cause. See Double vision (p. 39).

## Problems with seeing clearly

If there is nothing to suggest a problem with the eye surface (redness or stickiness) in the patient with blurred vision, then there may be a problem with the internal eye or with the optic nerve.

### Testing visual acuity: preferably standardized

It may not be necessary to measure vision accurately in all patients, but visual acuity is one important 'gold standard' in function (visual field is the other) and to assess how badly the vision is

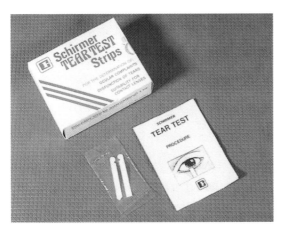

(a)

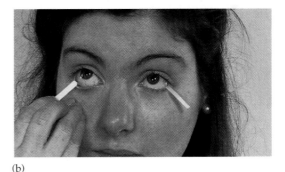

(b)

**Fig. 2.12** (a) Schirmer's test strips for dry eyes. (b) Strips positioned over the lower eyelid. The strip in the left eye is already half wetted.

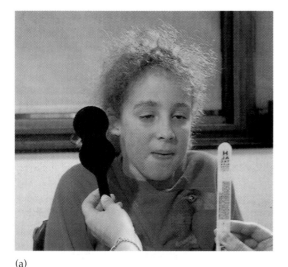

(a)

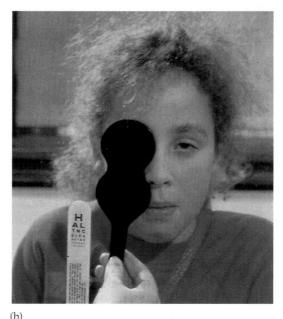

(b)

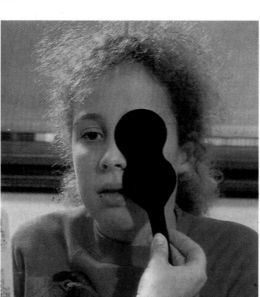

(c)

**Fig. 2.13** Cover test for squint. (a) Shows the right eye is convergent and the left is straight. (b) When the right eye is covered, the left eye does not move but stays straight, as it is already 'fixing'. (c) When the left eye is covered, the right eye is forced to 'fix' and moves out to look straight. This movement confirms that the right eye was squinting inwards. Reproduced from Taylor (1992) *Pediatric Ophthalmology* (slide atlas), Blackwell Scientific Publications, Cambridge, MA.

affected acuity should be tested. It is good practice to measure vision in any patient being referred to hospital (irrespective of urgency), and to record this in the referral letter. Vision is best measured using a standardized Snellen distance chart. A well-illuminated unfaded cardboard type can be hung on the wall and is inexpensive. The type is read at 6 metres (tape measure, counting floor tiles, or a clear red tape mark on the skirting board could show this). If a 6-metre distance is not avail-

able a smaller standard chart can be used at 3 metres. The patient should wear distance glasses if normally worn for TV or driving, and cover each eye in turn to test the vision of each one alone. Start at the top of the chart and work down until the patient falters. Encourage them to 'guess' if they can. Record the result as 6/the numeral of the smallest line they can read accurately. If there is an error (worse than 6/9) try again with the patient looking through a pin hole. The 6 numerator shows that the chart is at 6 metres for the test — in the USA the numerator is often 20 (for feet distant), and 6/6 is equivalent to 20/20.

> The standard Snellen's vision chart is used at 6 m distance

If the patient is unable to read the top 6/60 letter, distinguish between being able to count fingers (one or two reliably), often recorded as CF vision (Fig. 2.14), or see hand movements (HM). If this is not possible, decide if there is any perception of light (PL) or none (NPL). These may seem to be pedantic differences but in fact make a difference to likely diagnosis and to urgency.

Standardized near type, which is scored as an 'N' number, can be a convenient substitute for the Snellen type (Fig. 2.15), but acuity will depend on wearing suitable reading glasses in many cases. If no standard type is available a magazine or newspaper is a good functional test and allows at least comparison between the two eyes. It provides a better assessment of acuity than nothing so that some statement can be made about whether the patient can see tiny, small, medium or only largest type with each eye in turn.

## Poor focusing and the pin hole test: a simple but useful device

The commonest cause of blurring of vision is poor focusing (a refractive error) and it is worth asking whether the patient has visited an optician and if the problem is different at different distances. Short sightedness (with blurring in the distance) may be correctable by looking through a pin hole (Figs 2.16 and 6.5), and myopic patients may be impressed by this easy demonstration. Commercial pin hole devices are often available from eye drop manufacturers. Some patients will confess that their relative's reading glasses help when their own arms become too short to read the phone directory, and it is appropriate to refer these patients to the optician (see Chapter 6).

## Opacities in the eye media: difficult to see out and difficult to see in

The next common cause is lens opacities, and with

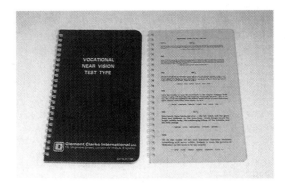

**Fig. 2.15** Standardized type to test near vision.

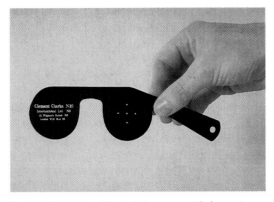

**Fig. 2.16** Occluder with pin holes on one side for testing distance vision if there is an error of focus.

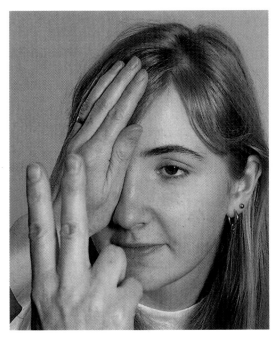

**Fig. 2.14** Testing the ability to count either one or two fingers in each eye.

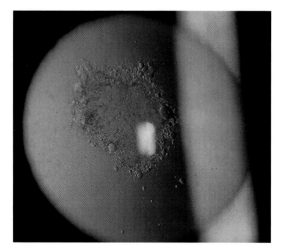

**Fig. 2.17** Lens opacity visible in the centre against the red reflex with the pupil dilated.

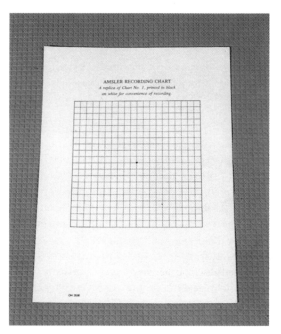

**Fig. 2.18** Squared Amsler chart for testing central visual loss or distortion. Graph paper would substitute.

practice these can be assessed with the ophthalmoscope. Firstly, the view of the retina will be blurred. Secondly, the opacity will be seen against the red reflex if the ophthalmoscope is focused forwards onto the pupil margin (Fig. 2.17). Lens or vitreous opacities will show up, especially if the pupil is dilated. If vision is very poor acutely and the red reflex is very poor or blacked out, suspect a vitreous haemorrhage or retinal detachment, especially in diabetics or after significant trauma.

### Testing central vision: try to define central defects with a simple squared chart

The patient who describes a 'patch' in the vision should be asked to define this—whether it is in one or both eyes and which part of the field is affected. The patch may be dead centre, off to one side or affecting the top or bottom of the field. The patient who can draw the affected area on a small squared (Amsler type) chart (Fig. 2.18) will usually have a retinal problem. The other important symptom which may be associated with the patch is distortion of straight lines which implies distortion of the retina, usually by oedema, and calls for dilating drops and the ophthalmoscope to examine the fovea. Patients rarely volunteer this important symptom, so ask about it specifically especially if the patient is elderly or diabetic.

### The fovea (sometimes referred to as the macula): the most important part of the retina if vision is affected

Problems with the retina will only reduce vision if the fovea is affected, and so it may be important to look at this area specifically. To do this properly the pupil must be dilated with drops. Tropicamide 1%, available as minims, works quickly (within 10–15 minutes but more slowly with a dark iris) and lasts about 2 hours. Warn the patient that their reading vision will be blurred for much of the rest of the day, and that they should drive only when they judge that their vision is 'safe' again, which may be an hour or so. This may apply even if only one eye is dilated. Look at the macula with the ophthalmoscope on the brightest setting, with the largest white filter in position. Remember that the macula is temporal to the optic nerve head on each side. It is the relatively avascular area enclosed by the major vessel arcades above and below (Fig. 2.19). The most sensitive central spot is the fovea. Ask the patient to look directly into the light to locate the fovea. Look for haemorrhages, exudates, scarring or pigment abnormality near

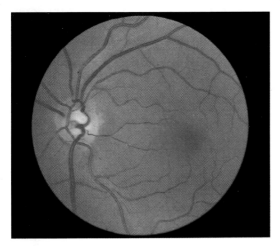

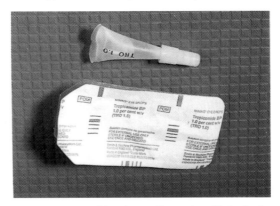

**Fig. 2.20** Drops to dilate the pupil—tropicamide in single-dose disposable minim form.

**Fig. 2.19** Normal fundus of the left eye, showing the optic nerve head (disc) and the macula to its right, with the redder central fovea.

the fovea. If you have difficulty with using the ophthalmoscope, revise your technique or consider changing your instrument (see below).

## Ophthalmoscopy: practice is the key to success

Many doctors feel unconfident in using the ophthalmoscope, perhaps because they have never mastered the technique, perhaps through lack of practice or because they use a poor instrument.

### Drops to dilate the pupil

Using dilating drops to see in properly is neither dangerous nor poor practice, and no opthalmologist will give an opinion on the retina without using drops. It is usually possible to see the optic nerve head without resorting to drops, but it is rarely possible to get a decent view of the macula without, as the pupil shuts down further when light falls on the central fovea. Modern drops such as tropicamide 1% are rapidly acting and wear off within hours (Fig. 2.20). Minims can conveniently be stored at room temperature and have quite a long shelf life. It is not necessary to reverse the drops. It does mean sitting the patient outside until the next case or two has been seen in a busy surgery, and warning them about blurring of reading vision and driving only when they feel safe again. Drops should not be used if the patient has an acute neurological problem (particularly head injury or coma), as an important sign will be obviated. Patients with iris-clip intraocular lens implants are rarely seen in general practice, but it is worth checking from cataract surgery patients if they have been given dilating drops in the hospital clinic since their operation. Every doctor who gives dilating drops should be aware of the symptoms and signs of acute glaucoma (see p. 81 and Diabetic eye screening, p. 145) but the risk of precipitating an attack with short-acting drops is extremely small.

### The ophthalmoscope

Ophthalmoscopes come in many shapes, sizes and prices (Fig. 2.21). Get the most expensive you can afford, but only if it feels comfortable to use. Being familiar with one particular model of instrument is important. Some pocket models are excellent value and are good for the bag. If screening diabetic patients it is best to have a model with a bright halogen bulb and a red-free (green) filter. In the surgery it may be best to have a rechargeable model and group practices might invest in a continuously charged or mains-operated type to be shared, even one fixed to the wall. Someone should be responsible for checking and servicing the scope regularly.

Use the ophthalmoscope to best advantage (Fig. 2.22). It is important to have dim surroundings, so on a sunny day if curtains are inadequate it may be necessary to find a passageway dimmer than the

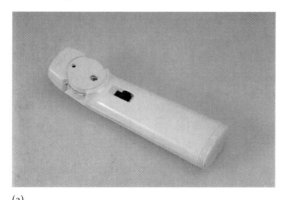

(a)

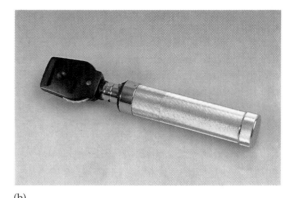

(b)

**Fig. 2.21** (a) Pocket ophthalmoscope, which is ideal for most occasions. (b) Full-sized ophthalmoscope, needed for specialist work and preferred for diabetic screening.

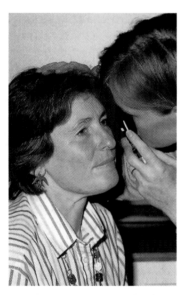

**Fig. 2.22** Using the ophthalmoscope. The observer is quite close, but ideally would be even closer. If the observer is tall, it may be better for the patient to stand.

consulting room. This is true even if drops are given. Position the patient comfortably at the best height and looking in the right direction. If the doctor is tall and the patient short, get the patient to stand up. Vice versa, ask them to sit down. Explain that they should look straight across the room into the distance and keep their gaze steady ('like a soldier on parade'). They should not hold their breath (nor should you). Use your right hand and right eye for the patient's right eye, and swap both eye and hand for the left, although this always feels awkward without practice.

> Keys to using the ophthalmoscope:
> - get a good instrument
> - position the patient with their gaze directed
> - make the room dark
> - get close

Choose the spot size of the beam and the focusing lens and be sure to have read and understood the leaflet which explains these with a new model before you need to use it. With undilated pupils use the smaller white beam. With dilated pupils use the larger white beam (which will cause the reactive pupil to constrict too much). If looking for small red haemorrhages or vascular abnormalities, especially in diabetics, use the red-free (green) filter (Fig. 2.23). Many models have a fixation target or a slit beam—in practice these are of little help. Some manufacturers might be persuaded instead to fit a cobalt blue filter, which is useful for assessing fluorescein staining of the cornea, but these are rarely standard. Practice using the scope without glasses if you wear these and ask the patient to remove theirs, unless either of you has a large focusing error.

> Use drops to dilate the pupil unless:
> - there is an acute neurological or neurosurgical problem
> - the patient has a rare type of iris clip lens implant
> - you do not know the features of acute glaucoma

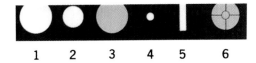

1. Wide Angle
2. Intermediate
3. Red Free
4. Macula
5. Slit
6. Eccentric fixation on Red Free background

**Fig. 2.23** Filters in the ophthalmoscope of different size and colour. Red-free is useful for diabetic work.

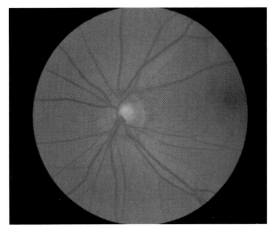

**Fig. 2.24** A normal optic nerve head is flat with a pink rim of nerve fibres and a pale central cup.

Select the starting focusing lens in the scope according to your own correction (will be near **0** if you don't wear glasses continuously or if you wear contact lenses). Experiment with the scope lenses until you are sure of your error, as different manufacturers have different lens notation. Correct also for the patient's focusing by trial and success. Some scopes have a lever for − or **0** or + position which puts an extra lens into the system: for most patients this should be in the **0** position, so this can be a pitfall for the unwary.

Approach the patient from the side at about 15 degrees to the straight-ahead axis, and you should come near to the optic nerve head on which you can focus best. If you find a blood vessel, follow the 'arrows' made by the branches as they point centrally to the disc. The most common cause of lack of success is not getting close enough to the patient. All the gaps between you, the instrument and the patient should be as small as possible, the scope should be jammed against your brow and nose, and your hair will often touch the patient's face. Check that the patient is still looking straight ahead steadily if you still can't find the disc. Once the nerve head is found and focused, ask yourself if the nerve head is normal (Fig. 2.24), of if it could be swollen (Fig. 2.25), pale (Fig. 2.26) or cupped (see Fig. 7.3). To look at the macula and fovea, move your view out to the temporal side of the disc, about 2.5 disc diameters away, where the retina is relatively featureless as there are no blood vessels. This will entail swinging your head and the scope slightly towards the patient's nose. Or, ask the patient to look straight into the light if you

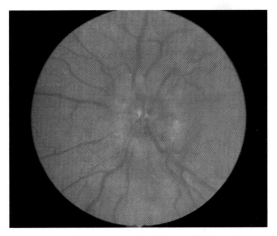

**Fig. 2.25** Swollen optic nerve head — papilloedema from raised intracranial pressure.

have used dilating drops. Ask yourself if there could be haemorrhage, exudate or scarring at the fovea.

Finally, if you still can't get a clear view it may be that there are opacities in the way, so look at the red reflex. Back off a bit from the patient and focus forwards until the pupil margin is sharp, and tilt the scope until light bounces back, giving the red reflex. Lens opacities will show up as black dots, spokes or discs. Vitreous opacities are black strands which may float slowly with eye movements. Loss of red reflex so that it remains black suggests dense lens opacities or vitreous haemor-

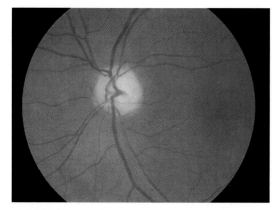

**Fig. 2.26** Optic atrophy with a pale neural rim and a normal cup (though this is more difficult to define).

rhage. Of course corneal opacities will also impair the reflex, but should be seen if the front of the eye has been examined carefully first.

## Neurological problems

### Testing visual fields

If there is no apparent abnormality with the eye itself, or with the optic nerve head, there may be a neurological problem 'further back'. In this case the most important test is to do confrontation of the visual fields as rapidly and accurately as possible, to avoid missing an 'obvious' defect — the patient may not give you the clue to a large homonymous defect as they may be unaware of it. There are several methods of doing this, but the principle is to learn one method and stick to it in order to have an idea of the size of the normal field. Always test each eye separately, otherwise you will miss the rarer but important chiasmal problem. Important patterns of visual field loss are summarized in Fig. 2.27.

Recognize the following visual field patterns:
- homonymous
- bitemporal
- altitudinal (top or bottom)
- central scotoma
- blind spot size

Test with both doctor and patient sitting comfortably and fixating each other's eyes. For the peripheral field, test in the four quadrants, not in

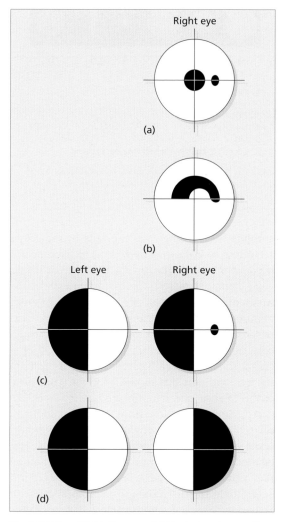

**Fig. 2.27** Visual field diagrams. (a) Central scotoma with normal blind spot with right optic neuritis. (b) Altitudinal (arcuate) scotoma with glaucomatous damage to the right optic nerve head. (c) Left homonymous hemivisual field loss with a right hemisphere stroke. (d) Bitemporal pattern.

the horizontal or vertical axes. If you have little confidence in your technique, try using the finger count method and practice on colleagues first. Ask the patient to cover one eye with the palm of their hand. Show the patient that you will hold up either one or two fingers with the tips close together and that you want them to detect this 'out of the corner of their vision', rather than looking to the target (which is considered 'cheating'). If they don't see the fingers at first they should wait until they can detect how many and then say either 'one' or 'two'. The doctor brings his or her hand in slowly from the limit of the field in each quadrant in turn, with the tips pointing inwards and the other fingers and thumb tucked away. When the patient responds the fingers can be presented in random fashion, one or two, until the response is reliable. In this way you can be sure that the target is seen and there is less room for misunderstanding than if just movement of the target is the stimulus. The method sounds complicated, but is simple after a bit of practice, and will reliably pick up bitemporal or homonymous problems—which are the most important—even if confined to one quadrant.

Detection of central or blind spot problems may need a red pin, traditionally of the hatpin type—about 8 mm diameter. With a bit of practice it is surprisingly easy to map the blind spot (about 15 degrees from fixation on the temporal side) and to know if it is enlarged—suggesting papilloedema if the optic nerve head is swollen but with normal visual acuity. Get the patient to fixate your eye and to say 'gone' when they can no longer see the pinhead. When the blind spot is located thus, ask them to say 'yes' as soon as they see the pinhead each time it appears, returning into the scotoma several times and thus mapping it from inside outwards in four directions. On the other hand, a swollen nerve head with poor vision and a central defect to the red pin (may fail to see the head at all at fixation, or may be only loss of colour here) suggests an intrinsic optic nerve problem such as optic neuritis. Such a patient should also be asked about colour sensitivity in each eye compared in turn using any available coloured object. The patient who describes dilution of colours in the affected eye could well have an optic nerve or macular problem.

### Input pupillary imbalance

If a problem with one optic nerve is suspected, it is important to look for imbalance in the response to light in the two eyes—the 'relative afferent pupillary defect' or 'swinging flashlight test' (Fig. 2.28). This is not just a fancy refinement but an important objective sign which needs care to elicit. Ask the patient to gaze steadily into the distance in a

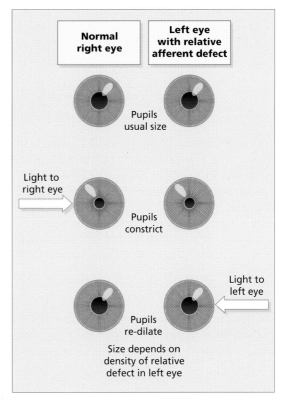

**Fig. 2.28** Testing for a relative afferent pupil defect. Pupils constrict to light shone into the right eye but react less well to light into the left eye if there is a relative defect in left afferent input. Swinging the light from one eye to the other makes the relative difference between right and left most obvious.

dim room. Use the ophthalmoscope on the largest and brightest setting. Concentrate only on the direct response, that is the reaction in each eye at the moment it is illuminated. Move the light from one eye to the other in turn, to and fro, shining the same light equally in the same way for the same time on each side. Normally the response will be equal or balanced in the two eyes, but if input down one optic nerve is impaired compared to the other (relative afferent pupil defect or RAPD) the pupil response to light falling on the impaired side is less and the pupil illuminated will dilate. If this is reproducible, even if slight, it is significant and is a very important finding to confirm a suspected acute or chronic optic nerve problem such as optic neuritis, ischaemic optic nerve or compression.

> Spend a few minutes to detect the obvious homonymous visual field defect which will otherwise be missed

> Compare the afferent pupil responses if the cause of loss of vision is unclear

Other neurological signs may be important, so it may be relevant to look for ptosis or pupillary inequality especially if there are problems with eye movements. Examining eye movements is discussed in the section on diplopia. Nystagmus is always a significant finding, but does not always imply a structural neurological lesion as there are many causes—anticonvulsant toxicity, for instance.

## Summary

To summarize, there are only a limited number of physical signs in ophthalmology and it is worth looking for them, though this takes some care and practice.

*If there is a problem with the eye appearance*
Look at both eyes carefully for redness, stickiness, swelling or lumps.

*If there is a problem with pain or discomfort*
Look at the cornea for brightness and stain with fluorescein. Look under the top lid for a foreign body.

*If there is a problem with vision*
• Measure visual acuity in each eye using distance or near targets (with a pin hole if distance vision is reduced).
• Test pupillary responses to alternating light if an optic nerve problem is possible.
• Look into the eye with the ophthalmoscope. Use dilating drops if this is difficult (test acuity and pupil responses before giving drops). Think about whether the media are clear, whether the optic disc is normal and whether there is a foveal problem.

*If there is no apparent cause so far*
• Assess the visual field in each eye using a squared chart or red pin if there is central blurring, and test peripheral fields with finger counting if there is no apparent ocular problem even if acuity is normal.
• Look for further neurological problems such as ptosis, pupils and abnormal eye movements in selected patients.

## Short guide to urgency of referral

For practical purposes, it is useful to have a summary guide to the urgency of referral for certain key disorders.

*Immediate without delay*
• Acute glaucoma
• Serious chemical burns
• Trauma if suspected foreign body inside the eye or penetration of its coat
• Perhaps central retinal artery occlusion—if onset less than 30 minutes ago.

*Very urgent within a few hours*
• Hypopyon—visible sediment of white cells in the front chamber
• Suspected giant cell arteritis.

*Urgent same day*
• Dendritic ulcer
• Zoster ophthalmicus with eye signs
• Acute iritis
• Suspected retinal detachment with vision reduced recently
• Vitreous haemorrhage if trauma or no previous diagnosed cause.

*High priority outpatient (mentioning the suspected diagnosis and findings)*
• Diabetic proliferative or maculopathy signs
• Retinal vein occlusion
• Suspected chronic glaucoma with pressure above 30 or visual field loss
• Macular degeneration with distortion
• Recurrent vitreous haemorrhage with previously diagnosed cause.

*Not to refer but to try and manage yourself*
• Blepharitis
• Dry eye

- Conjunctivitis
- Non-traumatic subconjunctival haemorrhage
- Subtarsal foreign body
- Corneal abrasion and simple corneal foreign body

- Meibomian cyst
- Arc eye
- Cataract with no handicap to the patient or if surgery is inappropriate.

# Chapter 3 **Disturbance of vision**

## Blurring of vision

When the complaint is blurring, it may be that neither patient nor doctor is quite clear what they are looking at! Despite this, by asking a few questions and performing some simple tests, much can be learnt about the likely cause, and the right management can be started.

The relevant questions are:
- Does it affect one or both eyes?
- How severe is the blurring?
- Does it involve the whole field of vision?
- How suddenly did it come on?
- Is it there all the time and at all distances?
- How long does it last, if intermittent?
- Is there associated pain or changed appearance of the eye—red, sticky or swollen?
- Are there any specific symptoms which may help narrow the field, such as glare, distortion, haloes, floaters or flashing lights?

The examination should include:
- Distance visions (*with a pin hole* if the vision is poor) or near visions with glasses.
- Looking at the front of the eye with a good light.
- Looking at the fundus with the ophthalmoscope, using dilating drops if necessary to look at the macula if the view of the retina is clear.

If there is no apparent cause *in the eye*, examine:
- Visual fields to finger count.
- Pupil reactions, looking for a *relative afferent pupil defect*.

The information can then be organized to make a diagnosis. Fortunately, understanding the mechanisms by which vision becomes blurred makes most diagnoses become clear!

To get a clear image to the visual cortex, five parts must function:
1 Light must pass within the eye without scatter.

2 Light must be focused onto the macula.
3 The macula must be intact.
4 The optic nerve must be intact.
5 The chiasm and central path must be intact.

With persistent and painless blurring of vision, some of the more likely causes are *within the eye* and some are changes you can see.

### Opacities within the eye

#### Corneal scars

Corneal opacity may occur from past trauma, grumbling herpetic scarring, or occasionally a dystrophy which might be familial. The past eye and family history will help and the changes will usually be visible with a bright light which shows focal or diffuse clouding. The view of the retina will be reduced. See Abnormal corneal appearances (p. 88).

#### Cataract

Cataract, or lens opacity, is best seen with the ophthalmoscope as a poor red reflex which gives a blurred view of the retina. Glare is a common symptom but may not be volunteered. Cataract is further discussed in Chapter 7.

#### Vitreous debris

Vitreous opacities are secondary to degeneration, to haemorrhage or to inflammation. This will usually cause floaters. Findings are similar to cataract. See Floaters (p. 36).

### Focusing problems

Poor focusing, or refractive error, is due to a problem with the size or shape of the eyeball, cornea or lens. Problems commonly start in adolescence or late middle age. Distance vision will improve with a pin hole which cuts out the need for refraction. The retinal view with the ophthalmoscope is clear with a correcting lens in place, unless astigmatism gives a distorted picture. Bilateral blurring of vision of slow onset without any other features should suggest a visit to the optician before going further. As many as one in 20 diabetics with acute problems of blood sugar control may develop a focusing problem or even present in this way. Refractive problems are discussed in detail in Chapter 6.

## Macular problems

Macular degeneration is common in the elderly. It may be subtle and best seen with the ophthalmoscope after pupillary dilatation. There are commonly scattered pale dots, spots or mottling at the macula (drüsen). Diabetic macular changes should be looked for, as diabetes can present with visual blurring. Hypertensive retinopathy occasionally causes this too—see Chapter 8 (p. 141). A haemorrhage or vascular occlusion involving the macula can cause persistent blurring perhaps with a specific patch of loss—this is discussed below in the section on Difficulty in reading. Oedema of the macula may occur after surgery inside the eye, particularly cataract surgery.

## Other causes

Glaucoma *rarely* presents with blurring, but should be borne in mind—so check for cupping of the optic disc. Swelling of the optic disc is rarely associated with persistent blurring (usually acute loss of vision—see Optic neuritis, p. 31) but paleness of the nerve head is very significant as it implies some persistent problem with the optic nerve and optic atrophy should be investigated further.

*Behind the eye*, neurological causes may not be obvious until the visual field is tested. Problems at the chiasm or behind may present in a number of ways, and it is important to check the visual fields of each eye if there is no other cause apparent for persistent blurring, as there may be a temporal or homonymous pattern of loss. Such a case needs further investigation, particularly for compression or stroke.

# Difficulty in reading

Reading is a very complex process, perhaps the most sophisticated one the eye and brain perform. It involves not only the eye, visual pathways and occipital cortex, but also other brain functions of perception, recognition and memory. Most reading problems arise from problems in the eye itself (Table 3.1). A smaller number are due to conditions affecting the brain.

## Focusing difficulty

This is the commonest cause in older patients. Near vision depends on the active process of accommodation, or changing of the shape of the lens by focusing for near (see Refraction, p. 111). The ability to focus for near declines from childhood to old age. At about the mid-forties, the presbyope finds prolonged reading tiring. Activities needing more magnification, such as threading needles and sewing or the performing of minor operations, from the removal of splinters upwards, are even more difficult. The problem is greater in low light, because of poor contrast and dilated pupils, and at the end of the day. Reading materials must be held further and further away. Eventually the arms are not long enough. The symptoms are described as blurring, 'letters running into each other', as well as a variable amount of 'eye strain' with discomfort in and around the eyes (Fig. 3.1). The treatment is with glasses (see Refraction, p. 114). In the interests of economy, many will be tempted to buy 'Ready-readers' (across-the-counter reading glasses) and they need to be reassured that wearing what might be the 'wrong' glasses will not do them any harm. At the same time it does need to be pointed out that they are missing out on an important opportunity for eye disease screening and they should be encouraged to have a formal eye test, including eye pressure

**Table 3.1** Some causes of difficulty in reading

| |
| --- |
| Poor focus |
| Cataract |
| Macular degeneration |
| Stroke with visual field defect |
| Dyslexia |

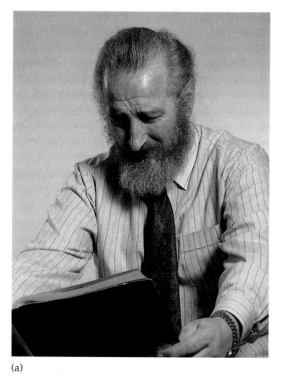
(a)

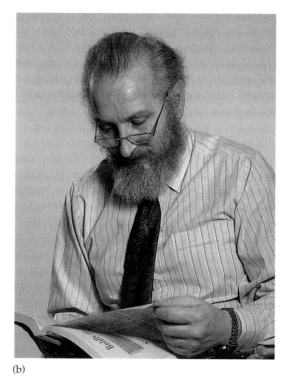
(b)

**Fig. 3.1** Reading the telephone directory becomes difficult at a certain age, and the patient may be much more comfortable with reading glasses.

measurement and test of visual field, at least every 2 years. Occasionally, diabetic patients find difficulty in focusing for several hours if their blood sugar changes rapidly, up or down.

### Other disorders of the lens

Early cataract can cause particular difficulty with reading, especially with bright light which causes glare. The patient will find a compromise level of lighting which suits. The problem is most common in those with central opacities, including steroid-induced.

### Problems with the retina

Age-related macular degeneration is particularly likely to be a cause in older patients. Ask about distortion in particular (see Distortion, p. 43) and, if the complaint is of a 'blob' near the centre of vision, see if there is an Amsler chart vision defect (see Chapter 2, p. 14) which makes a retinal problem likely. The changes at the macula can be difficult to see with the ophthalmoscope, even after

dilating the pupils. Look for scarring or haemorrhage. In diabetics, difficulty reading may be caused by early macular leakage so it is important to examine the macula for hard exudates (see Diabetic eye disease, p. 127).

### Problems with the brain

There may be a visual field defect (particularly homonymous), a problem with eye movements, or some disorder of sophisticated processing for recognition or language. If the problem is of sudden onset in someone at risk of stroke and the patient finds it hard to define, it is worth spending less than a minute to check the gross visual field (see Chapter 2, p. 18). With a brain problem, patients often say they get 'muddled' when trying to read.

### Problems with learning to read: dyslexia

Children with poor vision usually have surprisingly little difficulty with learning to read. On the other hand, the diagnosis of 'dyslexia' has become more common. This is defined as 'a severe reading problem not attributable to sensory or intellectual impairment or lack of opportunity'. It is likely that there are several types. Some may be due to an abnormality of fine eye movements, others to abnormal processing of visual information. There is sometimes a family history. Parents find it a frustrating experience trying to unravel the cause of the child's lack of success. If there is someone with an interest in dyslexia locally working in the NHS eye service (perhaps in an orthoptic department) it may be worth referring the child for an eye assessment, but warn the parents that there may be little practical outcome.

## Sudden loss of vision

Sudden loss of vision means anything from instantaneously to over the course of a week. Most episodes come on abruptly or perhaps overnight. A few of the conditions need urgent treatment (Table 3.2) and accompanying symptoms, as below, may help in diagnosis. Accurate diagnosis may well be difficult in a general practice setting and it is expected that, if there is doubt, patients would be referred to hospital.

### Symptoms that may help define the cause

• *Flashes or floaters* are classically symptoms of impending retinal detachment. Floaters on their own may also mean a vitreous haemorrhage or, much less commonly, inflammation within the back chamber (see below).

• *'A curtain coming up or down'* is also typical of retinal detachment but may occur in arterial occlusion in the retina or optic nerve.

• *Preceding episodes of transient visual loss* (amaurosis fugax) may occur before retinal artery occlusion, less commonly retinal vein occlusion or giant cell arteritis.

**Table 3.2** Important causes of sudden loss of vision

| |
| --- |
| Retinal vascular occlusion (venous or arterial) |
| Optic nerve ischaemia, including giant cell arteritis |
| Optic neuritis |
| Vitreous haemorrhage |
| Retinal detachment |
| Acute glaucoma |

• *Loss of part of the field of vision* is noticed remarkably rarely, for instance a homonymous hemianopia is easy to overlook and usually causes only rather vague symptoms. Does the problem affect one eye or both? Visual field loss, particularly of the top or bottom, may be noticed with a retinal detachment not involving the macula, or a branch retinal artery or vein occlusion. Ischaemic optic neuropathy, giant cell arteritis or a 'hemi' retinal vein occlusion all classically give an altitudinal (horizontal) half field defect. The field affected is the reverse of the part of the retina affected, so that loss of lower field is associated with death of the top part of the retina or optic nerve.

• *Central patch or distortion* are usually macular symptoms, but the central scotoma without distortion can also mean an optic nerve problem.

• *Pain* in the eye only rarely accompanies sudden visual loss. Giant cell arteritis in an elderly patient or optic neuritis in a younger person are possible causes. See also Acute glaucoma (below).

A familiar trap is the sudden discovery, as opposed to the sudden onset, of poor vision in one eye so that the suddenness is a red herring. A cataract is most often responsible, though chronic glaucoma can also, surprisingly, present in this way. Sudden loss in both eyes simultaneously is often of this type, the patient being unaware of the problem in the first eye until the second is affected. If genuine, acute bilateral visual loss suggests a basilar stroke, affecting the occipital cortex on both sides.

### Examination in sudden visual loss

Even quite a simple examination can provide useful diagnostic information. Check the *visual acuities*, using a Snellen or near chart. Test each eye separately, with glasses first and then also with a pin hole for distance. The pin hole is particularly useful if the glasses are old or have been left at home. A quick *visual field* check to confrontation is helpful, especially if there is any doubt as to whether the problem affects one or both eyes (see Chapter 2). Any acute bilateral problem will almost certainly arise from a disorder 'further back' than the eyes, orbits and chiasm, and so will need further neurological rather than eye assessment.

> In sudden loss of vision, check the relative pupil responses before dilating the pupils

> Expect a relative afferent pupil defect with:
> • central retinal artery occlusion
> • optic neuritis
> • giant cell arteritis
> • extensive retinal detachment

Before dilating the pupils, check for a *relative afferent pupillary defect* (RAPD). Swinging a light from the normal to the abnormal eye will result in dilatation of the pupil of the abnormal eye in a variety of problems (see Chapter 2, p. 19). These have in common a profound effect on retinal cells or the optic nerve. They include extensive retinal detachment, retinal arterial occlusion (but not most retinal vein occlusions unless very ischaemic), optic neuritis and ischaemic optic neuropathy (whether of arteritic origin or not). It is very helpful to be able to exclude these conditions when there is only a poor view of the retina, because of corneal scars, cataract or vitreous haemorrhage, none of which themselves will give a RAPD.

*Dilating the pupils* is highly recommended. There are very few absolute contraindications (see Chapter 2, p. 15), but do not dilate an eye with an iris clip type of intraocular lens, as it may dislocate. (This sort of implant is rarely used. The lens and two of its loops can be seen in front of the iris.) It will be safe to dilate eyes with any other sort of implant. The widespread fear of precipitating angle closure glaucoma is largely misplaced. It happens extremely rarely, and it can be treated (see Acute glaucoma, p. 81). Driving poses more of a problem, and is discussed in the section on Diabetic retinal screening (p. 146). The best dilating drop to use is 0.5% tropicamide, as it is short-lived and may not interfere with driving. If unavailable, 1% tropicamide (the usual strength) can be used.

*What you may see with the ophthalmoscope* through the dilated pupil is described in the following brief outlines of the commoner conditions likely to be responsible for acute visual loss.

## Retinal vein occlusion: a warning of vascular risk

This is quite common. It may be central (affecting all the retinal veins), hemisphere (affecting the upper or lower trunks) or branch (affecting a sector drained by the tributary). If the last, vision will only be affected when a temporal branch is involved which damages the macula.

*Symptoms.* Visual loss is usually fairly sudden and often discovered on waking, though there can be a 'stuttering' onset over about a week. The level of vision loss varies but is rarely total (this suggests an arterial event). The loss is unilateral, though it may be sequential in the two eyes.

*Findings.* The retinal appearance may be striking with grossly dilated, tortuous veins, masses of haemorrhages, cotton-wool spots, and swelling of the disc and macula (Fig. 3.2). Sometimes the signs are much less obvious, amounting to dilatation of the veins with scattered blot haemorrhages. In a hemisphere or branch occlusion there is a typical field of retina involved—either the top or bottom or a triangular sector fanning out from the occluded site at an arteriovenous crossing.

*Investigations.* Predisposing conditions are: widespread vascular disease (hypertension, diabetes, smoking), hyperviscosity syndromes and chronic glaucoma. The blood pressure should be checked and the following are useful investigations: FBC (look at the platelet count particularly); ESR; blood glucose; serum protein electrophoresis; and serum cholesterol. It is worth also considering ischaemic heart disease because these patients have a higher incidence, sometimes unexpectedly, so get an ECG checked.

*Management.* Management of the retina is directed at identifying significant ischaemia, as this may be complicated by formation of new vessels on the iris ('rubeosis') in central occlusion, or of the retina itself in branch occlusions. These can cause either thrombotic glaucoma or vitreous haemorrhage—both serious complications. Cotton-wool spots are an indicator of ischaemia, but a more reliable assessment can be given by fluorescein angiogra-

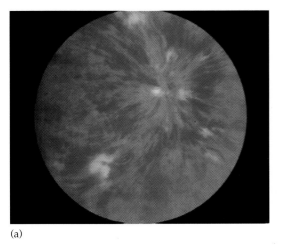
(a)

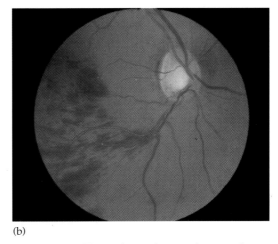
(b)

**Fig. 3.2** (a) Central retinal vein occlusion with typical 'bloodstorm' appearance. (b) Branch retinal vein occlusion with sector 'bloodstorm', arising from an arteriovenous crossing.

**Table 3.3** Risk factors for retinal vein occlusion

| | |
|---|---|
| Age | Haematological |
| Hypertension | High packed cell volume |
| Diabetes | High platelets |
| Hyperlipidaemia | Clotting tendency |
| Smoking | Paraproteinaemia |
| | Glaucoma |

phy. Laser treatment is needed to prevent these complications. Some patients may also benefit from laser treatment to control macular oedema if vision remains poor. Any glaucoma detected will need lifelong follow-up. Thus it is wise to refer patients with a retinal vein occlusion for specialist assessment and management.

The prognosis for vision is guarded. The risk to the other eye is not great, and is reduced by managing any risk factors. The ophthalmologist will normally appreciate the management of vascular risk factors (Table 3.3) by the patient's GP. The problem can occur in otherwise fit younger people, who need to be investigated carefully. The morbidity in this group is low if tests are normal, but they do have an increased risk of ischaemic heart disease at long-term follow-up.

## Retinal artery occlusion: a retinal stroke, usually irretrievable

This is much less common than retinal vein occlu-

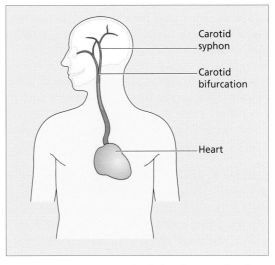

**Fig. 3.3** Common sources of emboli to the eye within the central retinal artery.

sion. It is a retinal stroke and carries the same warnings as a cerebral one. It is usually due to an embolus from the carotid arteries (less commonly, the heart), usually in a patient with background atheroma (Fig. 3.3). Very occasionally, retinal artery occlusion complicates other rare embolic disorders or it may be inflammatory, associated with giant cell arteritis (see below) or another systemic vasculitis such as systemic lupus erythematosus.

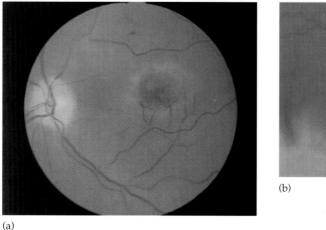

(a)

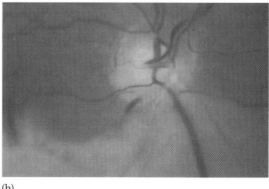

(b)

**Fig. 3.4**  (a) Central retinal artery occlusion several days after the event with pale retina, a yellowish pink fovea and narrowed arterioles. Vision is very poor in that eye. (b) Branch retinal artery occlusion with a pale embolus in the inferior branch artery, pale inferior retina and narrowed arteriole. There will be an upper half field defect in that eye.

*Symptoms.* There may have been previous episodes of amaurosis fugax (see Transient loss of vision, below). With a central occlusion, visual loss in the affected eye is profound, unless a cilioretinal artery is present which preserves a central island of vision. The patient may describe that a curtain has moved up or down or across the vision. As with retinal vein occlusion, only involvement of a temporal branch artery will affect central vision.

*Findings.* Expect to find a relative afferent pupillary defect, because the retina affected is dying or dead. Changes in the fundus are rather subtle and may be difficult to detect. Dead retina is rather pale, particularly around the macula, and there may be a 'cherry red spot' at the fovea itself (Fig. 3.4). The arterioles look narrow and irregular and if the vessels are carefully inspected a shiny white embolus may be seen at the disc or the bifurcation of a branch artery.

> Retinal changes in retinal artery occlusion may be subtle

Look for related features. Feel for the carotid pulses on both sides and listen for bruits. Examine the temporal arteries for tenderness, thickening and pulsation. Check for atrial fibrillation. Listen to the heart and measure the blood pressure.

*Investigations.* These are important. Although it is uncommon to get retinal arterial occlusion with giant cell arteritis, *in elderly patients an ESR and/or CRP is advised* to exclude it. Also check blood sugar and lipids, and an ECG. Referral to a physician for further cardiac and carotid investigations is usually only indicated in reasonably fit patients without obvious widespread vascular disease. In some it is worth investigating the carotid vessels with Doppler with a view to surgery on significantly stenosed vessels.

> In the elderly patient with retinal artery occlusion, look for a normal ESR to exclude giant cell arteritis (though this is unlikely)

*Treatment.* Treatment of central retinal artery occlusion *with onset within the previous hour* is an emergency, though, sadly, treatment rarely produces an improvement. Various measures can be tried to re-establish the retinal circulation including ocular massage, rebreathing and lowering the intraocular pressure with intravenous acetazolamide or possibly paracentesis of the anterior chamber with a needle. Aspirin is useful in the longer term, in reducing the risk of stroke. Advice on minimizing vascular risk factors such as smoking, diet and lifestyle is worth giving to the middle-aged, and control of blood pressure is im-

**Table 3.4**  Risk factors for retinal artery occlusion

| | |
|---|---|
| Age | Carotid stenosis |
| Hypertension | Atrial fibrillation |
| Diabetes | Mitral valve prolapse |
| Hyperlipidaemia | Endocarditis |
| Smoking | |

**Table 3.5**  Some possible clinical features of giant cell arteritis

Elderly

Headache

Acute visual loss, perhaps with top or bottom half of visual field affected

Temporal pain, tenderness, loss of arterial pulsation

Jaw claudication

Systemic features
  Unwell
  Anaemia
  Polymyalgia rheumatica

Pale swollen optic nerve head

Defective pupil response in affected eye relative to normal eye

Raised ESR or CRP

Positive temporal artery biopsy

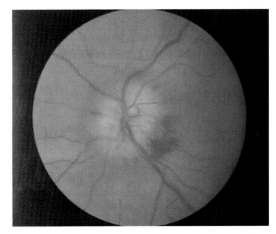

**Fig. 3.5**  Pale swollen optic nerve head of ischaemia, in this case secondary to giant cell arteritis. The erythrocyte sedimentation rate was 110 mm.

head may be infarcted. The retinal artery is a different branch of the parent ophthalmic artery and it lacks an elastic lamina, so is itself infrequently involved. GCA is most common in the elderly, especially women. If missed, the result can be bilateral irreversible blindness—so this is a particularly important diagnosis to make.

*Symptoms.* Symptoms of headache, pain in the jaw (especially on chewing) and scalp tenderness are characteristic (Table 3.5). In about half the cases visual loss (usually unilateral) occurs. There may be a history of malaise, weight loss and pain and stiffness of the shoulders or hips (polymyalgia rheumatica) to help in the diagnosis, but GCA often presents atypically and the diagnosis can be difficult.

> Refer immediately the elderly patient with acute visual loss if giant cell arteritis is suspected

*Findings.* The visual acuity may be reduced in one or both eyes. If involvement is uniocular, there will usually be a relative afferent pupillary defect. Check the field to confrontation as an 'altitudinal' or horizontal field defect is characteristic. The arteritis affects the posterior ciliary arteries which supply the optic nerve head, so *the affected disc is swollen and pale* sometimes with flame haemorrhages around it (Fig. 3.5). In five per cent of cases

portant (Table 3.4). Continued follow-up by the eye department is not usually needed, as long-term eye complications are rare. The prognosis for vision in that eye is poor, though in the other eye it is good and optimized by correcting risk factors.

> Patients with recent retinal artery occlusion should be referred urgently, but usually little can be achieved

### Giant cell (temporal or cranial) arteritis (GCA): a diagnosis not to be missed

This is an extremely important disorder for which GPs should have a high level of suspicion *in elderly patients with acute visual loss*. It is a disease of arteries possessing an elastic lamina, occurring throughout the body but with a predilection for arteries of the head and neck. The loss of vision is due to inflammation in the ciliary branch arteries that supply the optic nerve head, so the nerve

the central retinal artery is also affected and the fundus will then show the pale appearance of dead retina in addition to the disc changes. The temporal vessels may be thickened, tender or non-pulsatile, though these local signs are not invariable.

*Investigations. An urgent ESR is essential and a CRP estimation advisable* (Fig. 3.6). The ESR may be over 100 mm in the first hour and the CPR is invariably raised, so a normal CRP reassures that the problem is unlikely to be GCA (but it is not usually available urgently). A normal ESR does not completely rule out GCA and if the CRP is raised this adds to the suspicion. Temporal artery biopsy is attempted wherever possible to guide longer term management. Up to 48 hours of steroid treatment will not affect the result.

*Treatment.* Where there is a strong clinical suspicion, *treatment with large (80 mg) doses of oral prednisolone should be started as soon as the diagnosis is firm*, whilst making arrangements for temporal artery biopsy (Table 3.6). Intravenous hydrocortisone (1000 mg) or even methyl prednisolone (500 mg) may also be given if the vision of the second eye is already affected. The visual loss is irretrievable but the urgency is because, if left un-

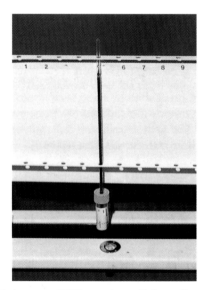

**Fig. 3.6** An urgent ESR is mandatory if giant cell arteritis is suspected. Many eye casualty departments are equipped to do the test on referral.

treated, there is a risk of total blindness with 75% chance of the second eye becoming involved, sometimes within hours of the first. Most patients will be admitted to hospital for a few days to ensure rapid control.

Successful control is shown by complete resolution of the headache and other symptoms and a fall in the ESR to normal. Good response to treatment provides a useful confirmation of the diagnosis. The dose of steroid can then be brought down rapidly, usually after the first week or two. Maintenance levels are determined by monitoring of symptoms and (probably less important) the ESR and CRP, aiming for 10 mg or less for control. Always aim to get the dose steadily down and the patient eventually off steroids unless clear relapse occurs. See also Chapter 4 (p. 52).

In many patients the disease will have burnt itself out in 2 years, but some will need prolonged treatment. It is in this context (of elderly people

**Table 3.6** Some principles in using steroids in giant cell arteritis

Start with a bold dose for an elderly patient
   As soon as the diagnosis is secure
   Before biopsy if this will delay starting, and biopsy within 48 hours
   Suggest enteric-coated prednisolone, 80 mg orally, as initial dose

Consider intravenous steroid if the second eye is involved

Use a high dose until symptoms and ESR are controlled

Thereafter the risk of acute visual loss is small

Tail to about 20 mg/day prednisolone, over the first 2–3 weeks if possible

Keep up pressure to reduce steadily unless recurrent symptoms or ESR prevent

Put up the dose for a few weeks to regain control then try again to reduce

Explain to the patient that 'trial and success' is necessary and relapse to be expected on trying to lower the dose, especially below 10 mg/day

Aim to stop steroids after 6 months of treatment or as soon after this as symptoms allow

Be prepared for 2 years of treatment, or more in some cases

Consider adding extra immunosuppressive, e.g. azathiaprine, to spare steroid side-effects in the long-term patient

Watch blood pressure and blood sugar and prevent osteoporosis early possibly with side-effects from the steroid) that the importance of the biopsy is realized, as a positive biopsy adds weight to the conviction that the diagnosis was originally correct and the treatment fully justified.

## Optic neuritis: a common cause of acute visual loss in younger patients

This is a relatively common and important cause of acute visual loss which can have repercussions for the patient in terms of the future. Inflammation of the optic nerve usually occurs in young adults, particularly women.

*Symptoms* (Table 3.7). Visual loss is initially accompanied or sometimes preceded by pain of variable degree in and around the eye, which may characteristically increase on eye movements. The visual loss usually takes the form of a central scotoma. Patients may also notice dulling of colours, difficulties in depth perception, or worsening of the vision on exertion or after a hot bath (Uthoff's sign). Optic neuritis rarely affects both eyes at the same time but can occur sequentially.

*Findings.* The *visual acuity* can vary from 6/5 to no perception of light (though this is unusual), depending on the severity of the attack and the stage at which the patient presents. Check the *visual field*, as an intact peripheral field should be demonstrable. Also check that the field of the other eye is normal. Looking for a *relative afferent pupillary defect* is vital as it may be the only sign, but patients with mild loss or a previous attack in the other eye may not show it. Colour vision as judged with the Ishihara plates is often reduced compared to the normal eye. The presence of *optic*

*disc swelling* depends on where the inflammation is along the course of the nerve. If the inflammatory plaque is 'retrobulbar', the disc is normal in the acute stages, later becoming atrophic. With inflammation at the nerve head itself, 'papillitis' occurs, with disc swelling (Fig. 3.7). Paleness of the disc of variable degree follows in all cases, within a month or so.

*Management.* Refer for confirmation of the diagnosis. Scanning to exclude a compressive lesion is only indicated in atypical situations. Reassure the patient that the usual course is for the pain to settle within a week although the vision may deteriorate during this time. In the second week vision should start to improve and this will continue for about a month. A difference in colour perception may well remain permanently. The acuity improves to a variable extent, sometimes to normal, and improvement is an important feature in the diagnosis. Analgesia is sometimes needed for the pain, but treatment with corticosteroids is usually only indicated if there is marked pain or bilateral involvement. Systemic steroids hasten but do not otherwise improve recovery.

The commonest cause of optic neuritis is multiple sclerosis (MS) and the optic nerve attack may well be the first manifestation of the disease. Widely differing estimates of the risk of progression to MS have been given in different studies (13% to 83%) but the risk is roughly 50%. Other,

**Table 3.7** Features suggesting an optic nerve problem

Loss of vision with a field defect
   Often maximal centrally
   Sometimes top or bottom part of field
Dulling of colour vision
Optic disc changes, either swelling or atrophy
A relative defect in afferent pupil response compared with
   the normal side
If acute and associated with pain, suspect optic neuritis or
   ischaemia, depending on age

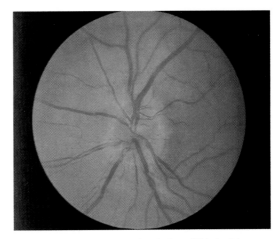

**Fig. 3.7** Swollen optic nerve head of papillitis, in this case from optic neuritis in a patient with subsequent multiple sclerosis.

uncommon, causes are preceding viral infection (especially in children), sarcoidosis and syphilis. A TPHA test for syphillis may be prudent in the occasional case. In discussion of the diagnosis it is debatable whether MS should be mentioned — probably not in the absence of previous neuro-logical symptoms or unless raised by the patient. A further episode of demyelination may after all never occur, be years away, or be mild.

A well-informed patient, wanting a definite diagnosis, may, though, request a magnetic reso-nance (MR) scan, in the knowledge that plaques of demyelination can be demonstrated by this sort of scan. As long as there is prior discussion about the possibilities of unexpected 'subclinical' lesions coming to light, it is only reasonable to grant the patient's wishes.

### Retinal detachment: check the peripheral visual field

This is another condition that often requires urgent referral.

*Symptoms.* Typically, the patient experiences flashes of light and a sudden shower of floaters in the affected eye. These are common symptoms of the vitreous moving forwards from the retina (posterior vitreous detachment, see Flashing lights and Floaters (below)) which may be associ-ated with pulling, producing holes or tears in the retina, particularly if there are pre-existing areas of weakness in the peripheral parts. These tend to occur in high myopia (10 dioptres or more) (Fig. 3.8) or in a variety of retinal degenerations, the commonest of which is called 'lattice'. Other risk factors are a family history of retinal detachment, a previous detachment in the other eye and aphakia (loss of the lens). Trauma is another cause, especially in children. If fluid in the vitreous then tracks through the tear or hole, the retina will separate within an embryological space. The rate of progress depends largely on gravity (Fig. 3.9). Holes and tears at the top lead rapidly to macular detachment and thus loss of acuity. Lower detach-ments progress much more slowly and may never rise up to the macula and the only symptom might be loss of the upper field as the lower retina sepa-rates. If progress is rapid, flashes and floaters are followed by visual loss, often described as a cur-tain being drawn across the field of vision.

Risk factors for retinal detachment are:
• high myopia
• previous detachment in either eye
• trauma
• cataract operation without lens implant

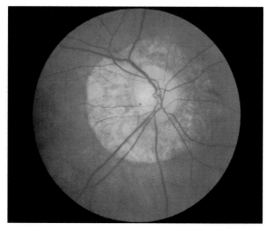

**Fig. 3.8** Optic nerve head with an atrophic crescent typical of a high degree of myopia. Highly myopic patients are at increased risk of retinal detachment.

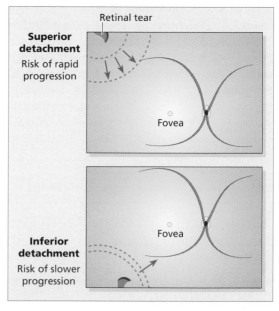

**Fig. 3.9** Effect of gravity on detachment of the superior and inferior retina.

Refer the highly myopic patient with acute visual symptoms to exclude a retinal detachment

*Findings.* Checking the visual field to confrontation gives an idea of the extent of the detachment. An extensive detachment, particularly if

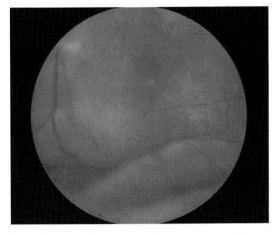

**Fig. 3.10** Retinal detachment with the lower part of the retina looking pale, out of focus and ballooned.

long standing, impairs the pupil response with a RAPD. Examination of the retina can be difficult, especially if the detachment is shallow or the patient highly myopic. The detached area of retina looks grey with dark blood vessels. Sometimes the retina may seem to balloon forwards (Fig. 3.10) or billow with movements of the eye. The underlying fundus geography is lost and a 'total' detachment can be confusing, as there is no normal retina with which to compare, but the vision will be very poor.

*Management.* Refer any suspected recent retinal detachment at once. A tear or hole without detachment can often be sealed by the laser or, if peripheral, freezing therapy. Otherwise, detachments need surgery (see Chapter 11, p. 176).

### Acute glaucoma: rare, but know the symptoms and signs

Acute glaucoma due to closure of the drainage angle is an important condition (Fig. 3.11) because, although it is not common, urgent treatment is vital to future good vision. It typically (but

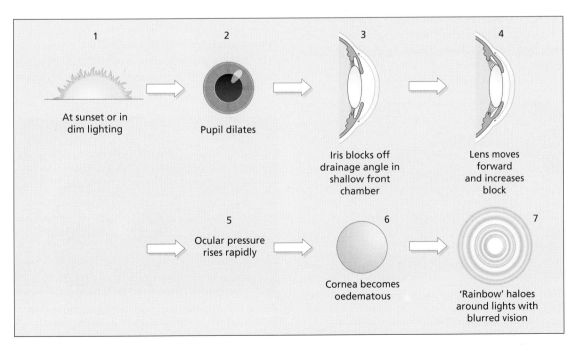

**Fig. 3.11** Mechanism of acute glaucoma with closure of the drainage angle. Note that increasing lighting, sleep and pilocarpine all tend to constrict the pupil and can abort an early attack at stage 3.

not exclusively) affects elderly long-sighted individuals. There may be a history of subacute attacks (see Haloes, below). Sometimes an attack is precipitated by emotion, the cinema or dilating drops given earlier in the day—although tropicamide alone is rarely responsible.

> - Acute glaucoma is an emergency
> - Refer without delay

*Symptoms.* These are of the rapid development of pain in and around the eye, which often becomes severe, with markedly reduced vision in the established attack. Nausea and vomiting may occur.

*Appearance.* The vision is poor, often reduced to counting fingers. The eye is congested, looking red especially around the cornea, with a purplish colour (Fig. 3.12). It is tender and very firm, like a cricket or golf ball. The cornea looks hazy because of oedema. The pupil is often oval, mid-dilated and inactive. It is usually difficult to assess the depth of the anterior chamber through the steamy cornea, so it is useful to look at the other eye. If the front chamber is shallow, there will be only a small space between the iris and cornea. It is difficult to be certain of this without experience of many normal chambers, so it may be an uncertain sign in the event.

*Treatment.* This is needed urgently, so refer as an emergency immediately. The intraocular pressure measured by slit-lamp confirms the diagnosis and is likely to be over 50 mm. Looking at the chamber angle with a contact lens device (gonioscopy) will show a closed angle and probably a very narrow angle in the other eye. If there is likely to be a delay in treatment of more than an hour, start Diamox (500 mg intravenously over several minutes), but still refer with minimum delay.

The eye pressure is lowered by intravenous acetazolamide (Diamox) plus topical timolol, both of which reduce aqueous production. Reducing the pressure can be difficult, particularly in established cases, and osmotic agents such as intravenous glycerol or mannitol may be needed. Once the pressure is falling and iris ischaemia relieved, pilocarpine drops have a chance of opening the drainage angle. It is important not to forget the other eye, which is treated prophylactically with pilocarpine from the outset. When the pressure is normal and the eye less inflamed, laser iridotomies (Fig. 3.13) or surgical iridectomies can be performed to both eyes to prevent further attacks (see Chapter 11, p. 175). Damage to the angle may cause chronic glaucoma needing long-term follow-up.

### Neovascular (rubeotic) glaucoma
Another condition giving a painful, red eye with poor vision and raised pressure is glaucoma from

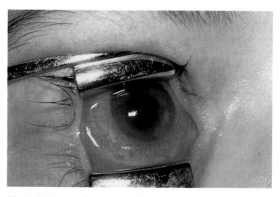

**Fig. 3.12** Acute glaucoma with a congested eye. Note that the eye is red and boggy with a steamy cornea and fixed semidilated pupil. The eye will feel cricket ball hard. Reproduced from Taylor (1990) *Pediatric Ophthalmology*, Blackwell Scientific Publications, Cambridge, MA.

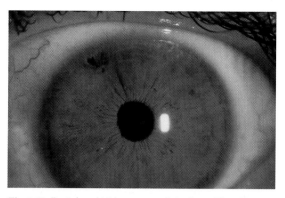

**Fig. 3.13** Peripheral iridotomy made by laser. There is a small hole in the iris at 11 o'clock. Note that the pupil is small from pilocarpine, used to treat an attack of acute glaucoma.

new vessels in the front chamber. This neovascular, or rubeotic, glaucoma is not rare and is usually found either in diabetics or after a central retinal vein occlusion. The onset is not as rapid as that of acute angle closure, symptoms developing over 1–2 weeks. The vision may have been already poor, depending on the reason for the ischaemia. Patients should be referred urgently if the eye is painful. Unfortunately, often all that can be done is to keep the eye comfortable with topical steroids and a dilating drop.

### Vitreous haemorrhage

The sudden onset of poor vision in one eye, perhaps with previous episodes of multiple small floaters, suggests a vitreous haemorrhage if the retinal view is poor using the ophthalmoscope. The red reflex is darkened and may be 'black' with a large bleed. The patient may, of course, be a known diabetic or could occasionally present thus. An alternative cause of vitreous haemorrhage is an associated retinal tear or detachment, past retinal vein occlusion or trauma.

## Transient loss of vision: amaurosis fugax

The Greek term means 'fleeting blindness'. A typical attack implies transient loss of blood supply and is an important form of transient ischaemic attack (TIA), perhaps heralding a stroke. If the symptom is in one eye this implies a problem with the carotid and retinal circulation on the same side. If the loss of vision is complete in both eyes, this may be a vertebrobasilar TIA affecting the occipital cortical circulation bilaterally.

*Usual clinical features.* True ischaemic attacks are brief and have a sudden onset. To be certain that visual loss is confined to one eye, vision in the other eye must be checked in an attack and found entirely normal. The loss may be total or partial and patients may describe a rapid onset like a curtain or 'blind' moving across or vertically. The episodes are painless and there is no impairment of consciousness. Visual loss persists for seconds or minutes, rarely up to an hour. Attacks lasting longer than an hour may not be true TIAs.

> Attacks of retinal ischaemia cause loss of vision which is:
> - brief (usually seconds or a few minutes)
> - in one eye only
> - often complete

Vision returns rapidly and usually becomes normal. Attacks may be recurrent, occurring in clusters over a period of days or weeks.

There may be associated features such as symptoms of transient cerebral ischaemia, perhaps hemiparesis or hemisensory, or dysphasia. If the attacks of blindness are total there may be symptoms of brainstem ischaemia such as intermittent vertigo or diplopia. The patient may have other vascular features or risk factors, such as angina, claudication, smoking, hypertension or hyperlipidaemia.

*Causes.* The retinal or cerebral TIA is usually due to a small embolus, arising from the proximal arterial vessels or heart (valves or chambers). Occasionally it is due to transient reduction in blood pressure, particularly if the cranial arteries are also stenosed. In children a cause is rarely found but they should be investigated by a cardiologist.

> Amaurosis fugax is a retinal transient ischaemic attack

*Look for related signs.* Check the pulse, particularly for atrial fibrillation, and heart sounds for murmur or mitral click. Check for a carotid bruit using the diaphragm lightly below the angle of the jaw bilaterally. Measure the blood pressure.

> In a retinal transient ischaemic attack, check:
> - blood pressure
> - if pulse is regular
> - heart sounds
> - carotid bruit

*Investigations* (Table 3.8). Initially, a full blood count, ESR, blood sugar and ECG should be done. Specialized tests include echocardiography, Doppler imaging of carotid vessels or formal angiography (Fig. 3.14). The last is reserved for candidates for carotid surgery.

**Table 3.8** Investigations in amaurosis fugax

Full blood count, ESR
Blood sugar, creatinine, lipid levels
Electrocardiogram
Possibly
   Echocardiography
   Carotid Doppler study

**Table 3.9** Causes of floaters

Vitreous debris from ageing and degeneration
Blood in the vitreous
  Retinal tear
  New vessels
    Diabetic
    Retinal vascular occlusion
    Sickle cell retinopathy
  Hypertension and macroaneurysm
  Trauma
  Subarachnoid haemorrhage
Inflammatory cells in the vitreous from uveitis

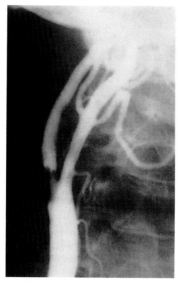

**Fig. 3.14** Carotid angiogram showing the common carotid artery branching into the internal (on the left) and external (on the right). The internal carotid artery is narrowed from atheroma near its origin — a common site. There may be a carotid bruit.

*Management.* Minimize risk factors such as obesity, smoking, raised lipids, diabetes and hypertension. Aspirin does have a significant effect in reducing the risk of major stroke, but carries significant risk of gastric bleeding. Carotid surgery is a specialized field. If there is doubt about the diagnosis refer to a neurologist or ophthalmologist. If the patient would be a candidate for cardiovascular surgery, refer to a cardiologist or vascular surgeon.

*Differential diagnosis.* Many episodes of transient visual loss have no identifiable cause. Patients with optic disc swelling (papilloedema) may have transient obscurations, but the disc appearance

is usually obvious. Migraine causes intermittent disturbance but there are usually characteristic associated visual features and headache. Intermittent blurring of vision of lesser degree may be refractive and an optician's assessment will be useful.

## Floaters

A floater is a dot of variable size and shape which moves with vision but seems to float as if suspended. The dot nearly always represents a piece of tissue which lies within the jelly-like vitreous in the main cavity of the eye. Floaters are extremely common and only occasionally indicate serious eye disease (Table 3.9). Sometimes they represent blood or inflammatory cells. Only refer those with a sudden onset or if floaters are numerous or rapidly increasing in number.

Isolated floaters are very common and seldom indicate serious eye disease

It is crucial to establish that a floater continues to move for some time after the patient's eye has stopped moving. If the abnormality in the vision is static the problem lies in the retina itself rather than in the vitreous and the patient is describing a scotoma or 'hole' in the vision.

Even young eyes are not optically perfect and observant individuals may notice tiny specks in their vision from time to time, particularly against a bright white background. These are called muscae volitantes (flitting flies) and are of no pathological significance. Larger floaters may appear

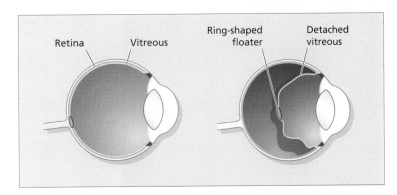

**Fig. 3.15** Floaters caused by vitreous detachment. A ring marking the attachment of the vitreous to the optic disc is a source of floaters when the vitreous detaches forwards.

suddenly in older people or in myopes and are variously described as spiders or cobwebs. They may seem so real that the patient reaches out to clear the imagined obstacle from in front of the eye before realizing the problem lies within it. Large floaters can sometimes be seen by the examiner using a direct ophthalmoscope. The size of floaters is not important but the sudden and numerous ones may be.

### Vitreous shrinkage

A sudden onset of floaters is often due to shrinkage and collapse of the vitreous jelly (Fig. 3.15). This event, known as posterior vitreous detachment, may also cause bright flashes of light to appear caused by the vitreous tugging on the retina as it collapses inwards (see below). Vitreous strands can occasionally (about one in 20 times) tear the retina and this is why the patient needs referral for careful examination of the peripheral retina. If a retinal tear is found laser treatment can usually be given to prevent progression to retinal detachment. Short-sighted people develop these degenerative changes at an earlier age and have a higher risk of retinal tear and detachment.

### Vitreous haemorrhage

Vitreous haemorrhage will also cause a sudden onset of floaters often described as a shower of 'midges' and vision is usually affected, sometimes being dramatically reduced. Once again, visualization of the retina may be difficult since the blood in the vitreous obstructs both the patient's and the examiner's view (Fig. 3.16). If the red re-

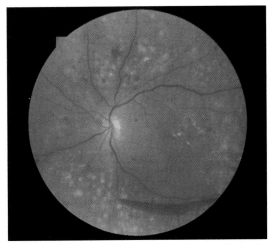

**Fig. 3.16** Haemorrhage in front of the retina, collecting below the fovea. This diabetic patient has bled from new vessels on the disc, despite laser treatment. The blood may move forwards into the vitreous itself.

flex is found to be black then vitreous haemorrhage is likely. Vitreous haemorrhage may result from any condition that causes proliferation of abnormal retinal blood vessels and easily the most common cause is diabetes. Rarer causes include retinal vein occlusion, sickle cell retinopathy and retinal arteriolar macroaneurysms. Vitreous haemorrhage is common with significant trauma and the red reflex is therefore important.

Refer floaters if:
• multiple and recent
• accompanied by flashing
• associated with myopia or trauma

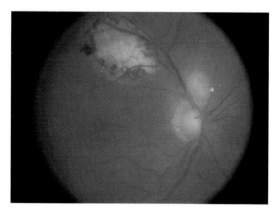

**Fig. 3.17** Cells in the vitreous causing floaters may come from a focus of inflammation in the choroid or retina. This patient shows the scar of an old *Toxoplasma* lesion above the fovea and a fresh focus above the optic nerve head.

## Uveitis

Inflammation within the eye (uveitis) is a rarer cause of floaters (Fig. 3.17) and in these circumstances the vision is often reduced. In general this is due to posterior uveitis rather than the more common anterior uveitis (iritis). Posterior uveitis can be secondary to diseases such as sarcoidosis or toxoplasmosis. Seeing the retina may be difficult because the inflammatory cells obscure the view. These patients should be seen by an ophthalmologist within a week or so.

## Flashing lights (Table 3.10)

This term means any visual sensation in the absence of an external stimulus. A careful history will distinguish between the brief flashes of light that can herald a tear of the retina and the longer lasting sensations that are the hallmark of classic migraine. In the former case referral is necessary without delay, whereas in the latter case referral is unnecessary.

> Retinal flashes are brief and unformed 'like lightning'

## Pulling on the retina

Collapse of the vitreous jelly within the eye occurs as a normal ageing phenomenon and the patient may suddenly experience floaters. If an abnormally strong attachment between vitreous and retina prevents a clean separation the collapsing

**Table 3.10** Causes of spontaneous flashes of light

| |
| --- |
| Retinal tugging |
| Retinal tear |
| Migraine |
| Optic neuritis or retinitis (rare) |

vitreous may tug on the retina and this mechanical retinal stimulation results in a flash. In nearly all cases the vitreous jelly eventually breaks free from the retina and the flashing lights disappear after some weeks or so. In a small number of patients the tugging continues and the retina may be torn (Fig. 3.18). This is why the sudden onset of flashing lights must be assumed to be due to a retinal tear until proved otherwise. Unfortunately this proof can't be obtained with a direct ophthalmoscope and referral to an eye department is necessary for a careful examination of the peripheral retina.

> Retinal flashes are often a tug, but sometimes a tear

## Migraine

The visual aura in a patient with classic migraine is unlikely to be confused with those described above but difficulties arise when the migraine attack is atypical. Sometimes migraine equivalents cause a visual aura not followed by headache (Fig. 3.19). The following features help to distinguish the aura. The visual sensation spreads from an initially small focus and may develop a pattern such as an expanding ring. The whole episode builds over some minutes before fading over 20 minutes or so. Though the patient may initially localize the sensation to one eye, it may really be homonymous. Finally, these patients may have a long history of similar episodes, and often in earlier years the attacks are more classically migrainous. There may be a family history of migraine. In older patients the attacks may represent small transient ischaemic episodes.

> Migrainous flashes are:
> • semiformed and may be zig-zag
> • last at least minutes
> • may follow previous similar episodes

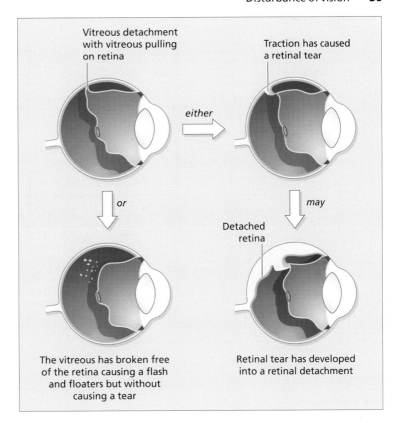

Vitreous detachment
with vitreous pulling
on retina

Traction has caused
a retinal tear

*either*

*or*

*may*

Detached
retina

The vitreous has broken free
of the retina causing a flash
and floaters but without
causing a tear

Retinal tear has developed
into a retinal detachment

**Fig. 3.18** Vitreous pulling on the retina may cause a tear.

## Double vision: diplopia (Table 3.11)

This is a specific and significant symptom, but there are some traps. Patients may complain that vision is double when it is merely unclear, so it is important to establish that there are distinctly two and only two images.

Most cases will be binocular—the doubleness arises when both eyes are used, and disappears when either eye is covered. It is due to loss of accurate alignment of the axes of the two eyes caused by some neuromuscular problem, so the eyes point in different directions. This results in a type of squint which may be present only in some eye positions.

Monocular diplopia, confined to one eye, can occur but is uncommon (discussed below). It is due to a disturbance of refraction within the eye, causing splitting of the light beam.

### Pattern of doubleness

The next step is to define the pattern of doubleness, as true binocular double vision can be logi-

**Table 3.11** Causes of double vision

| |
| --- |
| Neurological lesions of third, fourth and sixth nerves |
| Muscular lesions |
|     Thyroid eye disease |
|     Myasthenia gravis |
| Mechanical |
|     Trauma, especially blow-out fracture |
|     Inflammation in the orbit |
|     Tumour in the orbit |
| Breaking down of an old squint, previously controlled |

cally analysed. Is it constant or intermittent, does the pattern vary or has it worsened progressively, is it worse in the morning or evening? The pattern may be horizontal, vertical or tilted, or a combination of these, and will give important clues to the cause (Fig. 3.20).

> Double vision may have a characteristic pattern that suggests the cause

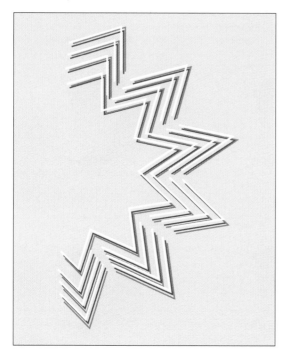

Fig. 3.19 Migrainous zig-zag flashing lights in the right hemifield.

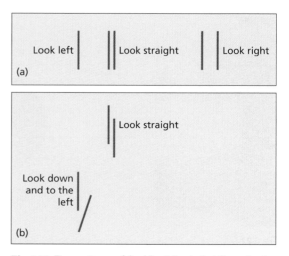

Fig. 3.20 Two patterns of double vision (what the patient will see). (a) Right sixth nerve palsy: the doubling is horizontal and worst on right gaze. (b) Right fourth nerve palsy: the doubleness is complex and worst on looking down and to the left.

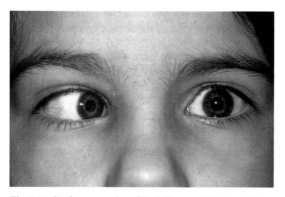

Fig. 3.21 Sixth nerve palsy of the left eye, which is unable to look left (in this child, traumatic in origin). Reproduced from Taylor (1997) *Paediatric Ophthalmology*, 2nd edn, Blackwell Science, Oxford.

For instance, absolutely horizontal and parallel double images, worse in the distance and on lateral gaze to one or to both sides strongly suggests weakness of one or both lateral rectus muscles. By far the commonest cause of this is a sixth nerve palsy, of one or both nerves (Fig. 3.21). Double

vision reading with a horizontal, vertical and tilt pattern suggests a superior oblique and therefore probable fourth nerve problem. Vertical diplopia which is worse on waking and on upgaze suggests thyroid eye disease. A variable pattern worse in the evening is characteristic of myasthenia.

## Associated symptoms

Important associated symptoms include pain or headache, ptosis or pupillary dilatation and facial numbness. These may suggest an intracranial cause for a nerve palsy, particularly if several nerves are affected. Many palsies are due to poor blood supply to the nerve associated with advancing age or diabetes, and diabetic palsies in particular may be painful. Acute onset of double vision with pain, ptosis and pupil enlarged could also be due to an intracranial aneurysm, enlarging to compress the third nerve (Fig. 3.22). This is a neurosurgical emergency, of course. A history of recent head trauma, usually enough to cause concussion, may be significant and is not always volunteered. Weakness of other muscles, particularly of eye closure (so that soap gets in the eyes easily), may suggest myasthenia. Symptoms of discomfort or lid puffiness may suggest a thyroid problem, so ask further about this.

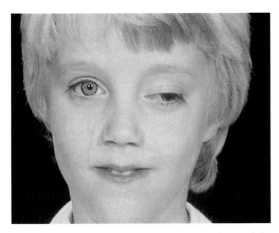

**Fig. 3.22** Third nerve palsy of the left eye with droopy lid, larger pupil and eye deviating down and outwards. Reproduced from Taylor (1992) *Pediatric Ophthalmology* (slide atlas), Blackwell Scientific Publications, Cambridge, MA.

*Signs.* Look at the full range of eye movements, beginning with the patient looking straight ahead. Where does the target look double: does this fall into a recognizable pattern? Are there associated signs of ptosis, pupil enlargement or reduced facial sensation? Is eye closure weak or is the double vision worse on sustained gaze, suggesting it fatigues? Are there signs of a thyroid problem? If the complaint is of doubleness when reading, is convergence weak?

*Managment.* Most cases need to be referred for hospital assessment, which may include an orthoptic review to document the pattern of eye movements. Recent onset double vision with neurological features should be sent promptly to a neurologist. Features of a third nerve palsy with pain needs urgent neurosurgical assessment because of possible aneurysmal enlargement which can be diagnosed from an angiogram. In the initial stages it is safe to suggest a patch over either eye or 'micropore' tape over one spectacle lens. Persistent double vision may be helped by spectacle prisms which can be supplied by an orthoptic department. Stable diplopia may be suitable for ocular muscle surgery or botulinum toxin injection.

### Monocular diplopia

If the patient insists that the double vision persists when looking with one eye alone, there may be an ocular cause. This includes abnormalities of the cornea, lens or retina (macula), best diagnosed using the slit lamp in an eye department. Rarely, patients with cerebral hemisphere problems may have true cortical polyopia, with multiple (often more than two) images.

### Squint without diplopia

Sometimes patients have an obvious squint or deviation of the two eye axes, but don't complain of double vision. There are a number of causes for this (see Squint, p. 126). The commonest is a non-paralytic squint of the childhood type in which one eye becomes 'lazy' and the brain never develops the ability to see both images together. The patient who has very poor sight in one eye will also fail to see double. Rarely, the condition may be due to a gradual steadily progressive ocular muscular weakness in which the brain gradually adjusts to 'seeing' one image only.

## Sensation of visual movement: oscillopsia

This is an uncommon symptom that the patient and doctor may find difficult to define, but certain features help to distinguish it. It is different from true vertigo, which is a sensation of rotation. Oscillopsia is a 'to and fro' sensation, a feeling that objects do not stay still but tend to bob about and be unstable. The symptom is worse when the patient is moving, as when walking or in a moving vehicle. An ambulance navigator found that he could not read his map until his driver pulled up. Bus numbers can only be read if the patient stops walking and stands still.

The problem lies in a defect of brainstem and cerebellar reflexes which normally stabilize vision. It is often associated with nystagmus, and there may be other brainstem features also, including diplopia. Tested in the clinic, the patient will be unable to read whilst shaking or nodding their head.

There are a number of causes, and the patient should be referred for neurological investigation. In some patients there will be the possibility of surgery to relieve compression at the craniocervical junction.

> A sensation of visual movement may suggest a disorder of the brainstem

## Haloes

Haloes, or circles around lights, may be white or rainbow-like. The coloured haloes are the more significant.

*White haloes* are fairly commonly noticed during the early stages of cataract development, before the visual acuity falls much. They may actually look more like spokes than circles. Permanent rather than intermittent, they are caused by irregular refraction from scattered lens opacities, which can also give rise to 'monocular polyopia', the appearance of one or more extra shadowy images, all arising from the same eye. As the cataract becomes more dense, these early symptoms give way to overall blurring.

*Rainbow haloes* are less common and potentially more important, being classically a symptom of episodes of rise in eye pressure, usually a warning of angle closure (see Acute glaucoma, p. 81). Just occasionally, haloes can occur from a build-up of mucus in the tear-film, noticeable on opening the eyes in the morning and clearing after blinking. This is quite common in patients with dirty contact lenses (Fig. 3.23). It may also occur after prolonged swimming in a pool containing detergent. The cause is refraction of light into colours by a hazy cornea.

### Warning attacks suggesting acute glaucoma is imminent

This is a rare phenomenon but it is necessary to know about it. Attacks of angle closure are monocular, typically occurring as it gets dark in the early evening, and in long-sighted subjects. There may be misting and a slight ache, as well as haloes. Resolution follows a few hours later after exposure to bright light or sleep. Seen in an attack, which is rarely possible, the signs are those of a mild attack of acute glaucoma. Between attacks, apart from a shallow front chamber, the eye would probably look normal, though repeated attacks could lead to pathological disc cupping. *These patients are particularly at risk of an acute pressure rise after dilating drops, so* **beware**.

> Rainbow haloes may signify attacks of acute glaucoma

*Mechanism.* Attacks of angle closure glaucoma occur in people with small eyes (long-sighted) and enlarging lenses (the elderly). Although only one eye tends to be affected on any one occasion, both eyes are at risk. As the pupil dilates in response to darkness, the passage of fluid drainage in the front chamber is obstructed (see Fig. 3.11). The intraocular pressure rises rapidly, causing oedema of the cornea which gives the symptoms of haloes and misting.

*Management.* If the attacks sound typical, prophylactic treatment with 1% pilocarpine drops four times daily should be started. The diagnosis is proven if the attacks stop whilst on this regime. Routine referral can then be made for assessment of the discs and visual fields. If there is doubt about the diagnosis, the ophthalmologist may perform a provocative test. Definitive treatment involves making an alternative route for fluid, bypassing the pupil. Laser iridotomy has largely replaced surgical iridectomy for this purpose (see Surgery, Chapter 11). If treatment is successful, long-term follow-up is not necessary. After the

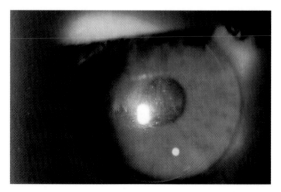

**Fig. 3.23** A dirty contact lens can give rise to haloes and glare.

hole in the iris is made there is no further risk from dilating the pupil, with drops or otherwise.

## Glare

Glare is a symptom often mentioned by patients that is sometimes significant. It is commoner in older people and to some extent is a normal ageing phenomenon. Glare is present when the brightness of a scene is so great that visual acuity falls.

Glare may be normal if a scene is very brightly lit as, for instance, when driving at night into oncoming traffic particularly if the windscreen is dirty. It may be abnormal, usually due to early cataract formation. This is because the cataract can cause light to be scattered within the eye, reducing contrast discrimination (Fig. 3.24). Paradoxically, patients with cataract often find that their vision is best in reduced lighting and they may use sunglasses or a peaked cap to cut down the light.

> • Glare may be an early symptom of cataract
> • Wearing dark glasses may help

Oedema of the cornea is a less common cause of glare but is again due to scattering of light within the eye as it passes through. The pattern is often that of coloured haloes around lights (see Haloes, above). Acute glaucoma is the most serious cause of corneal oedema but symptoms such as pain and nausea will probably dominate the clinical picture when these patients seek help. Contact lens wearers often get glare when their lenses need cleaning.

Glare should be distinguished from a discomfort from light called photophobia (see Photophobia, p. 54). Photophobia is characteristic of conditions such as corneal ulcers and iritis and is due to spasm or irritation of the internal eye muscles. Photophobia is a better indicator of eye disease but it is sometimes difficult to be sure whether a patient's aversion to light is based on difficulty with visual acuity or to discomfort. Patients who have had dilating drops may have both problems.

Examination of a patient complaining of glare is often unrewarding. Look at the cornea and lens. Dark areas in the red reflex may indicate early cataract formation and it may be difficult to see the retina clearly: clear images of the retina effectively exclude corneal oedema and significant cataract. Referral to a specialist is only necessary when an ocular abnormality has been detected or visual acuity has fallen. Simple measures such as sunglasses, hats and reduced room lighting help most patients.

## Distortion

Visual distortion is an important and specific symptom which implies a problem in the macular area of the retina. However, the patient may only complain of blurring and it is often only by asking specifically about distortion that the symptom is found. These patients need a careful look at the macula and fovea after dilating drops. Specialist referral is needed even if the cause is found as some patients will need prompt fluorescein angiography and may need urgent laser treatment.

> • Never ignore a complaint of distorted central vision
> • It signifies a retinal problem and warrants referral

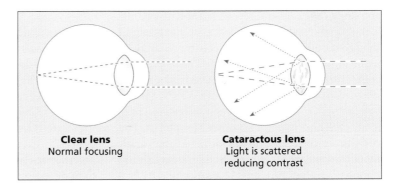

**Clear lens**
Normal focusing

**Cataractous lens**
Light is scattered reducing contrast

Fig. 3.24 Glare.

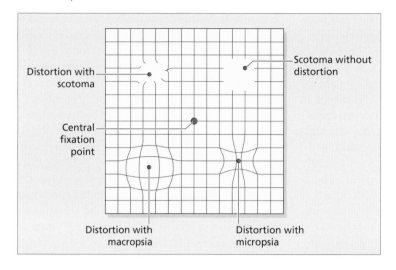

Fig. 3.25 Amsler chart patterns.

Distortion will cause everyday objects to alter their shape. Straight lines appear to kink or bend so that door or window frames will be twisted, and printed words will lean in different directions. Test for distortion by covering the unaffected eye and ask the patient to look at a sheet of graph paper on which a central fixation mark has been made. The patient keeps the tested eye still and attempts to define and draw the area around the spot which is distorted, since this can be directly correlated in size and position with the retinal area likely to show an abnormality (Fig. 3.25). In a hospital setting a 10 cm squared Amsler chart is used. When viewed at the normal reading distance this chart tests an area of retina extending 10 degrees from the centre of vision.

### Central serous retinopathy

In young people a condition of unknown aetiology called central serous retinopathy (CSR) is the commonest cause. CSR is usually unilateral though months to years later recurrences may be in the same eye or in the other eye. The patient will complain of blurred or distorted vision, and sometimes also of the images in the affected eye being smaller than in the normal eye (micropsia). There is no pain and usually no other symptoms. The condition is felt to be due to a localized abnormality of the cellular layer deep in the retina (retinal pigment epithelium) which allows underlying

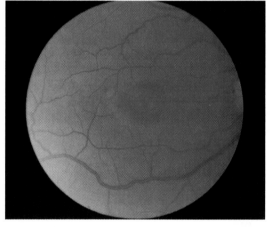

Fig. 3.26 Changes at the fovea may be subtle. This patient with central serous choroidopathy causing distortion of central vision shows a faint rounded area of oedema at the fovea.

choroidal fluid to leak through to the retina and lift it off. A bleb or cyst is produced, and may be seen clinically if the pupil is dilated and a stereoscopic instrument such as an indirect ophthalmoscope is used. However, it is often difficult to detect with the usual direct ophthalmoscope (Fig. 3.26). After initial deterioration over the first 2–3 weeks, the distortion may then remain static for some weeks, and the patient should be referred to an eye outpatient department during this time. Final recovery can take 6 months or more. Laser treatment is sometimes used to treat CSR, but not routinely because the condition nearly always resolves spontaneously and laser may have unwanted side-effects.

## Age-related macular disease

In older people the most common cause of distorted vision is age-related macular degeneration (ARMD) (Fig. 3.27). Patients with drüsen (white spots in the retina) are particularly predisposed to ARMD, which usually takes a slowly progressive course over many years, and is characterized by central visual loss bilaterally and without distortion (see also Chapter 7). The patient may experience further sudden visual loss in one eye and distortion may then be a prominent feature. The sudden change is due to the growth of abnormal vessels from the choroid into the macular area, which elevate and distort the retina (disciform macular degeneration). Clinical findings of ARMD such as drüsen and retinal pigment epithelial mottling will be found but, in addition, haemorrhage or exudate may be seen close to the fovea and the retina itself is raised. In these circumstances the patient should attend an eye department within the next day or two because it is sometimes possible to arrest further visual loss with laser treatment. Patients with ARMD who have already experienced this 'acute on chronic' pattern of visual loss may be asked to test themselves periodically for the presence or absence of distortion in the remaining eye, because if laser treatment is possible, it is only in the early stages of the disciform process. In the home, a tiled wall in the bathroom or kitchen may be an excellent alternative to providing the patient with an Amsler chart and this has the advantage of preventing the patient from panicking when they lose their chart!

## Other causes of distortion

Patients with diabetic retinopathy may have leakage of fluid out of damaged blood vessels in the macular area. If this tracks to the fovea it may cause distortion. These patients may need prompt laser treatment to leaking areas before the fovea is permanently damaged. Retinal vein occlusion affecting the macula may also cause oedema and distortion.

Patients with inflammation in the back chamber (posterior uveitis) may develop foveal oedema as a response to inflammatory mediators. This may respond to systemic (but not to topical) steroid therapy which is justified in selected cases.

Another condition causing distortion of vision is pre-macular fibrosis. This is fine fibrous tissue contracting and distorting the retinal surface. These changes may be difficult to detect with a direct ophthalmoscope. Surgical peeling of these membranes may be undertaken if vision is severely reduced, but the prospect for visual improvement is carefully weighed against the risks of surgery for each patient.

## Night blindness

Patients do not often complain of night blindness, but even so it is a significant symptom as it implies something wrong with the rods in the retina bilaterally.

Inability to see in dim surroundings suggests retinal degeneration, which may be familial

Patients notice that they cannot see properly in dim lighting conditions such as at the cinema, putting out milk bottles at night, or looking at the

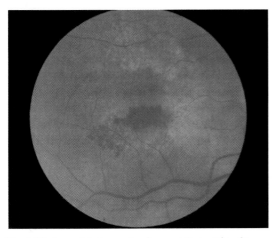

**Fig. 3.27** Age-related macular degeneration with pale scarring and recent bleeding, showing a disciform scar in the making.

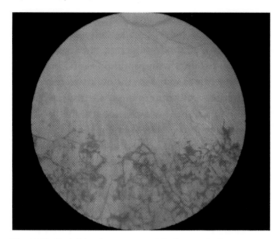

**Fig. 3.28** Retinitis pigmentosa with clumped pigment looking like bone patterns in the peripheral retina. This is usually a hereditary condition and is associated with night-blindness.

stars. Waking in the night, they are unable to see until the light is switched on. Driving at night becomes difficult.

The commonest cause is a degenerative retinal condition. Retinitis pigmentosa produces this symptom early on (Fig. 3.28). Diabetics who have extensive peripheral retinal photocogulation bilaterally will have poor rod function and experience night blindness. Other causes are rarer. Eating carrots might have improved night vision in rare cases of dietary vitamin A deficiency, but is not helpful in normal people nor in retinitis pigmentosa.

## Disturbance of colour vision

Disturbance of colour vision is found in some disorders of the retina and optic nerve. Congenital defects are common in the male population as an X-linked anomaly of retinal cones, leading usually to red/green confusion. The patient may not realize his defect until colour vision is screened, though his family may have remarked on his choice of clothing colour scheme or inability to match paint colours. The problem is of relevance to occupations requiring good colour discrimination (discussed under Screening children, p. 155).

Acquired disturbance is always relevant. The commonest cause is optic neuritis. The patient will notice that colours are less bright in the affected eye, looking 'washed out' or 'greyed' compared with the normal eye. The symptom may not be volunteered, so it is necessary to ask. In these patients it may be important to rule out optic nerve compression as an alternative diagnosis.

> Acquired disturbance of colour vision is common in disease of the optic nerve or central retina

If the problem is bilateral and progressive it may suggest a problem with retinal cones, usually of degenerative type and perhaps associated with age changes at the macula. Rarely, this is familial.

Patients with migraine may describe disturbance of colour perception acutely, and coloured spectra are a common migraine phenomenon.

Rarely, patients with cerebral lesions in specialized colour areas may lose the ability to name or to discriminate between colours. Occasionally they may have coloured hallucinations, sometimes very vivid. Coloured haloes arising from corneal disease are discussed under Haloes (above).

In looking for a defect in one eye of recent onset, the simplest rapid test is to ask the patient to compare colour impression in the two eyes separately, using objects around the room. Colour vision is better tested in a simple way using published Ishihara colour plates (Fig. 3.29a). These are designed specifically for congenital defects, but are of some value in comparing the two eyes or in detecting pronounced acquired defects. More formally, eye hospitals offer a 'Hundred-Hue' sorting test (Fig. 3.29b) which is accurate in defining both type and degree of impairment, though it takes about half an hour to complete.

## Bogus visual symptoms

Sometimes visual symptoms may not be genuine. The patient occasionally invents the whole episode, but more often may be elaborating a real problem. The suspicion arises if symptoms do not match signs, or if signs are inconsistent with each other. Unfortunately, some children are liable to exaggerate their symptoms, and 'blindness', blurring or diplopia may be difficult to evaluate.

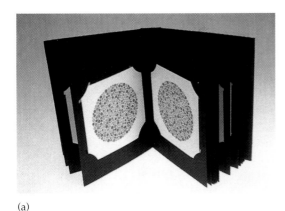

(a)

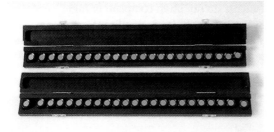

(b)

**Fig. 3.29** (a) Ishihara plates for a rapid assessment of colour vision. (b) Hundred-Hue test for colour vision — accurate but time-consuming. The upper set is randomized, the lower set sorted.

> The patient with a visual complaint may exaggerate it, but beware of some genuine underlying problem

There may be a history of a visual problem in the family or a friend, or problems with learning at school.

To take an extreme example, the patient who claims to be blind in one eye, with no perception of light, must have a corresponding defect of pupil light reflex on this side compared with the normal side. In patients with bogus visual defects the visual field plots may be very constricted and there are certain features which strongly suggest an artificial pattern. These include inconsistency in the plots on different occasions or using various methods, causing progressive spiralling or overlapping with different sizes of target or distance from the screen (Fig. 3.30).

The eyes themselves must be carefully examined, concentrating on the pupil responses and then the fundi and optic discs in particular after dilating the pupils. Skilful refraction and plotting of visual fields is helpful, and may need to be repeated over a period of time. Unfortunately, there are few tests of visual function which are relatively objective. Testing electrical responses from the retina (electroretinogram; ERG) or visual path (visual evoked potential; VEP) may be of help. It may be necessary to scan the visual path to exclude an intracranial problem. It should be remembered that problems in the visual

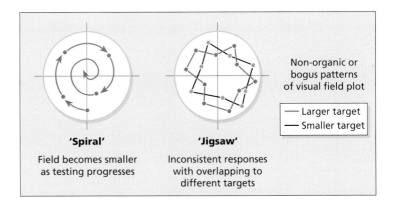

**Fig. 3.30** Patterns of visual field which cannot be genuine.

cortex may cause marked symptoms with normal pupil responses and normal VEP to standard technique.

Management of these cases requires careful serial assessment. Most cases improve, particularly in children, but careful follow-up is needed in case an organic problem emerges. If there are clear psychological features, psychiatric or educational assessment may be needed. It is helpful if those caring for the patient are open to each other about the doubt, but open also to the need for review.

# Chapter 4 **Pain and discomfort**

Eye pain is a common symptom. As with a symptom such as chest pain, it is critically important to define what exactly the patient means. The examination necessary depends on the way in which the history unfolds.

In general, pain around the eye can be divided into true pain or discomfort. Eye discomfort is described separately (see Discomfort of the eyes, below). True pain can be further divided on the basis of whether the eye is the cause of the pain or not. If the eye itself is painful, ask also about foreign body feeling as this may point to a corneal problem.

## Pain with an eye cause (Table 4.1)

True pain in or around the eye may be described as 'aching' or 'throbbing' and may be associated with photophobia. Ask if the pain is bad enough to need analgesics or to prevent sleep. The patient is sometimes unable to describe the pain accurately, and you need to ask particularly if the pain is due to a feeling of something being in the eye. If so the diagnostic possibilities lead down quite a different track, described below under 'Foreign body sensation with pain'.

*Look to see if the eye is red.* Established *iritis* will cause aching pain, the whole eye will be red and photophobia is usually prominent (and often alerts the experienced patient that a recurrence is brewing). *Acute glaucoma* will cause similar pain in the early stages, but it rapidly becomes much more severe, and vision is usually affected to a greater degree than in iritis. A *corneal ulcer* is painful, so look for opacities and stain with fluorescein. You may find the dendritic pattern of herpes simplex. All of these conditions have associated physical findings which help distinguish them, but the pain is essentially similar. See The

red eye (p. 57) for further details of these conditions.

> Conjunctivitis may be uncomfortable but not painful

> Beware the painful red eye in a contact lens wearer

If the eye is 'quiet' (not red or swollen) and the vision is normal, it is unlikely to be the cause of the pain and another source must be considered (see Pain without an eye cause, below). Moderately raised eye pressure found in chronic glaucoma is *not* a cause of eye pain and patients are frequently relieved to hear that pain around the eye does not mean they have 'ordinary' glaucoma.

> • Chronic glaucoma is painless
> • Acute glaucoma is painful

The concept of 'eye strain' is a common one but patients will not damage their eyes by using them and should visit an optometrist if their symptoms are brought on by close work. Optic neuritis is painful but there are usually other signs to suggest this diagnosis. A rare cause of pain, arising from the eye but with little in the way of eye signs, is scleritis of the posterior part of the eyeball, so if the patient is genuinely and persistently bothered by the pain it is worth referring for a specialist eye opinion even if the eye itself seems quiet.

## Foreign body sensation with pain

This symptom will be familiar to most people and is usually due to a foreign body like a piece of grit lodging somewhere on the eye surface or under the upper lid, or to a corneal abrasion or scratch. The discomfort may last for hours or even days,

**Table 4.1** Common causes of eye pain when eye signs are usual

| |
| --- |
| Corneal |
|   Abrasion |
|   Erosion |
|   Foreign body |
|   Arc eye |
|   Ulcer |
| Iritis |
| Optic neuritis |
| Giant cell arteritis |
| Acute glaucoma |
| Scleritis |

and there is often (but not always) a clear precipitating event. The eye may appear white if the patient is seen early on but will become red if the foreign body persists or the scratch fails to heal rapidly. Examination should include fluorescein staining and upper lid eversion (see Chapter 2, p. 9), when the offending foreign body or corneal scratch is usually identified, perhaps with a magnifying loupe. Some patients with in-turning lashes have extreme discomfort, relieved by removing the lashes. For management of corneal abrasion and foreign body, see pp. 167–168.

The acutely painful red eye warrants
• fluorescein staining of the cornea
• inspection of the everted upper lid

**Recurrent corneal erosion**

Recurrent corneal erosions are quite common and can cause a great deal of misery to those most affected. There is almost always a history of acute corneal abrasion at the outset. Some abrasions, those caused by babies' fingers or the edge of a newspaper being notorious, are more likely to lead to recurrent erosion than others. An occasional patient has an underlying corneal dystrophy with impaired epithelial healing.

The basis of recurrent erosion is thought to be that during the healing of a corneal abrasion the new epithelial cells do not adhere completely to the basement membrane, making them susceptible to loosening and shedding. During sleep the lids stick to the cornea slightly so when they are opened during the night or in the morn-

ing, the corneal epithelium is tugged, and in the poorly attached area the epithelium may loosen and be lost. This has been likened to newly laid turf before roots have grown down into the soil beneath.

*Symptoms.* These are the clue to the diagnosis, ranging from a mild pricking to severe pain and watering, and *classically occur on waking from sleep*. Often a full-blown recurrent erosion follows a long period of intermittent low-grade symptoms, the significance of which has not been realized.

Sharp pain on waking suggests a corneal erosion

*Appearance.* The appearance is that of a corneal abrasion—a red, watering, photophobic eye. There may or may not be fluorescein staining, depending on whether the epithelium is merely loose or has sloughed off. Using the slit-lamp, tiny cysts may be seen in the corneal epithelium (Fig. 4.1).

*Treatment.* Lubricate and pad until the epithelium has healed. Loose epithelium is often reluctant to 'stick' back and may need debridement at the slit-lamp to give the cornea a new start. Milder symptoms may just need lubrication, particularly at night. This is also the basis of prevention of further episodes. Lubricating the eye regularly every night is usually necessary for at least 1 month and often up to 3 months. Simple eye ointment or Lacrilube are recommended. The eye may be padded each night. A few recurrent erosions fail to heal with padding, and a soft 'bandage' contact lens can be helpful. In the most persistent cases, corneal micropuncture, carried out at the slit-lamp in the eye clinic, can prevent further attacks.

**Arc eye (welder's keratitis)**

A specific and extremely distressing cause of this type of eye discomfort is seen in welders. Should a welder be unwise enough to dispense with his protective glasses or mask, his eyes will quickly be exposed to excessive quantities of ultraviolet light, and this is absorbed in the cornea and causes acute inflammation of the epithelium. Numerous tiny areas of epithelial breakdown develop in 6–

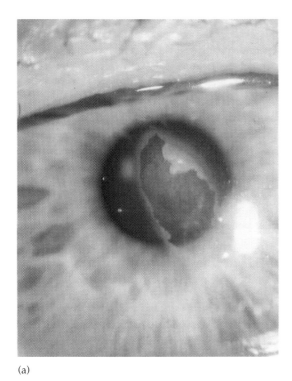

(a)

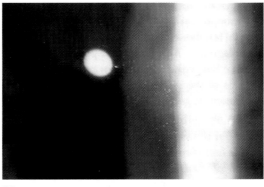

(b)

**Fig. 4.1** (a) Corneal erosion, causing recurrent pain from a poorly healed large abrasion. (b) The signs of a healing erosion may be subtle and best seen with the slit-lamp. Tiny white microcysts like dust are characteristic.

12 hours, so the unfortunate person is relaxing at home after his day's work before the problem becomes apparent, and little sleep will be had that night. Fortunately the condition resolves spontaneously in 24 hours, and treatment is directed toward easing patient discomfort, with ointment, padding or systemic analgesics. Topical anaesthetic drops should not be given as they delay healing. If the problem is unilateral, suspect instead a corneal or subtarsal foreign body, perhaps composed of slag. A similar problem to arc eye may occur in winter sports enthusiasts and is known as snow blindness, or in those who use a sunlamp without adequate eye protection.

When foreign body discomfort persists for days in the presence of ocular discharge and without any obvious cause, conjunctivitis should be suspected. Symptoms begin in one eye and may then spread after a few days into the other eye. The cornea may be involved in some viral cases and patients who do not settle quickly will need slit-lamp assessment. True pain and stickiness sug-

**Table 4.2** Causes of pain around the eye with a normal eye examination

| |
| --- |
| Giant cell arteritis (before vision or optic nerve head affected) |
| Migraine |
| Herpes zoster ophthalmicus (perhaps before onset of rash) |
| Trigeminal neuralgia |
| Intracranial aneurysm |
| Depression |
| Scleritis (if posterior eye) |

gest a more serious problem such as a corneal ulcer, particularly in a contact lens wearer.

## Pain without an eye cause

This can be a very tricky area as pain is a common symptom which quite often defies diagnosis, but sometimes there is one of a variety of treatable problems and some of these are urgent (Table 4.2). The non-specialist's job is to decide if the pain fits into any recognizable pattern and then whether to treat or refer.

## Cranial (temporal) arteritis

*This very important disorder must be borne in mind in any elderly patient with pain in the temple, scalp or around the eye.* (See also p. 29.) The diagnosis is suggested particularly if there is also acute visual disturbance, but pain may be the only feature initially. Ask particularly about tenderness of the scalp making it painful to brush hair or lie on the pillow, and about pain in the jaw perhaps when eating. Examine the temporal arteries for thickening, tenderness or loss of pulsation. The patient may also have proximal muscle symptoms suggesting polymyalgia rheumatica. If in doubt do an ESR and CRP (C-reactive protein, a component of the ESR response). If the diagnosis is suspected, either before or after the result is known, refer for a neuro-ophthalmic opinion. Ophthalmologists are probably more aware of the diagnosis and its threat to vision and eye casualty officers should be alerted to the likelihood. *In patients with visual loss the referral should be immediate as the need to start treatment is very urgent*; in patients with pain only, referral within days is acceptable. Patients may need to be admitted for starting systemic steroid treatment and for temporal artery biopsy within 48 hours of this. It would be justified for the GP to start treatment immediately if the diagnosis is clear, an ESR and CRP sent and there might be delay in getting to a hospital. It would still be prudent to arrange for biopsy.

> Visual loss with pain in an elderly patient is giant cell arteritis until proved otherwise

Management should be with initial boldness in choosing a starting dose of steroid, once the diagnosis has been established as far as possible, and then courage in reducing the steroids progressively once symptoms, signs and laboratory tests are showing control. A usual starting dose for the patient who already has visual loss would be 80 mg prednisolone orally daily in the enteric-coated form. If there is no response in symptoms after 48 hours, increase to 120 mg. If pain persists unchanged the diagnosis is likely to be wrong so consider further possibilities and brain scanning. Add an $H_2$-receptor blocker if there is past peptic

ulceration or if indigestion occurs and warn the patient to avoid aspirin and alcohol.

Intravenous steroids such as hydrocortisone 1000 mg or methyl prednisolone 500 mg may be justified in patients who already have evidence of ischaemic optic nerve involvement in the second eye. Control is usually established within a week or so; the ESR and CRP should be monitored every few days until the ESR falls below about 40 mm in the first hour and the CRP towards normal.

> Diagnosis and initial management of giant cell arteritis is urgent and precedes biopsy

Once under control steroids can be tapered, aiming for a reduction to 20 mg within the first month or so and monitoring both the symptoms and tests. Recurrence of symptoms is of more importance than a rise in ESR or CRP unless this is marked, but it is sometimes worth slowing the pace of reduction if both the ESR has risen above perhaps 50 mm and the CRP above its previous level. The long-term management of the condition can be very difficult and prolonged and it is wrong to be dogmatic about strategy, except that overall there should be a constant goal to get steroid dose as low as possible but to back-track the dose up if there is a really convincing relapse. The GP can have a very important part in management but most are happier with some sort of specialist overview, though if the strategy is agreed this need not be frequent. It is often very difficult to get the patient below 10 mg prednisolone daily as all their usual aches recur and the ESR tends to rise, so concentrate on the cardinal types of pain with tenderness suggestive of true recurrence.

### Sinusitis

This can cause pain around the eye which is usually associated with local tenderness. If in doubt scanning the sinuses will show opacification.

### Migraine

This can cause pain around the eye rather than headache. It is usually episodic but sometimes becomes almost continuous, although it occurs in phases. It may be severe and the episodes may be frequent, particularly in cluster headache.

Unlike trigeminal neuralgia (see below), it is never triggered by touch or by eating, though it may be precipitated by certain foods such as chocolate or cheese. It is worth asking about past attacks that might be more typical of migraine, and about a family history of migraine. If there is associated disturbance of vision with patterns of flashing or zig-zagging light then the diagnosis springs to mind, but if it is a recurrent or persistent boring pain around the eye it may only be by a trial of antimigraine treatment, perhaps with beta-blockers, that the problem can be helped. Cluster headaches, or migrainous neuralgia, are a particularly virulent form of migraine around the eye. This needs to be assessed urgently by a neurologist and may respond to ergotamine treatment.

### Trigeminal neuralgia

This springs to mind if the pain has a paroxysmal and shooting quality, particularly if it is triggered by touching the face or by eating. It is usually in the cheek and very rarely in the forehead, always unilaterally. There is no loss of facial sensation. The patient should be referred to a neurologist who may begin management with carbamazepine.

### Atypical facial pain

This is an unsatisfactory diagnosis which does not have specific treatment. It is better to use the term undiagnosed facial pain.

### Herpes zoster ophthalmicus (Fig. 4.2)

This is an important problem as far as eye complications are concerned. These are discussed elsewhere (see Corneal inflammation and ulceration, p. 73). The diagnosis is usually self-evident except early in the attack before the skin vesicles appear or if these are sparse. Patients with recent severe pain around the eye should be asked about increased sensitivity to touch and warned about reporting any rash suggestive of shingles so that treatment with acyclovir can be considered early.

> With unexplained acute eye pain remember:
> - zoster ophthalmicus
> - intracranial aneurysm

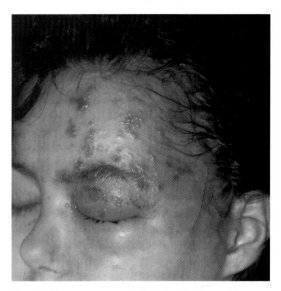

**Fig. 4.2** Herpes zoster—ophthalmic shingles—with typical distribution of skin vesicles and upper lid involvement. The eye beneath must be carefully checked. Reproduced from Taylor (1990) *Pediatric Ophthalmology*, Blackwell Scientific Publications, Cambridge, MA.

### Intracranial aneurysm

It is possible for an intracranial aneurysm to cause pain in the trigeminal distribution without any other neurological features although these must be looked for very carefully, particularly lid, pupil, eye movement or facial sensory disturbance. The pain is usually of sudden onset and may be very distressing, though it varies in severity.

### Depression

Headache and pain around the eyes are common in patients who are depressed, and if the pain defies all attempts to pigeon-hole a diagnosis it may be justified to try a course of treatment with low dose amitriptyline 25–50 mg at night, to see if the pain improves within a matter of weeks. Some patients with true migraine are helped by adding a similar low dose of tricyclic to their antimigraine regime. Some patients particularly fear that they may have an eye disease such as glaucoma (which is on the contrary usually painless) or a brain tumour and may need specific reassurance. In anxious patients tension may be associated with pain around the eyes.

## Discomfort of the eyes

Eye discomfort is a very common complaint and it is worth trying to find a limited number of recognizable causes which have a specific treatment. In contrast to acute causes of discomfort, chronic discomfort is often harder to diagnose and to treat.

### Dry eyes

Dry eyes are common in the elderly, either on their own or associated with systemic conditions such as rheumatoid arthritis (Sjögren's syndrome). A gritty discomfort is characteristic—like sand in the eyes—and patchy dotted staining of the cornea, because of drying of the epithelium, may be evident with fluorescein and magnification (Fig. 4.3). Schirmer testing (see p. 11) is crude but worth while to confirm a suspicion of dryness and, as with many tests, it will detect the definitely abnormal and definitely normal, leaving a number of patients in the middle with an indeterminate result. Strangely enough, if a patient volunteers that the uncomfortable eye waters from time to time this does not exclude a dry eye, as basal tear secretion may be inadequate even though reflex tearing in response to a stimulus is retained. Dry eye symptoms can occur even when tears are copious, due to inadequacy of the overlying oily layer that is produced from the lid margins. Treatment of dry eyes is with tear substitutes in the first instance. There are several formulations of these (see Appendix 1) and it is worth trying different preparations to find one which suits. If the problem is severe, refer for a specialist opinion.

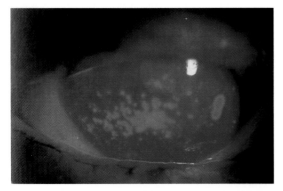

**Fig. 4.3** Dry eye stained with fluorescein to show uptake in the exposed zone between the eyelids.

An eye that can water may still be dry much of the time

### Blepharitis

Chronic inflammation of the lid margins (blepharitis) is also common in elderly patients and frequently coexists with poor tear production. The lid margins may be swollen and red, and crusting around the lashes is common. Treatment is aimed at removing the crusts and, using an antibiotic or combined antibiotic–steroid ointment, to suppress inflammation in the meibomian glands (see Blepharitis, p. 84).

### Other lid and lash problems

Deformed eyelids, either turning out (ectropion) or in (entropion), particularly if lashes are in contact with the cornea, can cause eye discomfort. The treatment is to remove offending lashes and to consider lid surgery (see Minor surgery around the eyes, pp. 184 and 190).

### Photophobia

Literally meaning 'fear of light', the symptom is best described as discomfort or pain in the eye due to light exposure. It is believed to be caused by a reflex resulting in histamine release in the iris and ciliary muscles. It is common in inflammatory eye conditions such as keratitis (cornea) and iritis, but also occurs in migraine, subarachnoid haemorrhage and meningitis. In milder cases it may be difficult to distinguish from glare or dazzle, which are of much less clinical significance (see Glare, p. 43).

Permanent dislike of bright lights may occasionally suggest a retinal problem, in particular albinism. Photophobia is frequently associated with watering and excessive blinking, both of these functions probably being reflexly stimulated at the same time as the ciliary muscle since they are all supplied by the ophthalmic division of the fifth cranial nerve. Patients may ask if light can damage their eyes and the answer is usually 'no' unless they gaze directly at the sun. There is as yet no evidence that using a VDU can cause damage. Patients with macular degeneration or retinitis pigmentosa may reasonably be advised to avoid bright light.

When it is due to inflammatory eye conditions, photophobia may be relieved by dilating drops which paralyse the iris and ciliary muscles. This is one of the mainstays of treatment of acute iritis. Photophobia that is central in origin (subarachnoid haemorrhage or migraine) is not relieved by dilating the pupil.

Photophobia in a baby or child could rarely signify glaucoma, discussed in the next section on watering, which may also occur.

## Watering

A watering eye may be due to something obvious like a foreign body, in which case it is acute and of course resolves with treatment of the underlying cause. However, chronic watering of one or both eyes is common in the elderly, and is usually associated with disease of the eyelids. Quite often patients with thyroid eye disease complain of watering eyes, so bear this diagnosis in mind, especially in younger patients. Persistent watering of one or both eyes in a baby or child may very rarely be associated with childhood glaucoma (called buphthalmos) so it is important with this symptom to look carefully and decide whether the cornea and eyeball look normal, or if either could be enlarged or the cornea could be cloudy. There may also be dislike of bright light.

If the eye is quiet without an obvious abnormality that might account for watering, there is probably a drainage problem. Look at the position of the lower eyelids, particularly the inner parts where the openings of the drainage channels lie—these pin-point holes are the puncta and they lead into the tear ducts or canaliculi (Fig. 4.4). If the puncta are not turned slightly inward so as to catch the tears as they build up at the inner canthus then the tears will eventually brim over. Outward turning of the lower lid (ectropion) is common in the elderly, and may cause watering in this way (Fig. 4.5). A vicious circle may then be set up, because the patient rubs the eye when it waters, and may mechanically drag the lid downward in the process and aggravate the ectropion. Also prolonged wetting of the eyelid skin may cause it to become soggy and swollen, which again aggravates the ectropion. Surgical correction of the ectropion should be curative and is described in the minor ops section.

### Syringing tear ducts for patency

If the lid position is normal, the next step is to see if the lacrimal drainage system is open. This is done by passing a fine, blunt-tipped cannula into the punctum and gently injecting saline (see Minor surgery around the eyes, p. 184). Normally, the patient feels saline passing into the back of the throat, and this shows patency of the drainage system. If not, there is likely to be a blockage somewhere. A blocked lacrimal drainage is amenable to surgical correction, dacryocystorhinostomy, but the operation is comparatively major, and is carried out under general anaesthesia. It is sometimes difficult to recommend the operation if the

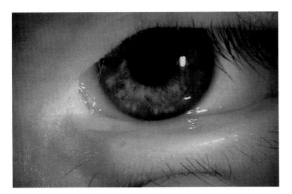

**Fig. 4.4** The lower lacrimal drainage punctum is seen when the lower eyelid is everted.

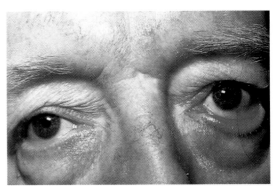

**Fig. 4.5** Ectropion or drooping of the lower eyelid, like a bloodhound, may cause watering of the eye.

patient is elderly and the watering eye is only a nuisance and it is perhaps best reserved for those who are finding watering a major problem, particularly if work is proving difficult.

## Itching

Sudden onset of itching around the eyes is most commonly due to acute allergic conjunctivitis and often occurs in the setting of previous episodes and an atopic predisposition with hay fever, asthma or eczema. The conjunctiva will be swollen or boggy looking and there is sometimes a mucus discharge which is characteristically 'stringy', in contrast to the purulent discharge of infective conjunctivitis (see Conjunctivitis, p. 60).

The conjunctiva and skin around the eye may be sensitized by an external allergen, resulting in conjunctival swelling and redness, and periorbital dermatitis. Topical medications such as atropine and neomycin are frequently to blame. Occasionally the problem can be traced to cosmetics, shampoos, jewellery, etc. The treatment, of course, is to remove the offending allergen, and it is sometimes prudent to prescribe a weak steroid skin cream to accelerate resolution of the dermatitis.

Chronic itching around the eyes in elderly people may be a non-specific symptom associated with conditions such as dryness of the eyes or blepharitis. Treatment of these may not always result in complete clearing of the symptoms. The chronically uncomfortable and itching eye in the absence of obvious pathology is a frustrating state of affairs for patient and doctor alike!

# Chapter 5 **Abnormal eye appearances**

## The red eye

Red eyes are common. Diagnosis and management depend on identifying the less common but more serious intraocular inflammations from the much larger number which are due to some sort of conjunctival problem (Table 5.1). Treating conjunctivitis effectively means finding the cause which is not always easy. Identifying the red eye due to something more serious means being alert to certain key clues. In this book we have opted to use the term 'iritis' to describe what a specialist would probably call 'anterior uveitis' (see below).

### Relevant features in the history
- *Trauma* suggests scratches and the possibility of foreign bodies.
- *Contact lens* wearing suggests corneal damage with risk of infection.
- *Previous* red eyes suggests episcleritis, iritis or herpes simplex corneal ulcer.
- *Contact* with other red eyes suggests infective conjunctivitis.
- *URTI* (upper respiratory tract infection), current or recent, suggests viral conjunctivitis.
- *Cold sores* suggests herpes simplex corneal ulcer.
- *Systemic* conditions such as atopy or joint disease.

### Accompanying symptoms (and their likely relevance)
- *Irritation, sore, gritty*: conjunctiva, episclera, dry eye.
- *Foreign body feeling*: cornea, lash, subtarsal foreign body.
- *Burning*: dry eye, blepharitis.
- *Pain or aching*: cornea, iritis, zoster, scleritis.
- *Itching*: allergy, blepharitis.
- *Photophobia* (a very useful symptom): cornea, iritis.
- *Watering*: non-bacterial conjunctivitis, cornea, iritis.
- *Discharge* (pus): bacterial or chlamydial conjunctivitis.
- *Discharge* (stringy, mucous): viral or allergic conjunctivitis, dry eye.
- *Visual problem*: cornea, iritis, acute glaucoma (Table 5.2).
- *Lid swelling*: infection, allergy, tear sac or gland.
- *Lid margin lump*: stye, molluscum.
- *Lid position abnormal*: entropion, ectropion.
- *Rash*: zoster, simplex, rosacea.
- *Headache, malaise, fever*: zoster, orbital cellulitis.
- *URTI*: adenoviral conjunctivitis.
- *Vomiting*: acute glaucoma.

### Examination
It is not intended that the suggestions given below for examining the red eye should be followed in their entirety on every occasion. Be guided by the history. A good bright torch or ophthalmoscope is invaluable, particularly if it has a blue filter for using with fluorescein. Fluorescein shows up areas of epithelial loss of the cornea and also of the conjunctiva. It is available as impregnated paper strips which can be moistened, preferably by sterile saline or water. The tiny strips that come in books like matches are not big enough — 'Fluorets' are recommended (see Fig. 2.5). Fluorescein washes out quickly, and in the presence of much watering the 2% minim ampoules are better. They are also easier to use for the examination of small children. Prepare for the yellow dye to get everywhere, but it washes out easily. A magnifier or loupe will allow smaller problems to be seen and foreign bodies to be removed.

### Lids
Is the lid position normal or does it roll in (entro-

**Table 5.1** Important causes of the red eye

Conjunctivitis
  Bacterial
  Chlamydial
  Viral
  Allergic
  Caused by trichiasis or sutures
  Dry eye or irritant medication
  Contact lens overwear
Subconjunctival haemorrhage
Episcleritis (less commonly scleritis)
Corneal problem
  Abrasion
  Erosion
  Foreign body
  Ulcer
Lump on the eyeball
  Pinguecula
  Pterygium
Iritis
Acute glaucoma  } less common

**Table 5.2** Vision in the red eye

Normal in conjunctivitis
Mildly affected in iritis
Variably affected in corneal problems
Severely affected in established acute glaucoma

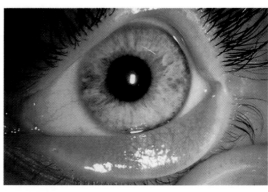

(a)

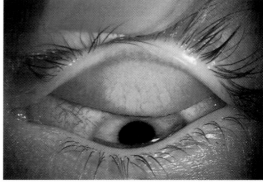

(b)

**Fig. 5.1** Learn to evert the lower lid by pressing it up and over your fingers (a). The upper lid is everted as shown in (b) and Fig. 2.8.

pion) or out (ectropion)? Entropion can be latent so first ask the patient to screw the eyes up tightly. Look for swelling, redness, tenderness and 'cellulitic' appearance suggesting infection, or just puffy (possibly with flaky or fissured) skin suggesting allergy. How many lids are affected? If there is gross lid swelling make sure the eye underneath is not pushed forwards or sideways. Are there lumps in the lid or on the margins? Are the lid margins inflamed, red, flaky or ulcerated suggesting blepharitis? Is there a rash suggesting zoster, simplex or rosacea? Are the lashes all pointing away from the eye?

*Eversion of the upper lid*
Evert the upper lid if a foreign body beneath is suspected. This is easily done by asking the patient to look down, gripping the lashes firmly with one hand whilst holding a glass rod or cotton bud (or match or paper-clip) against the lid near the upper part of the tarsal plate, about 7 mm up from

the lid margin (Fig. 5.1). Downward pressure on the tarsal plate with lifting of the lashes will hinge up the lid, showing the conjunctiva lining it (see also p. 9). As well as finding foreign bodies, any gross conjunctival reaction in the form of lumps such as follicles or papillae (see Conjunctivitis, below) may be found, most easily seen with a loupe. Pull down the lower lid while pressing upwards to roll the lower lid out over the fingertips to examine the lower lining conjunctiva.

> Both corneal ulcer and iritis can cause identical symptoms

*The eyeball or globe*
Assess the extent and nature of the redness. Is it dense and uniform, obscuring the vessels like a subconjunctival haemorrhage (Fig. 5.2)? Are the

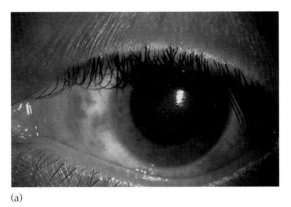

(a)

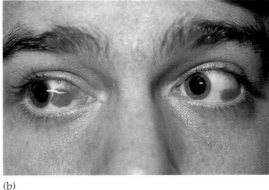

(b)

**Fig. 5.2** Subconjunctival haemorrhage of different degrees. If spontaneous this may be innocent, but beware if it is secondary to trauma where it may mask a penetrating injury (a). (b) Following 'Bunjee' jumping with a sudden increase in venous pressure.

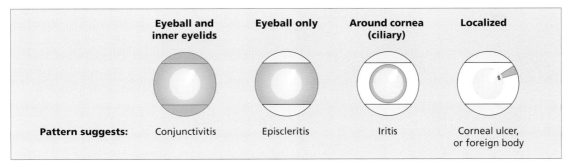

**Fig. 5.3** The pattern of redness suggests the possible diagnosis.

vessels most red in the depth of the fornix, as is typical of conjunctivitis, or around the cornea, as classic in iritis (Fig. 5.3)? A leash of dilated vessels next to the cornea often points to a corneal ulcer or foreign body. A localized area of redness may surround a degenerating pingueculum (see p. 83) or, especially if it takes the form of a nodule, be a sign of episcleritis. An active pterygium will extend onto the cornea at 3 or 9 o'clock. Small lumps on the surface of the eye which may accompany inflammation include limbal follicles (collections of white cells)—creamy swellings whose centres may stain with fluorescein. These may be part of a follicular conjunctivitis which is due to staphylococcal hypersensitivity and are seen almost exclusively in teenagers. Pingueculae are often noticed by patients for the first time when the surrounding eye is red. Occasionally they are responsible for low-grade inflammation. To see which coat of the eye is involved, look at the pattern of the dilated

vessels; the deeper episcleral vessels run radially. A purplish colour is characteristic of congestion as in acute glaucoma but also occurs in iritis and scleritis (see Fig. 5.21). Staining of the conjunctiva occurs in alkali burns. Consider less common causes such as toxicity to topical medication (especially gentamycin) (Fig. 5.4), and rarely self-inflicted injury. Oedema of the conjunctiva covering the eyeball is typical of an allergic reaction (Fig. 5.5) but also occurs in thyroid eye disease and severe conjunctival infections, sometimes producing a balloon-like appearance.

### Cornea
The cornea is normally bright, with a shiny reflex. Clouding of the cornea can be due to oedema or infiltration by white cells. Infiltrates tend to be small and may cluster round a foreign body or be due to infection or staphylococcal hypersensitivity. Consider a herpes simplex infection or a severe iritis.

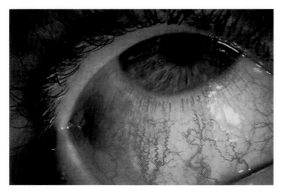

**Fig. 5.4** Red eye from gentamicin toxic conjunctivitis.

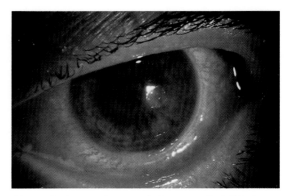

**Fig. 5.6** Red eye with a corneal ulcer at 3 o'clock. This is easy to miss unless the cornea is stained with fluorescein.

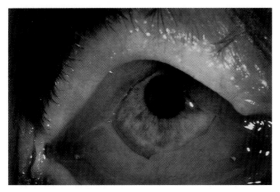

**Fig. 5.5** Acute allergic reaction of the conjunctiva with swelling and redness. The eye is usually very itchy.

Oedema is classically found in acute glaucoma. Precipitates, collections of white cells adhering to the back surface of the cornea, may be visible in iritis (see Fig. 5.43). Corneal abrasions and some ulcers (such as a dendritic ulcer—Fig. 5.6) are difficult to detect without the use of fluorescein. Scratches on the upper cornea should suggest a subtarsal foreign body.

> Beware infection in the soft contact lens wearer (oddly, especially if the disposable type)

*Pupil*
A small pupil is often found in iritis and irregularity due to adhesions to the lens may be seen when dilating drops are given (see Fig. 5.29). In acute glaucoma the pupil is classically oval, mid-dilated and unreactive (see Fig. 5.30).

*Vision*
Check the distance vision with and without a pin hole if the patient says it is blurred. A slight reduction is common in iritis. Central corneal oedema, abrasions and ulcers of any sort will affect the acuity, but it will often correct up to normal with the pin hole. The vision is very poor in acute glaucoma.

*Pre-auricular nodes*
The nodes in front of the ear are enlarged and tender in classic adenoviral and chlamydial conjunctivitis.

## Conjunctivitis
Inflammation of the conjunctiva is a common reaction to a variety of agents which include infection, physical conditions such as dryness and contact lens wear, and exposure to toxic materials ranging from preservatives in drops to industrial chemicals. It is therefore important to identify anything relevant in the history. Factors most often overlooked include *contact lens wear* (all sorts of problems, see the section on contact lenses), *prior drop treatment* (toxicity or hypersensitivity) and *previous cataract surgery* (broken or loose sutures).

*Symptoms* of conjunctivitis depend on the cause. Irritation, soreness, grittiness or foreign body feeling are common. If the cause is infection, discharge or stickiness is usual. Itching, burning, watering and swollen lids may occur. Secondary corneal changes may give *slight pain, photophobia and visual blurring, but these are not prominent symptoms in conjunctivitis, so turn to an alternative diagnosis if they are pronounced.*

> Stitches from cataract surgery may first cause irritation years later

> Red eye plus pain or photophobia is usually serious

### Bacterial conjunctivitis (Table 5.3)

This is the commonest sort of infective conjunctivitis and is usually bilateral. There may well be a history of contact with other cases. Conditions predisposing to bacterial infection include dry eyes, lid margin disease (blepharitis), obstruction to tear drainage and trauma to the conjunctiva. The most frequent organisms isolated are *Strep. pneumoniae*, *Haemophilus* species or *Staph. aureus*, although culture is often negative. A particularly sticky eye is occasionally produced by *Branhamella* (*Neisseria*) *catarrhalis*. Ophthalmia neonatorum (neonatal conjunctivitis) was traditionally caused by *Neisseria gonorrhoeae* but now results mainly from maternal *Chlamydia trachomatis* infection (see below).

*Symptoms* of bacterial infection are sore, red, sticky eyes (Fig. 5.7). Patients usually present to their general practitioner and uncomplicated cases are rarely seen in hospital practice.

*Appearance* is of reddening of the conjunctivae both inside the lids and on the eye itself, maximally in the fornices, with discharge in the lower fornix or stuck to the lashes.

Taking cultures is rarely indicated in the first instance, but may be useful if treatment fails. If so, leave for 48 hours without treatment before swabbing.

*Treatment* (Fig. 5.8) is not invariably necessary, as many bacterial infections are low grade and self-limiting. The topical treatment of first choice is *chloramphenicol*, as it has a broad spectrum, low toxicity (to the eye), a low rate of sensitivity reactions and is cheap. Drops should be instilled 2 hourly for the first 2 days, then four times

**Table 5.3** Features suggesting bacterial conjunctivitis

| |
| --- |
| Red + |
| Sticky ++ |
| Sore – or + |
| Usually bilateral |

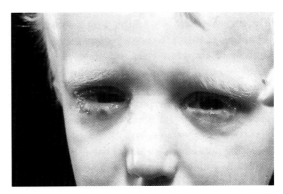

**Fig. 5.7** Bacterial conjunctivitis with sticky crusts on the lid margins. Reproduced from Taylor (1992) *Pediatric Ophthalmology* (slide atlas), Blackwell Scientific Publications, Cambridge, MA.

daily for 3 days. Additional ointment at night is not really necessary. Ointment is useful in children and in situations where frequent applications are difficult, but many adults find it blurring and ointments are also best avoided in dry eyes. It should be applied four times daily for 5 days.

Fucidin ointment has the advantage of patient acceptability with its comparatively non-viscous nature and twice daily use, but the disadvantage of a narrow spectrum limited to staphylococci. Neomycin has no advantages apart from its price and it is a frequent cause of hypersensitivity. Sulphacetamide is obsolete.

A good rule for general practice is never to substitute a second antibiotic if the first seems ineffective. It is likely that either the first treatment wasn't used, or is causing toxicity, or that the diagnosis needs to be revised. Gentamicin used as a second agent is especially prone to cause necrosis of the conjunctiva (see Fig. 5.4). Never be afraid to stop the treatment and observe or take swabs.

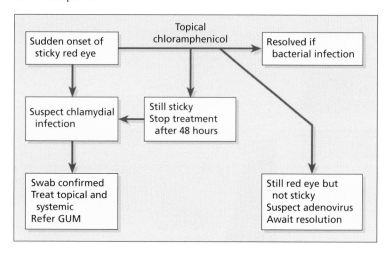

**Fig. 5.8** Management of infective conjunctivitis.

---

• In conjunctivitis, do not give a second antibiotic if the first has not worked
• In conjunctivitis, never be afraid to stop treatment that is not working

---

Any underlying problem such as dry eye or blepharitis should be sorted out once the bacterial infection is under control.

### Chlamydial conjunctivitis (Table 5.4)

*Chlamydia trachomatis* is responsible for two different patterns of conjunctivitis. Serotypes A, B and C cause trachoma (see below), whilst serotypes D to K produce an acute conjunctivitis with follicles known variously as 'inclusion', 'TRIC', or 'chlamydial' conjunctivitis. The infection is sexually transmitted, and occurs typically in younger adults, as well as being a cause of conjunctivitis in the newborn.

---

*Chlamydia* is a cause of ophthalmia neonatorum (in the first week of life)

---

*Symptoms*. A sticky, red, sore eye is usually unilateral. There may be slight blurring and photophobia. Other effects of chlamydial infection—vaginal discharge, urethritis or joint pain or swelling—may be revealed, but, unless volunteered, a sexual history is probably best left until infection is confirmed. It may be a shock to be told

**Table 5.4** Features suggesting chlamydial conjunctivitis

| |
| --- |
| Red ++ |
| Sticky +++ |
| Sore + |
| Usually unilateral |
| Swollen lid |
| Follicles |
| Enlarged preauricular node |
| Baby or sexually active young adult |

that a sexually transmitted disease is the cause of sticky eye.

*Appearance* is of a very red eye, with lid swelling and a lot of sticky discharge. The tarsal conjunctiva looks bumpy due to enlargement of follicles, best seen with a magnifying lens (or slit-lamp, see Fig. 5.11). In the upper lid, these can give a slight ptosis. The pre-auricular gland is often swollen and tender. There may be associated punctate erosions, especially of the upper cornea, though these are hard to see without a microscope.

*Treatment*. Referral is needed if chlamydial conjunctivitis is suspected, as conjunctival smears on a glass slide and/or a dry swab have to go to the laboratory in a special transport medium, for cytology or an ELISA test. Whilst awaiting confirmation of infection, treatment should be started at all ages with topical tetracycline ointment five times daily, continued for 3 weeks. *Systemic treatment is also necessary.* In adult patients, this is best left to the GUM clinic, who will want to take swabs before starting oral tetracycline 250 mg four times daily for 14 days, or doxycycline 100 mg daily for 10 days. Infants can be prescribed oral erythromycin, 30 mg/kg daily in two to four divided doses, for 3 weeks. Refer both parents, if possible, to the GUM clinic.

> Reserve swabbing the conjunctiva for:
> * treatment failure
> * suspected *Chlamydia* infection

> If chlamydial conjunctivitis is confirmed refer to the GUM clinic

Chloramphenicol inhibits, but does not cure chlamydial infections. Prior use reduces the likelihood of a positive swab result, so you must have the right index of suspicion to pick up these cases at the beginning, or follow the rule of swabbing after 48 hours off treatment if the infection persists or recurs.

Chlamydial and adenoviral conjunctivitis have many features in common and it can be impossible to make a definite diagnosis on some occasions. The main difference is a more purulent discharge in chlamydial infection. The clinical course, together with any swab results, then has to be watched. Untreated, adenoviral infections eventually resolve whereas chlamydial ones get worse. Adenovirus is more likely to cause an outbreak of contact cases as spread is non-sexual.

### Sticky eye in babies (Table 5.5)

Sticky eyes in a neonate (within the first week) may be ophthalmia neonatorum (Fig. 5.9), the commonest cause of which is now *Chlamydia trachomatis.* Conjunctival swabs should therefore be taken for chlamydial isolation as well as for bacterial culture. If chlamydia are found, the baby should receive tetracycline ointment five times daily for 3 weeks and erythromycin 30 mg/kg daily in two to four divided doses also for 3 weeks. If confirmed, the mother and her sexual partner must be referred to the genitourinary clinic.

Sticky eyes in babies after the first week tend to accompany URTIs and will often be self-limiting. Cultures are seldom worth while. If treatment is needed, chloramphenicol ointment four times daily for 5 days is adequate.

A recurrently sticky eye or eyes, with watering sometimes noticeable between attacks, is likely to be due to a failure of opening of the lower end of the nasolacrimal duct. This should happen by, or soon after, birth, but often fails. Treatment with topical antibiotics has only temporary benefits and it is best to rely on simple cleaning of the eye.

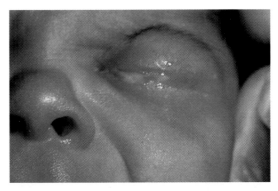

**Fig. 5.9** Sticky and swollen eye in a neonate with ophthalmia neonatorum. Nowadays in developed countries, chlamydial infection is the most common cause, and the eye should be swabbed to confirm this. (Courtesy of Mr A. Shun-Shin.)

**Table 5.5** Conjunctivitis in babies

| Age | Cause | Swab | Action |
|---|---|---|---|
| First week | Pyogenic | No | Chloramphenicol (topical) |
| | Chlamydial | Yes | Refer to eye and GUM departments |
| Older | Upper respiratory tract infection | No | Chloramphenicol (topical) |
| Recurrent | Blocked duct | No | Chloramphenicol (topical) and refer at 9 months |

The chances of spontaneous opening of the duct in the first year of life are high, and probing is not usually carried out until the age of 12 months. If the eye continues to be watery and sticky, consider referral at about 9 months, to allow for plans to be made. Probing occasionally needs to be repeated, but after 18 months it is less likely to be successful. The child will not suffer from repeated short courses of topical antibiotic but try to get the parents to accept some compromise.

> Refer a suspected blockage of the tear duct at age 9 months

### Trachoma

Trachoma, the world's most common cause of preventable blindness, is endemic in many parts of the world, particularly in rural communities with inadequate supplies of clean water. Infection is spread from eye to eye, with discharge-seeking flies playing an important role. Severe disease is most common in the poorest in any community. Recurrent episodes of keratoconjunctivitis, starting in early childhood, lead to scarring of the tarsal conjunctiva which causes the lashes to turn in towards the eye and rub on the cornea (trichiasis). This causes scarring of the cornea. In less severely affected eyes a characteristic sign is 'pannus', vascularization with slight opacification at the top of the cornea. Treatment of active disease is with topical tetracycline, as for other chlamydial conjunctivitis. Regimes have been devised for the treatment of populations of schoolchildren in hyperendemic areas, involving intermittent courses of tetracycline. Lid surgery and corneal grafting can be useful where it is possible to offer them. Prevention and control of reinfection will only be achieved by improvement of living conditions.

### Viral conjunctivitis (Table 5.6)

Viral conjunctival infection is most commonly caused by adenovirus (several types) and herpes simplex. Conjunctivitis can also complicate various systemic viral illnesses such as chickenpox and mumps, and it is characteristic in measles. Finally, remember the occasional case of molluscum contagiosum (see Fig. 5.13).

### Adenoviral conjunctivitis (Fig. 5.10)

This is an acute, usually unilateral, infection sometimes associated with an upper respiratory tract infection. It is highly contagious and other members of the household may have been affected. Epidemics of conjunctivitis due to types

**Table 5.6** Features suggesting viral conjunctivitis

Red ++
Sticky – or +
Sore + or ++
Usually unilateral, but may be sequential
Follicles
Enlarged pre-auricular node
Often epidemic

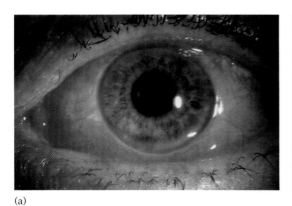
(a)

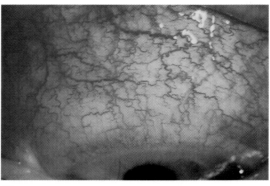
(b)

**Fig. 5.10** Viral conjunctivitis with red and swollen conjunctiva, but little discharge. Adenovirus was isolated by culture from a conjunctival swab.

8 and 19 are often based on workplaces—some of which have received such delightfully graphic names as 'shipyard-worker's eye'—and eye departments ('eye-hospital patient's eye'?) but can also occur sporadically. Needless to say, adenoviral conjunctivitis is an occupational hazard especially of ophthalmologists and can cause havoc in the eye department, so try to avoid referring these patients if possible! Transmission is by hand to eye, the fingers of members of the family or staff, contaminated by an infected patient, inoculating the eyes of others. Thorough cleaning of the hands and slit-lamp between each patient is the only way of preventing further spread and this is almost impossible in the family setting.

*Symptoms.* These are often florid, and are of sudden onset with a red, swollen, watering, uncomfortable eye characteristically without sticky discharge.

*Appearance.* The eye is often very red, possibly with conjunctival swelling and a slightly droopy lid. This is due to enlargement of follicles of the upper lid conjunctiva. Follicles of both lids may be visible with the naked eye as a generalized lumpiness, like porridge (Fig. 5.11). There may be preauricular lymph node enlargement. In early and uncomplicated cases the cornea will be clear. Distinguishing adenoviral conjunctivitis from that due to chlamydia can be difficult, as mentioned above (see Chlamydial conjunctivitis). Adenoviral infection can occur at any age, whilst chlamydial infection is unlikely outside the younger adult age group and the newborn. Otherwise, the relative absence of sticky discharge is often the helpful feature to favour a viral infection.

> Adenovirus is the most common cause of viral conjunctivitis

*Investigation.* Unless the diagnosis is unusually clearcut, particularly without an established epidemic, it is sensible to take swabs on presentation, for viral and chlamydial culture. Unfortunately, adenoviruses take a long time to 'grow', although some laboratories can provide a rapid identification based on a smear.

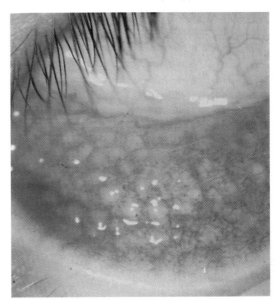

**Fig. 5.11** Follicles in conjunctivitis—the pale lumps are collections of white cells. There are a number of possible causes. Reproduced from Taylor (1992) *Pediatric Ophthalmology* (slide atlas), Blackwell Scientific Publications, Cambridge, MA.

The conjunctivitis takes 1–2 weeks to settle, but a keratitis may follow, initially consisting of many small corneal erosions (not usually visible without the slit-lamp), evolving into scattered corneal infiltrated opacities which should be visible with a loupe. These corneal problems cause mild visual blurring and photophobia and can last for *months*.

*Treatment.* At present *there is no treatment for adenovirus infections*. If bacterial infection cannot clinically be ruled out, topical antibiotics such as chloramphenicol drops will do no harm, and they may be soothing. The most useful action is to try to limit the spread of infection. As transmission is largely by hand to eye, handwashing before any contact with others is essential. People working in institutions where there is close contact with other people really need to stay at home. At home, sensible hygienic measures should be carried out. Once the eye is no longer red further virus shedding will no longer be a risk. *Occasionally*, if blurring and photophobia due to corneal opacities follow the resolution of the conjunctivitis, topical steroid such as prednisolone 0.5% four times daily is useful in suppressing the corneal infiltrates. This will suppress the symptom but will not hasten recovery, which may take months, so the course may extend for a long time; steroid treatment should only be given under slit-lamp observation. The risk involved in giving steroid to a viral conjunctivitis is particularly high as the conjunctival infection could be due not to adenovirus but to herpes simplex and steroid could precipitate corneal herpetic ulceration.

*Herpes simplex conjunctivitis*
Infection of the *conjunctiva*, as opposed to the cornea, occurs mainly as a primary exposure. It is therefore usually found in children and young adults, presumably from contact for the first time with someone with a 'cold sore'. It is almost always unilateral. (See also Corneal inflammation and ulceration, p. 73.)

> Eyelid infection in a young child may be herpetic

*Appearance.* There may be vesicles or small ulcers on the skin around the eye (Fig. 5.12), as well as pre-auricular node enlargement. With magnification, some follicles may be visible, but there is no lid swelling (unlike adenovirus and chlamydia) unless the lid itself is involved, and the eye is

not so floridly red. Small branching (dendritic or stellate) corneal ulcers may be visible on staining with fluorescein.

*Treatment* is with acyclovir ointment to the eye, five times daily. Any skin lesion will resolve spontaneously, though eczematous children (eczema herpeticum) may need topical or even oral treatment for the skin. Refer if there are symptoms of blurring or photophobia. *Steroid treatment of any strength should **not** be given in herpetic infection as this may precipitate a corneal ulcer.*

> Beware, herpes simplex corneal infections can still blind

*Molluscum contagiosum* (Fig. 5.13)
This is an occasional cause of conjunctivitis, particularly in childhood. Typical umbilicated lesions on the lid margin (see Lumps around the eye, p. 92) shed virus into the eye, resulting in a chronic conjunctivitis with follicles, resistant to all medication. Once the skin lesion has been curetted or expressed, the conjunctivitis will settle.

**Varieties of allergic conjunctivitis**
This is likely to be the most common eye problem managed in general practice, though it competes with blepharitis for this honour. Sometimes it is the sufferer who decides on their own treatment using self-medication, as 'hay fever' is by far the commonest type of allergic conjunctivitis. Other forms of conjunctivitis involving immune re-

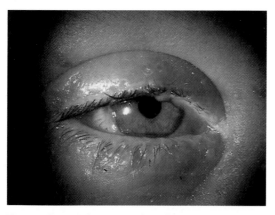

**Fig. 5.12** Primary herpes simplex infection with vesicles on the eyelids in a child. A red painful eye suggests an associated corneal lesion, which should be stained with fluorescein.

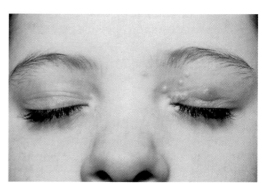

**Fig. 5.13** Molluscum contagiosum of the eyelids—multiple pearly lesions in a young patient. (Courtesy of Mr A. Shun-Shin.)

**Table 5.7** Types and origins of immune conjunctivitis

| Type | Most common origin |
| --- | --- |
| Seasonal allergic (hay fever) | Pollen |
| Perennial allergic | House dust |
| Acute allergic | Plants |
| Vernal catarrh | Pollen? |
| Giant papillary | Contact lens wear |
| Atopic keratoconjunctivitis | Adult atopic |
| Contact hypersensitivity | Eye medication, metals |
| Phlyctenular | *Staphylococcus* |
| Cicatricial pemphigoid | Autoimmune |

**Table 5.8** Seasonal allergic conjunctivitis

Bilateral
Episodic
Seasonal
Plant pollen allergen often
Younger atopic patient
Hay fever symptoms common

Treat with topical mast cell stabilizer plus topical or oral antihistamine

sponses are a variation on the theme but may need different management and have a different prognosis. These include a number of conditions with confusing names, but it is worth getting to grips with the differences, as they each describe a different clinical pattern (Table 5.7).

> Suspect allergic conjunctivitis if the eye is itchy

*'Hay fever' or seasonal allergic conjunctivitis: the most common type* (Table 5.8)
This is due to a type 1 immediate immune response involving histamine release. It is particularly common where there is a personal or family history of *atopy* and is *seasonal*, being at its worst in Great Britain from April to July—with a peak in May—as grass pollens are the commonest precipitants. The weather also plays a part, affecting the rate of release of pollen into the atmosphere. Hay fever is worse in the young, tending to improve with age. At a rough estimate, it affects one person in every ten at some time.

*Symptoms* affect both eyes and are of *intense itching*, watering, intermittent lid swelling and mucous discharge. They fluctuate through the season depending on exposure to allergens. Ocular symptoms are usually accompanied by sneezing, rhinorrhoea and, less often, wheezing.

*Appearance.* There may be lid swelling and conjunctival redness, but usually the symptoms are out of proportion to the signs, with the eyes looking normal between acute bouts.

*Investigations* are only occasionally indicated. Eosinophils are found in 50% of conjunctival smears. IgE levels are usually raised in the blood. Skin prick testing will often demonstrate the responsible allergens but may offer no practical solution.

*Treatment.* In most patients, symptoms can be controlled, with varying degrees of success, by a topical mast cell stabilizer, used regularly. As well as the well-established sodium cromoglycate (Opticrom), there are now nedocromil (Rapitil) and lodoxamide (Alomide). Cromoglycate and lodoxamide are used four times daily, and nedocromil is used twice daily. It is important to stress to the patient that the drop regime will not suceed unless it is used very faithfully and that it is no use expecting it to work if used just when symptoms occur. It blocks the histamine response but cannot work 'after the event'. It is up to the patient to decide if the trouble is really worthwhile. For more acute use, levocabastine and emedastine may be useful. These newly developed topical antihistamines are much more effective than the long available antazoline (Otrivine). An oral antihistamine such as loratadine (Clarityn) 10mg daily may be particularly helpful if nasal symptoms are also present. Loratadine, cromoglycate and levocabastine can all be bought in small supplies across the counter. Topical steroids are very rarely necessary and often cause problems in prolonged use with rebound phenomena. Desensitization is now rarely used due to the risk of anaphylaxis. The patient may wish to follow advice about pollen counts, but most of us cannot avoid going outdoors on certain days. It is wise for car windows to be shut on high count days.

**Table 5.9** Perennial allergic conjunctivitis

Bilateral
Episodic
All the year
Household allergen, especially house-dust mite
Younger atopic patient
Eczema common

Treat with topical mast cell stabilizer, maybe topical or oral
    antihistamine

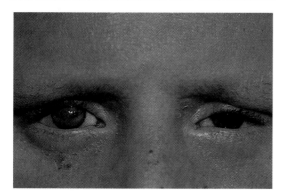

**Fig. 5.14** Atopic subject with perennial conjunctivitis and
eczema of the eyelids. This young patient also has a right
corneal ulcer.

*Perennial allergic conjunctivitis: discouraging for
patient and doctor* (Table 5.9 and Fig. 5.14)
This gives symptoms and signs similar to hay
fever, but *throughout the year*. A common cause is
house-dust mite allergy, demonstrated by raised
specific IgE levels in the tears and serum of those
affected. Other precipitants are moulds, pollens,
animal danders and chemicals such as food
preservatives.

*Treatment* is with topical cromoglycate, nedocromil or lodoxamide and is very boring and
discouraging for the patient. Few manage to use
the drops reliably enough. Reducing allergen
exposure may help. Topical or oral antihistamines may be tried. Occasionally patients develop an allergy to the preservative in the drops;
preservative-free cromoglycate is available, but
difficult to obtain.

*Acute allergic conjunctivitis: alarming but harmless*
(Table 5.10)
This rapidly follows exposure to an allergen

**Table 5.10** Acute allergic conjunctivitis

Acute
Often unilateral
Single or sporadic episodes
Not necessarily atopic
More common in summer
Plant allergen likely
Chemosis ++

Treat with reassurance

**Table 5.11** Vernal catarrh

Grumbling
Usually seasonal, in spring
Not always atopic
Papillae
Secondary corneal changes may occur

Treat with topical mast cell stabilizer, sometimes topical
    steroid

which is usually not identifiable but is commonly
a *plant*. Ragwort is sometimes to blame—Oxford
is the home of ragwort and every summer there
is a seasonal flood to eye casualty of unsuspect-
ing residents and visitors who were enjoying an
afternoon on the river at the onset. It is often, strangely, unilateral. The onset is sudden, with itching,
lid swelling, conjunctival redness and swelling,
which often balloons the conjunctiva out between
the swollen lids (see Fig. 5.5). The whole picture
looks most alarming, but fortunately it resolves
very quickly and spontaneously, *without treatment*, though oral antihistamine may be given.

*Vernal catarrh: look under the top lid for 'cobblestones'*
(Table 5.11)
This is a disease affecting *young atopes* and is commoner in boys than in girls, usually presenting before the age of 10. As its name suggests
(*verna* = spring), it has a *seasonal* pattern, symptoms starting in the spring and continuing
through the warmer months, though in some it is
perennial. Both eyes are affected, often asymmet-
rically. No specific allergens have been implicated. Infiltration of the conjunctiva by lymphocytes,
plasma cells and eosinophils leads to the formation of *giant papillae of the conjunctiva lining the
upper lid* (Fig. 5.15) and limbal follicles. The cornea

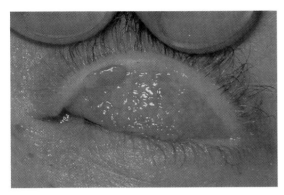

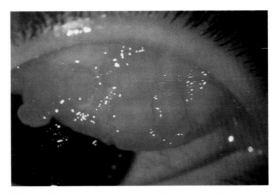

**Fig. 5.15** Papillae beneath the upper lid in vernal conjunctivitis, looking like cobblestones. Reproduced from Taylor (1997) *Paediatric Ophthalmology*, 2nd edn, Blackwell Science, Oxford.

**Fig. 5.16** Giant papillae of the conjunctiva, with particularly large 'cobblestones', in a soft contact lens wearer. Reproduced from Taylor (1992) *Pediatric Ophthalmology* (slide atlas), Blackwell Scientific Publications, Cambridge, MA.

can also be affected, with erosions and plaque formation.

*Symptoms* are of intense itching, foreign body sensation, watering, sticky discharge and drooping of the upper lids. If the cornea is involved, there will be photophobia and possibly blurred vision.

*Appearance.* A mechanical ptosis due to the papillae is common. If the lid can be everted, the '*cobblestone*' like papillae will be found. The lower lid usually looks normal. The eye may be red, with follicles around the edge of the cornea looking like grains of rice. Corneal erosions will stain with fluorescein, and any plaque will be seen as a flattened, opaque area of cornea.

*Treatment.* Topical sodium cromoglycate, nedocromil or lodoxamide are the mainstay of treatment. Topical steroids may also be needed for exacerbations. Hospital outpatient clinic supervision is advisable. The disease tends to remit after 5–10 years.

*Giant papillary conjunctivitis: especially in soft contact lens wearers* (Table 5.12)
This is quite common in *contact lens* wearers, an ever-growing band, and occasionally following eye surgery. Friction between the contact lens, or sutures, and the conjunctiva lining the upper lid provokes the growth of papillae and a 'cobble-

**Table 5.12** Giant papillary conjunctivitis

| |
| --- |
| Contact lens wear or surgical eye sutures |
| 'Cobblestones' |
| Often unilateral |
| Treat by stopping contact lens wear or removing sutures |

stone' appearance similar to that seen in vernal conjunctivitis (Fig. 5.16). The eye is itchy, watering and may have a slight ptosis. There is usually poor tolerance of contact lens wear. It is commonest in soft contact lens wearers, probably because soft lenses are larger than rigid lenses and also because mucous deposits on the surface of the lens may be allergenic. Interestingly, the eyes may be affected in a highly asymmetrical manner.

*Treatment.* If due to sutures, these can be removed. Contact lens wear often needs to be suspended altogether until the symptoms settle, which may take months. If the lenses are worn again advise getting a new pair; lens hygiene should be scrupulous and wearing times reduced to a minimum. Changing lens material, perhaps from soft to 'gas-permeable' may prevent recurrent problems. Topical cromoglycate is occasionally useful. It is possible for the patient to be sensitive to the preservative in one of their lens solutions so it is worth trying preservative-free solutions if lens wear is tried again.

**Table 5.13** Atopic keratoconjunctivitis

Chronic
Often severe
Adult atopic patients
Lichenified skin

Treat with topical mast cell stabilizers and steroids,
    sometimes antibiotics
Complications common and often severe

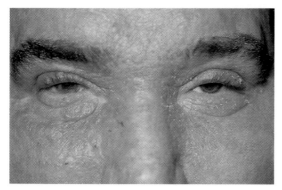

**Fig. 5.17** Adult atopic with eyelid eczema and
conjunctivitis. There is a high risk of secondary
complications.

*Atopic keratoconjunctivitis: a serious threat to vision
in adults* (Table 5.13)
This is a severe chronic disease, fortunately rare,
occurring in adult atopes (Fig. 5.17). It is often
associated with cataract and keratoconus. Eye
rubbing may play some part. As well as a giant
papillary reaction of the upper lid and corneal
plaques and scarring, there are meibomian gland
abnormalities.

*Symptoms* are similar to vernal catarrh. Vision is
more likely to be affected, however, due to corneal
scarring and cataract.

*Treatment* is with topical cromoglycate and
steroids, with topical or systemic antibiotics for
any lid infections. This must be undertaken by a
hospital clinic as the condition is obstinate and
persistent, and complications are serious.

*Contact hypersensitivity* (Table 5.14)
Contact hypersensitivity or 'allergic contact dermatitis' is a type 4, lymphocyte-mediated delayed

**Table 5.14** More common causes of periocular contact
dermatitis

Topical
    Eye medication, especially neomycin, atropine and
        dorzolamide
    Cosmetics applied to the eyelid
Spectacle frames
Match heads
Resin adhesive
Cosmetic or perfume applied elsewhere
Nickel

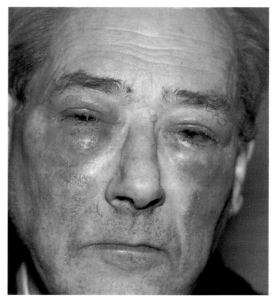

**Fig. 5.18** Contact sensitivity of skin around the eye,
usually secondary to eye medication. (Courtesy of Mr A.
Shun-Shin.)

immune response requiring previous sensitization. Reactions involving the eyes and lids are
frequently caused by substances applied to them.
Neomycin, atropine, dorzolamide and preservatives such as benzalkonium are particularly likely
culprits. In other instances, contact with the allergen may be remote from the eyes, such as metals,
match heads, resins or perfumes, which tend to be
rubbed off the fingers once the cycle of itching
starts. There is no seasonal pattern. One or both
eyes may be affected (Fig. 5.18).

*Symptoms* of itchy, watering eyes with swollen
lids take at least 48 hours to develop from expo-

sure to the allergen. With time, the lid swelling gives way to established thickening of the skin.

*Appearance.* The skin changes of the lids are characteristic, with a dusky colour and firm thickening or roughness (lichenification). Swelling is variable but never gross. There may be a velvety papillary reaction and slight redness of the conjunctiva.

*Treatment.* This is essentially of identifying the allergen and, wherever possible, avoiding it. In the case of eye drops this should be straightforward. Patch testing may be helpful in more obscure cases. Topical steroids and cromoglycate are *not* helpful and steroids may be harmful.

### Phlyctenular conjunctivitis

This is an unusual conjunctivitis occurring in children and teenagers, and is probably also an example of a delayed immune response. It was originally described as being associated with tuberculosis, but is now thought to be a reaction to staphylococcal infection. The usual picture is of a sticky, red eye which fails to respond to topical antibiotics. The *phlycten* is a small, raised, creamy lesion, the top of which stains with fluorescein. It is usually seen on the conjunctiva near the edge of the cornea, but may rarely be found on the cornea itself.

*Treatment.* Phlyctenular conjunctivitis responds rapidly to topical steroid, such as betamethasone 0.5% drops four times daily for 1 week. The prob-lem may recur if the staphylococcal infection persists, so treat the associated lid blepharitis (see below).

### Cicatricial pemphigoid (benign mucous membrane pemphigoid) (Fig. 5.19)

This is not at all benign, though it is fortunately rare. The diagnosis should be considered in any patient with recurrent eyelash problems (trichiasis). Patients with cicatricial pemphigoid often have soreness and ulceration of other mucous membranes, particularly the mouth and in women the vulva, though rarely the blistering skin lesions of bullous pemphigoid. Deposition of antibody in the conjunctiva may have a role in causing the disorder but the damage is done by chronic inflammation. It is a chronic disease of later life, more often in women, invariably bilateral. Stevens–Johnson syndrome is similar but has an acute damaging event at the onset (see Eye problems in skin disorders, p. 139).

*Appearance.* The eyes are affected by conjunctival scarring which leads to symblepharon—adhesions between the lids and the eyeball—and to deformity of the lid margins with folding in of the lashes and poor lid function. The eyes may become dry and the cornea scarred and vascularized from exposure and lash damage.

*Treatment* has not been effective in halting the scarring process, even with topical steroids. Symptoms may be improved by lubrication, electrolysis

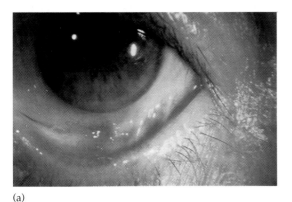

(a)

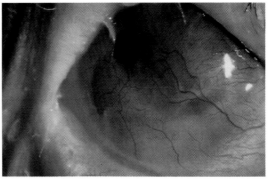

(b)

**Fig. 5.19** Cicatricial pemphigoid, a rare autoimmune conjunctivitis, which may cause corneal scarring and blindness.

**Table 5.15** Episcleritis

Common
Redness of all or part of the eye coat
Uncomfortable
Occasionally an identifiable systemic cause, infective or
  inflammatory

*Treatment*
Try to avoid any cause
Try non-steroidal anti-inflammatory drugs, topical or oral

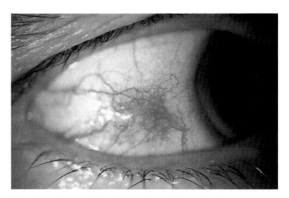

**Fig. 5.20** Episcleritis with a red nodule, which is uncomfortable but not painful. (Courtesy of Mr A. Shun-Shin.)

**Table 5.16** Scleritis

Uncommon
Redness of all or part of the eye coat
Swelling of the eye coat
Painful
Often an identifiable underlying systemic cause which
  may be severe
Most commonly an autoimmune vasculitis, e.g.
  rheumatoid arthritis or Wegener's syndrome

Treatment by a specialist

and entropion surgery. However, immunosuppressive drugs may be necessary.

### Episcleritis (Table 5.15)

*Epi* is Greek for 'next to' and the episclera lies beneath the conjunctiva, wrapped round the white coat of the eye. Episcleritis is a common inflammation of the eyeball, of unknown cause, occurring mostly in healthy young adults. It is often recurrent. Occasionally there may be a systemic problem, so ask about general health.

> Episcleritis causes a red and uncomfortable eye

*Symptoms* are of redness and perhaps some discomfort. If the eye is painful, suspect something else, such as scleritis. The eye is not really sticky, unlike many types of conjunctivitis.

*Appearance.* The deeper radial episcleral vessels are dilated, together with the overlying conjunctival vessels. This is usually localized though it may be diffuse. If localized, there is often a nodular swelling in the area (Fig. 5.20). The lids and their lining conjunctivae are *not* inflamed and vision is normal. The cornea is clear and non-staining.

*Treatment* is not necessary if the eye is merely a bit red, as episcleritis often settles spontaneously. Otherwise, use topical steroids such as betamethasone 0.1% drops four times daily, reducing soon on improvement to twice daily for a few days. It is often necessary to tail off the steroids to avoid a 'rebound' attack. An alternative treatment, which avoids the use of steroids, is an oral non-steroidal anti-inflammatory such as ibuprofen 400 mg three times daily.

### Scleritis (Table 5.16)

Scleritis can be mistaken for episcleritis, but there are crucial differences. Scleritis is much less common but more severe. It is due to closure of episcleral capillaries supplying the underlying avascular sclera and so is an ischaemic process.

*Symptoms* are more pronounced, with eye pain which can be severe, and sometimes with blurring of vision due to iris or optic nerve head involvement. Scleritis is commonest in the middle-aged and elderly, frequently in association with a connective tissue disorder, usually rheumatoid arthritis.

> Scleritis causes a red and painful eye

*Appearance.* The eyeball is diffusely or locally inflamed. There may be a nodule of thickened sclera

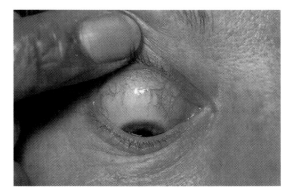

**Fig. 5.21** Scleritis with a bluish-red eye, which is painful.

and oedema of the eyeball locally. The very deep vessels are involved, giving the eye a purplish look (Fig. 5.21). Recurrent attacks thin the sclera leaving dark patches.

*Treatment.* Patients with suspected scleritis should be referred urgently as they may need systemic steroids to control the disease. They respond poorly to topical steroid, some respond to systemic non-steroidal anti-inflammatory drugs, but treatment must be carefully monitored by a specialist to minimize the risk to the eye.

## Corneal inflammation and ulceration:
### keratitis (Table 5.17)

It is important to identify these conditions because of the risk of permanent damage to sight from corneal scarring. Scars are a common reason for corneal grafting. Perforation of the eye can also occur, though fortunately this is rare. Whatever the cause, the symptoms are similar: pain, photophobia, watering and often some blurring of vision, which varies depending on the area of the cornea affected. The eye is usually red. Additional symptoms, such as a sticky discharge or rash may be helpful in establishing the cause. The cornea can also be involved in some types of conjunctivitis, and in lid margin disease. These will be described with the parent condition.

Although there are many types of corneal ulcer, only five are common enough to be of concern to the non-specialist:
- Marginal
- Herpes simplex and herpes zoster
- Bacterial

**Table 5.17** Features of keratitis (many shared with iritis)

Red eye
Pain
Watering
Photophobia
Sometimes reduced vision
Sometimes rash, e.g. herpes simplex, herpes zoster or
  rosacea

- Neuroparalytic, due to poor closure
- Rosacea associated.

Symptoms of corneal ulcer are:
- pain
- watering
- photophobia
- blurring of vision

Risk factors for corneal ulcer are:
- dry eye
- contact lens wear
- insensitive eye
- blepharitis
- herpes viruses — zoster or cold sore

### Marginal keratitis: the most common

As the name suggests, this occurs near the edge of the cornea. It is probably the commonest keratitis. It consists initially of a cellular infiltrate, over which the epithelium may then ulcerate. It typically affects the middle-aged and elderly who have lid margin disease (blepharitis) and is thought to be due to hypersensitivity to staphylococci lurking in the lid margin. It can affect either eye and has a strong tendency to recur.

*Symptoms* are of redness, irritation, pain (not usually severe), mild photophobia and watering. There is rarely real discharge, but the lid margins may be crusty from blepharitis.

*Appearance.* The lid margins will look red, crusty and irregular if there is associated lid margin disease. The eye is red, and this is often localized adjacent to the corneal ulcer. The ulcer itself is an oval creamy opacity, sometimes spreading circumfer-

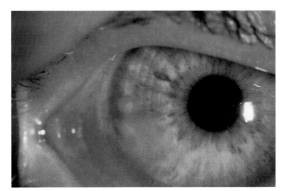

**Fig. 5.22** Marginal corneal ulcer with local redness and an opaque oval lesion at 8 o'clock on the edge of the cornea. The surrounding haze is an infiltrate of white cells.

**Table 5.18** Herpes simplex corneal ulcer

Usually unilateral but there may be past attacks in the other eye, sometimes bilateral scarring
Rash uncommon on the eyelid and suggests primary infection
Dendritic pattern common, but others possible
Often recurrent
Corneal sensation sometimes reduced
Complications other than corneal scarring uncommon

Treat with topical antiviral
Topical steroid contraindicated in the acute attack

entially shaped in the form of a crescent, very near to the corneal edge (Fig. 5.22). It usually stains with fluorescein. It is important to differentiate the marginal ulcer from a peripherally located herpetic ulcer.

*Treatment.* Marginal keratitis responds very well to a short course of topical steroids, such as betamethasone 0.1% drops, four times daily for 1 week. In typical (recurrent) cases treatment can be given without referral, warning the patient to stop treatment and to return if symptoms worsen or do not completely settle. Healing often leaves a small scar, which can be an aid to diagnosis on future occasions. Being in the periphery of the cornea, scarring will not affect vision. Treating lid margin disease may reduce the rate of recurrence though a course of systemic antistaphylococcal antibiotic may be necessary (see Blepharitis, below).

### Herpes simplex keratitis: look for a dendritic staining pattern (Table 5.18)

*Primary infection with type 1 herpes simplex virus*
*This is uncommon* as the virus is usually acquired first at a site other than the eye. It can occur in children and teenagers as a result of contact with a 'cold sore', usually giving a vesicular rash on the lids and a conjunctivitis with follicles (see p. 65). It is also a cause of ulcerative blepharitis in children. If the eye is watering and photophobic, with the child preferring to keep it shut, corneal involve-

ment should be suspected. This takes the form of multiple tiny epithelial erosions or small dendritic ulcers. These stain with fluorescein, but may be difficult to see without a slit-lamp. The child may be unwell and have an enlarged pre-auricular node.

> Eyelid infection in a young child may be herpetic

> Beware, herpes simplex corneal infections can still blind

*Treatment.* Although the attack is usually self-limiting, it is best to treat the eye and skin with a topical preparation of acyclovir eye ointment, five times daily—for 5 days to the skin and for up to 3 weeks to the eye if there is a keratitis. Because of the small risk of recurrent infection, the parents should be advised to report any subsequent red eye, as this may be a reactivation.

*Recurrent herpetic infection (which represents 95% of cases)* (Fig. 5.23)
*This is due to reactivation* of virus lying dormant in the trigeminal ganglion. An attack can be provoked by factors such as sunlight, illness and trauma, although most patients cannot identify any such stimulus. The classic lesion is the branching dendritic ulcer, but deeper (more serious) stromal infection can also occur.

A variety of modified patterns can follow a typical dendritic. A neglected dendritic ulcer, or particularly one treated with topical steroids, may develop an 'amoeboid' shape. 'Disciform' kerati-

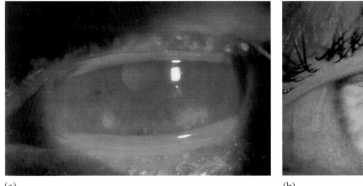
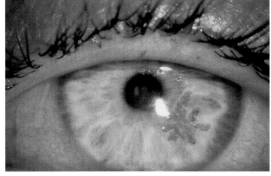

(a)                          (b)

**Fig. 5.23** Dendritic ulcers stained with (a) fluorescein and (b) rose bengal, typical of secondary herpes simplex keratitis. (Courtesy of Mr A. Shun-Shin.)

tis, in which there is a disc of central corneal oedema, is also not due to active infection, but probably represents an immune response. It is comparatively common. All these secondary forms can be especially troublesome.

*Symptoms* are of pain, photophobia, watering and redness. The amount of blurring of vision will depend on the site of ulceration and is always prominent in the disciform type.

*Appearance.* The eye will be red, maximally around the cornea, and frequently with a localized patch 'pointing' towards the ulcer. The *dendritic ulcer* is usually surrounded by clear cornea and is thus not obvious until the cornea is stained with fluorescein. The cornea may look hazy with oedema or with scarring from a previous episode. Stromal keratitis gives a localized creamy opacity. Disciform keratitis usually also has iritis, and keratic precipitates may be visible. Recurrent herpetic infections interfere with corneal sensation, so testing with a wisp of tissue is helpful (compare with the other eye as some normal patients have reduced sensation).

*Treatment* is the same as for the primary infection, with a *topical* antiviral. Acyclovir eye ointment five times daily is the treatment of first choice and will heal the majority of ulcers in 2 weeks. In a clear-cut case, particularly with access to a slit-lamp, this treatment could be carried out in prac-

tice, referring in the event of an inadequate response. Acyclovir is not likely to give side-effects unless used in the long term, when the effect of the ointment base on the tear film, especially in dry eyes, can produce multiple corneal erosions which may be mistaken for a lack of response to treatment. Debridement of a dendritic ulcer, in addition to acyclovir, can speed healing but should be done at the slit-lamp.

Other antivirals such as idoxuridine, vidarabine and trifluorothymidine ($F_3T$) are occasionally used. Disciform keratitis responds to low dose topical steroids, although they may be needed for prolonged periods of time to avoid relapses, and these patients *will require slit-lamp supervision*. All patients except those on the tiniest doses of topical steroids will need topical antiviral 'cover' as well.

The risk of recurrent dendritic ulceration is quite high, with a rate of 25% within 2 years of a first attack and 40% after subsequent attacks. Recurrent herpes simplex can be very aggressive and defy every effort at treatment. Fortunately it is bilateral in only 6% of individuals, mostly atopes who also have some of the most severe disease. In selected cases with scarring, corneal grafting can provide a useful improvement in vision, which will be most appreciated if the other eye sees poorly. Complications are unfortunately common, with recurrent infection possible in the graft, and a high risk of rejection in eyes with corneal vascularization.

*Herpes zoster keratitis: beware patients with ophthalmic shingles* (Table 5.19)

Herpes zoster of the ophthalmic division of the trigeminal nerve (herpes zoster ophthalmicus or HZO) accounts for 7% of all shingles attacks. The elderly and immunocompromised tend to have the most severe outbreaks. Ocular involvement, usually but not invariably forecast by vesicles on the nose, occurs in 50% of cases. *This is a potentially serious threat to sight and the eye must always be examined carefully in ophthalmic shingles.*

> • Ophthalmic shingles is a potentially blinding condition
> • Refer if the eye is red or vision has fallen

An attack starts with *unilateral head pain* followed by a vesicular rash in the distribution of the

**Table 5.19** Herpes zoster corneal ulcer

Always unilateral
Rash on face, nose and eyelid
Seldom recurrent
Dendritic pattern unusual
Corneal sensation often reduced
Other complications common with iritis, glaucoma, cranial nerve palsies

Treat with topical and systemic antiviral
Topical steroid may be needed in the acute attack, only with slit-lamp supervision

ophthalmic branch of the fifth cranial nerve. The pain may precede the rash by several days and cause diagnostic difficulties. With the rash can come gross *periorbital swelling*, sometimes bilaterally, in which case the patient needs to be reassured that the infection is not spreading to the other side. A *purulent discharge* may occur. If it is possible to open the lids, *vesicles* may be seen on the lid margins or on the eye surface and the involved eye will look red.

Corneal involvement at the onset consists of *epithelial lesions*—punctate, stellate or 'dendriform' in shape. Later manifestations include small, hazy 'nummular' lesions and disciform keratitis (see Herpes simplex keratitis, above). *Diminished corneal sensation* is a very significant finding as secondary neurotrophic keratitis may follow 3–6 months later. Punctate erosions develop in the middle of the cornea, sometimes leading to frank ulceration. The corneal lesions of HZO are peculiarly prone to lipid deposition, giving them an eventual bright white appearance that has cosmetic as well as visual effects.

The *iritis* of HZO usually develops about 2 weeks after the onset of the rash (Fig. 5.24). Quite often it causes *secondary glaucoma*. Secondary iris atrophy is also seen, characteristically in a sectorial pattern, probably due to ischaemia. *Cranial nerve palsies* are not uncommon, but usually settle spontaneously. In the long term,

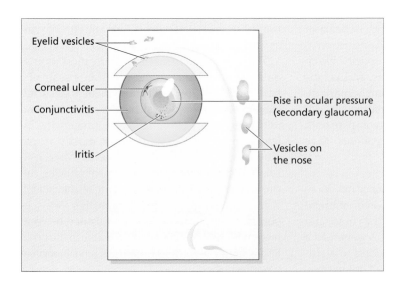

**Fig. 5.24** Ophthalmic herpes zoster should be borne in mind.

**Table 5.20** Treatment of ophthalmic shingles

No eye involvement: no extra treatment
Early to moderate eye involvement: add topical acyclovir
  ointment five times daily
Severe eye involvement: admit for intravenous acyclovir
  plus topical acyclovir with or without steroid

**Table 5.21** Bacterial corneal ulcer

Unilateral
Associated causes
  Trauma or contact lens wear
  Dry eye
  Insensitive eye
  Eye already blind and painful
Red ++, particularly local to the ulcer
Pain ++ (beware—no pain in the anaesthetic eye)
May be hypopyon
Refer immediately for culture before treating
Urgent topical treatment
High risk of complications and permanent visual loss

post-herpetic neuralgia can cause much misery.

*Immediate treatment* (Table 5.20). If presenting within 48 hours of onset, it is reasonable to use *oral* acyclovir 800 mg five times daily for 7 days, unless the attack is only mild, as the drug has been shown to alleviate the initial symptoms. Longer term benefits, such as reducing post-herpetic neuralgia, are not so well established. Analgesia is also usually needed. If the eye seems at all involved, add acyclovir *ointment* five times daily and refer for slit-lamp assessment within the next few days. Only if the eye is comfortable, certainly uninflamed and seeing normally, is referral not necessary. Severely affected people (as the very elderly often are) may benefit from admission to hospital where intravenous acyclovir can be given.

*Long-term treatment.* After 2–3 weeks the lid swelling, conjunctivitis and any superficial corneal lesions will be settling and the topical acyclovir can be stopped. Iritis, disciform and nummular keratitis may need topical steroids, with control of pressure if there is secondary glaucoma. It is not uncommon for any of these complications to become chronic or recurrent over the course of some years, requiring repeated courses of topical steroids. Glaucoma may become chronic as well. Also in the long term, neurotrophic keratitis caused by poor corneal sensation may need treatment with lubricant drops, ointments and padding. Bacterial infection must be watched for and vigorously treated. Ulcers are at risk of becoming indolent and central tarsorraphy is sometimes the only way to get the cornea to heal.

### Bacterial keratitis: a hazard in injury or contact lens wear (Table 5.21)
This is not common in healthy eyes unless they are subject to *trauma*, of which *soft contact lens* wear (particularly on an extended basis) is a potent cause. Otherwise, bacterial infection may occur in a dry or insensitive eye or one with pre-existing corneal disease. Beware *agricultural* or *gardening* injuries, where fungi may also be present.

Pathogens most often implicated include *Staphylococcus aureus* and *Streptococcus pneumoniae*. Soft contact lens wear predisposes to infection with *Acanthamoeba* and *Pseudomonas aeruginosa*. *Pseudomonas* is an especially feared pathogen as it can cause rapid corneal perforation. Contact lens contamination unfortunately can occur despite good hygiene.

Beware infection in the soft contact lens wearer (oddly, especially if the disposable type)

*Symptoms* are of pain, photophobia, watering and redness. A sticky discharge, though expected, is not universal. The site of the ulcer will dictate the amount of blurring, although a severe infection anywhere on the cornea will affect vision. A history of a predisposing factor should be asked about specifically.

*Appearance.* The eyeball is reddened to a variable extent. In severe infections the eye will be very red, with conjunctival swelling. Mucopus may be present in the lower fornix. Infiltration of the cornea is visible as a creamy opacity, staining with fluorescein, which may be surrounded by hazy, oedematous cornea (Fig. 5.25). Some degree of secondary iritis is to be expected, even a

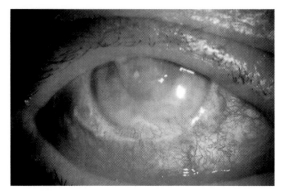

**Fig. 5.25** A bacterial corneal ulcer, with which there may be white cells infiltrating the cornea. This central ulcer shows hazy fluorescein uptake.

collection of white cells at the bottom of the chamber (*hypopyon*).

*Treatment.* Whenever there is a possibility of bacterial infection of the cornea, the patient should be *referred immediately* for microscopy and culture of scrapings from the ulcer, done at the slit-lamp. Whilst awaiting identification of the organism, treatment will be started with very frequent broad-spectrum topical antibiotics (often two types, though a quinolone alone may be sufficient in milder cases) plus a dilating drop. Admission for continuing assessment may be needed, especially if the patient lives far from the hospital. Topical steroids are often added once the infection is under control. Healing takes from 2 to 6 weeks. The cornea may be left scarred with permanently reduced vision and corneal grafting is then needed to improve sight, though as bacterial keratitis is prone to occur in the already damaged eyes of elderly people, grafting is often inappropriate.

### Neuroparalytic (exposure) keratitis

The commonest cause of this is a Bell's palsy. Inadequate lid closure and poor blinking due to deficient facial nerve function will result in a variable amount of corneal exposure depending on the efficiency of Bell's phenomenon—the upward rolling of the eye on attempted lid closure (Fig. 5.26). It also appears that some people sleep with their eyes a bit open. Drying of the surface of the cornea leads to erosions of the lower cornea, initially punctate but becoming a confluent ulcer if

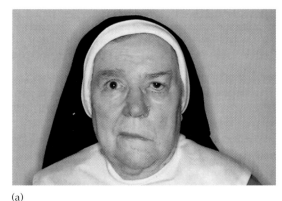

(a)

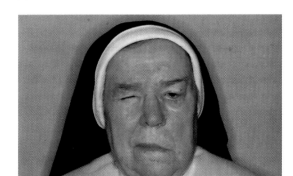

(b)

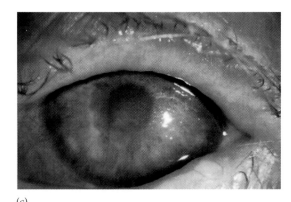

(c)

**Fig. 5.26** (a, b) In the eye with a facial palsy, the cornea may be exposed if blinking is poor (as on the left side). (c) Shows hazy cornea from exposure damage.

neglected. The eye may also water, as some ectropion of the paralysed lower lid is often seen with displacement of the punctum. The problem may be secondary to leprosy in parts of the world where this is endemic. Corneal exposure can also occur in a proptosed eye as in thyroid eye disease. The risk of ulceration is greater if the cornea is also insensitive (neurotrophic ulcer).

*Treatment* (Table 5.22). Refer any patient with inadequate lid closure. In the short term, as whilst awaiting recovery from a Bell's palsy, the eye should be kept lubricated by putting in artificial tears frequently during the day, with ointment or liquid paraffin (Lacrilube) at night. Taping the lids shut at night may also be helpful. Occasionally, injecting botulinum toxin into the upper lid to cause a temporary ptosis can be useful. If there is no recovery, or the facial paralysis is known to be permanent (as after removal of an acoustic neuroma), a lateral tarsorrhaphy should be done. This gives much greater protection to the cornea although it can be cosmetically unsightly.

### Rosacea keratitis
Corneal ulcers are seen in some patients with acne rosacea (Fig. 5.27), in whom blepharitis is very common. The ulcers start at the edge of the cornea

**Table 5.22** Management of the exposed eye

| |
| --- |
| Lubricate |
| Tape at night |
| Consider |
|    Botulinum toxin to lower the upper lid |
|    Surgical tarsorrhaphy |

with infiltrates which leave scarring, thinning and vascularization as they heal. Vision falls if the centre of the cornea is affected. Perforation can result from extreme thinning.

*Treatment* is with short courses of topical steroids and a trial of long-term oral tetracycline, starting with a dose of 250 mg four times daily for 1 month and reducing to 250 mg for at least 6 months. Repeated courses are often needed.

### Iritis
This means inflammation of the iris. It is a term which ophthalmologists rarely use because in their jargon it is called 'anterior uveitis', to distinguish it from 'posterior uveitis'. From the non-specialist's point of view 'iritis' is the more concise and descriptive term. Inflammation of the iris may complicate other conditions producing a red eye such as corneal ulcer, including herpes simplex and zoster ophthalmicus.

Iritis is not a specific diagnosis as many different conditions may be associated with it. Isolated 'idiopathic' iritis is quite common in otherwise fit young patients in whom there must be a cause but we are so far unable to find one. It may be associated with systemic diseases, particularly those associated with joint involvement, such as ankylosing spondylitis (Fig. 5.28), Reiter's syndrome, sarcoidosis, Behçet's syndrome and juvenile chronic arthritis (see p. 137). The yield from

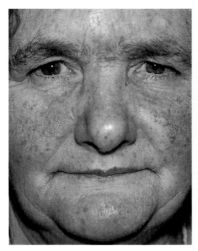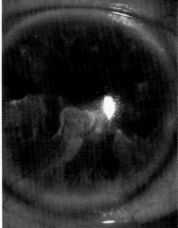

**Fig. 5.27** Rosacea may be associated with corneal ulceration and scarring.

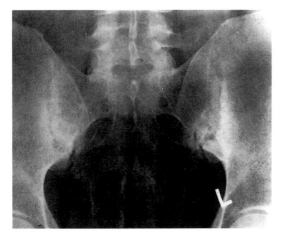

**Fig. 5.28** Ankylosing spondylitis, with sacroiliitis on radiography, may be associated with iritis.

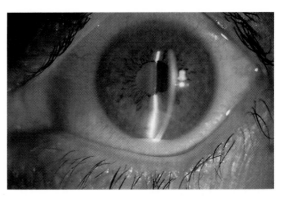

**Fig. 5.29** Iritis with a red eye. Cells in the front chamber (visible with the slit-lamp) have sedimented to the bottom. The iris is stuck to the lens in places, causing a small irregular pupil. (Courtesy of Mr A. Shun-Shin.)

**Table 5.23** Features of acute iritis (many are shared with corneal ulcer)

---

Unilateral more often than bilateral
May be recurrent
Pain + to ++
Photophobia
Mildly reduced vision
Red + to ++ around edge of cornea
Variably turbid aqueous with cells and protein (usually seen only using slit-lamp)
Corneal precipitates — may be hypopyon if severe
Small pupil perhaps with festooning
Ocular pressure usually low, but sometimes high

---

investigating first attacks of uncomplicated unilateral iritis is very low, particularly if there are no systemic symptoms as clues. Iritis tends to be recurrent and may become chronic and it may then be worth investigating further.

> In iritis, ask about:
> • back and joints (thinking about ankylosing spondylitis)
> • skin and chest (thinking about sarcoid)

*Symptoms* of acute iritis are what usually present to the GP (Table 5.23). There is rapid onset of *aching or pain* which may spread into the forehead if the attack is severe. If milder, the pain is often worse on near vision due to involvement of the ciliary body. The eye is almost always *photophobic and waters*, but there is *no sticky discharge*. Vision is usually only slightly blurred.

*Appearance.* Classically there is redness around the corneal edge (called 'ciliary injection'). If the iritis is more advanced the whole eye can look very red. The eye is often tender. The cornea is bright but precipitates of white cells appear on its internal surface and are occasionally visible with a magnifying lens (see Fig. 5.43). The slit-lamp is invaluable for seeing these and other features, in particular the cells which are diagnostic of iritis. If the cell response is profuse the cells may sediment at the bottom of the chamber in a small crescent (hypopyon) which is a signal for immediate referral (Fig. 5.29). The pupil in iritis is small, and after dilating drops may show irregularity or 'festooning' from abnormal anchorage points to the lens behind (posterior synechiae). Spots of pigment on the surface of the lens, the result of previous attacks, may be visible. With the slit-lamp, white cells in the anterior chamber are seen and their density estimated. Leakage of protein into the aqueous causes turbidity of the fluid in the front chamber (flare). Ocular pressure must be measured — it is usually normal or low but some forms of iritis (particularly zoster ophthalmicus) can cause glaucoma.

*Investigations* are not usually very useful unless there are symptoms of associated diseases. If attacks are recurrent and severe, everyone feels happier with negative investigations which would include a full blood count (FBC), erythrocyte sedimentation rate (ESR), chest X-ray and HLA typing looking for HLA type B27. It might be worth a specific hunt for sarcoid. In children, a positive ANA may suggest juvenile arthritis (see Chapter 8). Children with iritis and adults with recurrent attacks need a specialist assessment.

> In iritis, investigations are not worth while if the patient is otherwise well

*Treatment* entails suppressing the inflammation with *topical steroids* and relieving or preventing iris adhesions with a *dilating drop*. The strength and frequency of the drops used depends on the severity of the attack and the response to treatment, and should only be done under slit-lamp supervision. For most cases a standard regime might be dexamethasone 0.1% drops 2 hourly at first (for a few days until symptoms are controlled) then four times a day, with betamethasone ointment at night. The standard dilating drop is cyclopentolate 1% three times daily. The regime is tapered when the slit-lamp signs have cleared. Severe inflammations may need subconjunctival injections of steroid mixed with a dilating agent.

The paralysis of iris and ciliary muscles with dilating drops helps to relieve pain but also, of course, produces tiresome blurring of near vision. In mild attacks dilators need not necessarily be used, enabling patients, who are usually young, to continue to work. Again, the slit-lamp is invaluable in making this decision. Dilators are vital in children with iritis. *Atropine should only be used under hospital supervision at any age*, as it has such a prolonged duration of action.

> In iritis, dilate the pupil early in the attack

Rarely, an episode will not respond to topical treatment and treatment with systemic steroids is needed. Follow-up in hospital clinics is continued until the iritis has settled. The steroids, whether topical or systemic, need to be reduced gradually to lessen the risk of a 'rebound' inflammation. A

small number of people who carry the gene for chronic simple glaucoma respond to topical steroids with a rise in intraocular pressure. Extra care then has to be taken to monitor the effects of treatment, in particular the *eye pressure*.

It seems reasonable that a GP should prescribe topical steroid and dilating drops if the diagnosis is suggested by previous attacks defined as iritis. The first attack is more tricky, as most symptoms are shared with herpetic keratitis, so slit-lamp confirmation is necessary before starting treatment.

### Acute glaucoma: known the symptoms, signs and initial management (Table 5.24)

Acute glaucoma due to closure of the drainage angle is an important condition because, although it is not common, urgent treatment is vital to future good vision. It typically (but not exclusively) affects elderly long-sighted individuals and may be precipitated by emotion, the cinema or dilating drops given earlier in the day (Table 5.25). There may be a history of subacute attacks (see Haloes, p. 42).

*Symptoms* are of the rapid development of pain in and around the eye which often becomes severe, with markedly reduced vision in the established attack. Nausea and vomiting may occur.

*Appearance.* The vision is poor, often reduced to counting fingers. The eye is congested, looking red especially around the cornea, with a purplish

**Table 5.24** Acute glaucoma

Usually elderly, may be long-sighted
Usually unilateral, though both eyes may be at risk
May be previous less severe attacks
Pain + to +++
Markedly reduced vision
Nausea and vomiting common
Red and congested eye
Cornea steamy
Pupil dilated and may be oval and fixed
Eye is 'golf or cricket ball' firm to pressure
Ocular pressure usually more than 50 mmHg (using slit-lamp)
Front chamber shallow (using slit-lamp)

**Table 5.25** Precipitating factors in acute glaucoma

Dilatation of the pupil
   Dim light
   Emotion
   Drops or systemic medication
Old age with forward shift of the lens
Short eyeball with long-sighted eye (hypermetropia,
    convex spectacle lens)
Trauma
Some forms of iritis

**Table 5.26** Treatment of acute glaucoma

*Immediate*
Refer
Intravenous acetazolamide, 500 mg
Topical timolol and pilocarpine

*Casualty*
Osmotic agents
Iridotomy by laser or surgery

*Long term*
Iridotomy to other eye as preventive measure
Follow pressure and field for at least 3 months

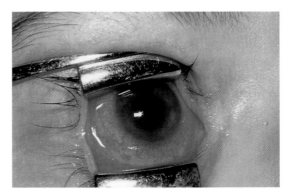

**Fig. 5.30** Acute glaucoma with a congested eye. Note that the eye is red and boggy with a steamy cornea and fixed semidilated pupil. The eye will feel 'cricket ball' hard.

colour (Fig. 5.30). It is tender and feels very firm, like a golf or cricket ball in comparison with the normal eye (like a squash ball). The cornea looks hazy because of oedema. The pupil is often oval, mid-dilated and inactive. It is usually difficult to assess the depth of the anterior chamber through the steamy cornea, so it is useful to look at the other eye. If the front chamber is shallow, there will be only a small space between the iris and cornea (it is difficult to be certain of this without experience of many normal chambers, so it may be an uncertain sign in the event).

- Acute glaucoma is an emergency
- Refer without delay

*Treatment* is needed urgently, so refer as an emergency immediately. The intraocular pressure measured by slit-lamp confirms the diagnosis and is likely to be over 50 mm. Looking at the chamber angle with a contact lens device (gonioscopy) will show a closed angle and probably a very narrow angle in the other eye. If there is likely to be a delay

in treatment of more than an hour, start Diamox (500 mg intravenously over several minutes), but still refer with minimum delay (Table 5.26).

The eye pressure is lowered by intravenous acetazolamide (Diamox) plus topical timolol, both of which reduce aqueous production. Reducing the pressure can be difficult, particularly in established cases, and osmotic agents may be needed. Once the pressure is falling and iris ischaemia relieved, pilocarpine drops have a chance of opening the drainage angle. It is important not to forget the other eye, which is treated prophylactically with pilocarpine from the outset. When the pressure is normal and the eye less inflamed, laser iridotomies or surgical iridectomies can be performed to both eyes, to prevent further attacks (see Glaucoma surgery, p. 175). Damage to the angle may cause chronic glaucoma needing long-term follow-up. In children, glaucoma with corneal oedema is the rare condition known as buphthalmos.

*Rubeotic glaucoma is another condition* giving a painful, red eye with poor vision and raised pressure, which is glaucoma from new vessels in the front chamber, sometimes visible with a bright torch. This glaucoma (Table 5.27) is not rare and is usually found either in diabetics or after a central retinal vein occlusion. The onset is not as rapid as that of acute angle closure, symptoms developing over 1–2 weeks. The vision may have been already poor, depending on the reason for the ischaemia.

**Table 5.27** Rubeotic glaucoma

Associated with retinal ischaemia from diabetes or retinal
  vein occlusion
Presents with redness and pain
Eyeball is hard and tender
Blood vessels visible on iris (usually only with slit-lamp)

Treatment with oral or intravenous acetazolamide, topical
  steroid and atropine
May benefit from retinal laser treatment

**Table 5.28** Causes of subconjunctival haemorrhage

Usually spontaneous, circumscribed and benign, though
  may be recurrent
Traumatic or sport associated (beware if haemorrhage is
  extensive as it may indicate serious eye damage or a
  skull fracture)
Hypertension
Certain types of conjunctivitis, usually viral
Pertussis
Bleeding tendency or underlying vascular anomaly (rare)

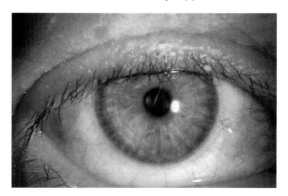

**Fig. 5.31** Pinguecula, common innocent fatty lumps on the white of the eye.

### Red lumps on the eye

True tumours of the eye surface are rare. Malignant tumours are even more rare; they usually enlarge rapidly and may bleed. Patients with a lump on the exposed part of the 'white' of the eye can therefore be reassured. Usually the lump will be near the edge of the cornea and is *likely to be either a pingueculum or a pterygium*—Latin and Greek terms which sadly have no familiar English equivalents.

### Pingueculum (Fig. 5.31)

These creamy lumps to either side of the corneal edge, in the central area, are due to collagen degeneration resulting from ultraviolet light exposure. They are almost universal in older people. They can become inflamed, causing a sore, red, watering eye without discharge or photophobia, and must be distinguished from episcleritis. The surrounding redness makes the pingueculum stand out, and this often draws attention for the first time. A short course of topical steroid, such as prednisolone 0.5% three times daily for a week, will usually settle the inflammation. Excision is very occasionally needed for repeated episodes of inflammation but the lump often recurs. The swelling may interfere with the tear film and give dry eye symptoms. Artificial tears are usually helpful then.

### Pterygium (Fig. 5.32)

This is another consequence of ultraviolet light exposure and is much commoner in the tropics than

Patients should be referred urgently if the eye is painful. Unfortunately, often all that can be done is to keep the eye comfortable with topical steroids and a dilating drop.

## Miscellaneous causes of red eyes

### Subconjunctival haemorrhages

These are the cause of a strikingly red eye in which the onset is usually painless, though there may be pricking sensation (see Fig. 5.2). The vast majority occur spontaneously, mostly in otherwise healthy people (Table 5.28). It is worth checking the blood pressure. As the bulbar conjunctiva is lax, the blood can track widely. This can cause great alarm to onlookers though the patient is often unaware that anything is wrong until they look in the mirror. Resolution takes 1–2 weeks.

*Trauma* (varying from an insignificant abrasion to an orbital fracture) may also cause subconjunctival bleeding (see p. 59). A traumatic haemorrhage in which a posterior limit cannot be seen should arouse suspicion of serious trauma, as it may have tracked forwards from bleeding behind the eye.

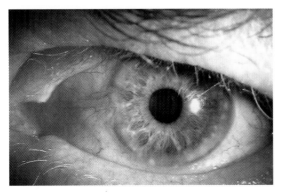

**Fig. 5.32** Pterygium with blood vessels extending from the conjunctiva onto the peripheral cornea.

in northern Europe. A pterygium is an overgrowth of vascular conjunctiva onto the cornea associated with destruction of the superficial layers of the cornea. It is always found in the exposed zone mid-way between the two lids. A rather similar appearance can be seen in a 'pseudopterygium' where a fold of conjunctiva adheres to the peripheral cornea following an ulcer. This can occur anywhere around the edge of the cornea. Pterygia tend to have periods of active growth, giving rise to symptoms of a sore, red eye, which may be eased by a short course of topical steroid such as prednisolone drops 0.5% three times daily for 2 weeks.

In the absence of symptoms or encroachment onto the visual axis, a pterygium is best left alone, as recurrence following excision is common.

## Blepharitis: a common cause of red eyelid margin (Table 5.29)

Lid margin disease is very common, and blepharitis is probably the most frequent eye diagnosis in general practice, competing with allergic conjunctivitis for this honour. Blepharitis comes from the Greek and means 'inflammation of the eyelids'. Usually the lid margins are the only part of the lid to be affected. Another term, meibomianitis, refers to inflammation of the meibomian oil glands in the lids. These are modified sebaceous glands embedded in the tarsal plates, about 30 in each lid, which produce the oily component of the tear-film.

Meibomian gland disease and blepharitis are

**Table 5.29** Blepharitis

Red lid margins
Stickiness, crusts or flaking among eyelashes
Itching
Thickened lids
Loss of lashes
Complications
    Recurrent conjunctival inflammation or infection
    Conjunctival cysts and concretions
    Meibomian cyst formation
    Trichiasis with lashes irritating the eye

commonly found together. The lid margin problem is usually a mixture of seborrhoeic and infective components. Blepharitis is common in 'seborrhoeic' individuals with skin scales and dandruff, and in those with acne rosacea. Interestingly, lid disease is not associated with common acne. Blepharitis often worsens the symptoms of dry eyes and is a common cause of contact lens intolerance. Ulcerative blepharitis, once common in undernourished children, is now rarely seen and is usually due to herpes simplex infection of the lid margin.

*Symptoms* are of irritation, itching, burning and crusting. The eyes may look red-rimmed and the patients complain that they always look tired and bleary. The eyes may water slightly, or feel dry. They may be difficult to open in the mornings, though not actually glued together by discharge (which suggests an acute infection).

*Appearance.* The lid margins may look uneven or notched and reddened (Fig. 5.33). In chronic inflammation telangiectasia form. Crusts adhere to the bases of the lashes; partly flakes of dandruff, partly exudate. The lashes may thin, whiten and fall out.

### Associated features and complications

A low-grade conjunctivitis is often present with blepharitis, leading to the appearance of concretions and conjunctival 'cysts', both of which may concern the observant sufferer. *Concretion* is seen on the tarsal conjunctiva as a small white chalky deposit (Fig. 5.34); it is of no significance unless, rarely, it erodes through the epithelium and rubs

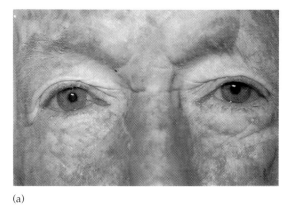
(a)

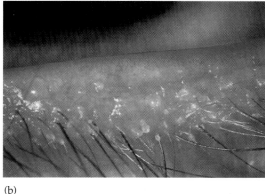
(b)

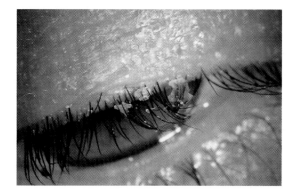
(c)

**Fig. 5.33** (a) Blepharitis showing reddened lid margins.
(b) Blepharitis with scales adhering to the lashes.
(c) Blepharitis with larger crusts.

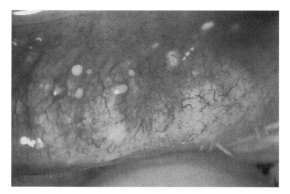

**Fig. 5.34** Yellow or white conjunctival concretions are
common, harmless and often associated with blepharitis.

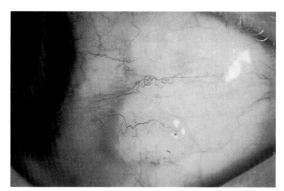

**Fig. 5.35** Conjunctival cysts with clear fluid may form on
the eye surface or inside the lids.

on the eye surface. If so, it can be removed with a
needle. Most can be safely left alone. *Conjunctival
cyst* is a clear retention cyst of a mucus goblet cell
or accessory lacrimal gland (Fig. 5.35). It may be
punctured with a needle and the patient reassured. *Trichiasis* can result from distortion of the

lid margin so that the lashes turn inwards to the
eye surface.

### Meibomian cyst (chalazion)
This is the most common and troublesome complication and usually occurs on a background of

low-grade lid margin disease. It is often a granuloma rather than an abscess. Usually the lumps develop gradually as small firm pea-like nodules in the substance of the lid, just behind the lid margin (Fig. 5.36). Some also produce a small fleshy lump on the inner surface of the lid. Symptoms (other than cosmetic) from an uncomplicated cyst are uncommon, unless one in the upper lid presses on the cornea to cause astigmatism. A third of meibomian cysts (Fig. 5.37) resolve spontaneously and it is best to wait for several weeks before resorting to surgery, especially in children, who will need a general anaesthetic (see Removal of a meibomian cyst, p. 186). Topical antibiotics are not indicated for an uninflamed chalazion, but for those unfortunate individuals plagued by repeated eruptions, it is worth trying oral tetracycline 250 mg four times daily initially (reducing to twice daily) for at least 4 months.

> The simple meibomian cyst needs no treatment except time

*Meibomian abscess.* This arises from acute infection in a meibomian gland. Sudden diffuse swelling of the whole lid localizes and may then point and discharge, either inwards through the conjunctiva, or outwards through the skin. Such abscesses often resolve after spontaneous discharge. Incision, preferably from the conjunctival side, is sometimes helpful, followed by a course of topical chloramphenicol.

> A single inflamed eyelid is usually due to an inflamed meibomian gland

*Treatment of blepharitis* (Table 5.30). People with blepharitis need to know that they have a chronic condition which is difficult to cure but to be reassured that their sight is not threatened. As with

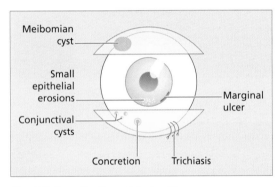

**Fig. 5.36** Complications of blepharitis.

**Table 5.30** Treatment plan for blepharitis

| |
|---|
| Regular lid cleaning |
|   Heat |
|   Massage |
| Intermittent topical |
|   Antimicrobial |
|   Weak steroid |
| Treat underlying |
|   skin or scalp problem |
|   dry eye with tear supplements |

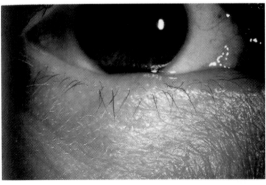
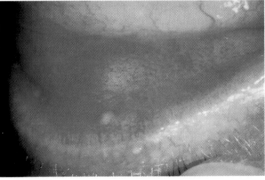

(a)                                                    (b)

**Fig. 5.37** Meibomian cyst is the most common cause of a lid lump. (a) Outside appearance. (b) Appearance from inside the everted lid.

other chronic or recurrent problems, insight into the nature of the disease is particularly useful in helping to cope with it. They need sympathy in coping with a depressing cosmetic problem. Patient 'information sheets' may help (see Appendix 4). There are *three principal elements to treatment* (the three Ts).

*Toilet to the lid.* The crusts must be cleaned from the base of the lashes with a wet cotton bud dipped into a solution of sodium bicarbonate (a teaspoon in a teacup of boiled water). The cotton bud is rubbed along the lid margins. This should be done morning and night. It will be most effective when there is a lot of crusting in patients prepared to take the time and trouble to do it. Applying heat to the lids may help, using a clean face cloth wrung out in water as hot as can be tolerated, repeated for a minute or so twice a day.

*Tear supplements.* Blepharitis is often associated with a poor quality tear-film with inadequate wetting. Artificial tears, of which there are many formulations (none, unfortunately, anywhere near as good as tears), are often helpful. First try hypromellose drops four times a day, reducing frequency once symptoms are under control. More viscous lubricants, such as carbomer 940 (Geltears and Viscotears) or liquid paraffin (Lacri-Lube) are preferred by some people.

If the eye is dry, avoid ointment

*Topical treatment to the lid margin.* Antibiotic and steroid mixtures such as chloramphenicol 1% plus hydrocortisone 0.5% as ointment can be rubbed into the lid margins (not into the eye) using a finger tip or cotton bud. This is done after lid toilet, or just at night. Ointments affect tear-film stability, and these patients should therefore use the preparation sparingly and try to avoid getting ointment into the eye itself. By confining steroid to the lid margins, side-effects should be avoided but it is wise to use them only in courses of a few weeks at a time rather than continuously. 'Trial and success' is usually needed to find the treatment most helpful to each patient.

*Trichiasis.* This can be dealt with by pulling out the lashes repeatedly (see Minor surgery around the eyes, p. 184). Sometimes patients' relatives become very adept at this. It is also something a practice sister could usefully do, armed with a loupe and a good pair of epilation forceps. The offending lashes may be very fine. Electrolysis or cryotherapy may offer more permanent relief.

### Stye and cyst of Moll
Other glands in the lids are the glands of Zeiss (the sebaceous glands of the lash follicle) and the glands of Moll (modified sweat glands) which open into the lash follicle or onto the lid margin. Cysts of Moll (Fig. 5.38) are commonly seen as tiny translucent swellings on the lid margin. They can be punctured or deroofed. Infection in a gland of Zeiss produces a stye, a tiny abscess on the lid margin. Resolution of these is spontaneous, but it can be hastened by hot compresses and by pulling out the lash of the affected follicle (see also Lumps around the eye, below).

### Infestation of the lashes (Fig. 5.39)
Infestation of the lashes by *Phthirus pubis* (crab-lice) can produce symptoms resembling blepharitis, often with ulceration and bloody discharge. Sometimes they are a chance (and rather un-nerving) finding on slit-lamp examination. The lice are best removed with forceps. The eggs or nits, if more adherent, can be loosened by

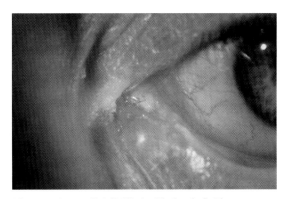

**Fig. 5.38** A cyst of Moll, filled with cloudy fluid, at the inner margin of the lower lid. (Courtesy of Mr A. Shun-Shin.)

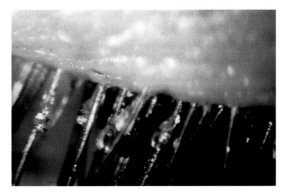

**Fig. 5.39** Nits (egg cases of pubic lice) attached to the eyelash base—an occasional surprising finding.

**Table 5.31** Types of sticky eye

| |
| --- |
| Pus |
|     Bacterial |
|     Chlamydial infection |
| Stringy mucus |
|     Allergic conjunctivitis |
|     Suture reaction |
| Crusts or flakes |
|     Blepharitis |

**Table 5.32** Associated factors of sticky eye in elderly patients

| |
| --- |
| Blepharitis |
| Poor tear drainage, either blockage or lid malposition |
| Dry eye |
| Sutures of cataract surgery |

greasing the lashes with ointment, following which they should drop off. The pubic hair needs to be treated with insecticide lotions such as malathion or pyrethrin. A bit of subtle detective work in contact tracing is necessary.

## The sticky eye

The commonest cause of pus around the eye is *bacterial conjunctivitis*. The discharge may be profuse, particularly on waking. Stickiness can also occur in *blepharitis*, when most of the crusting discharge clings to the lashes, and the lid margins are sore and red. Stringy discharge, which stretches like melted cheese, is characteristic of *allergic conjunctivitis*. It is therefore worth being clear about the type of stickiness the patient describes (Table 5.31).

Mild stickiness can accompany irritation of the eye and in a patient with previous eye surgery may be a symptom of a broken suture, which should be removed (Table 5.32). Beware particularly sticky eye in a contact lens wearer in whom the organism can be atypical and minor trauma from the lens predispose to serious corneal infection. Unusual infections causing a particularly pus-filled eye include *Chlamydia*, *Branhamella*, *Gonococcus* and *Actinomyces*.

Not all sticky eyes need to be swabbed. Reserve this for particularly severe or recurrent cases and for some neonates within the first week, or in adults, if you suspect chlamydial infection specifically (see Chlamydial conjunctivitis, above).

Not all sticky eyes need antibiotic treatment, but some need specific agents. (See under Conjunctivitis, above.) Many small children have sticky eyes with an upper respiratory infection. This needs no treatment if the discharge is scanty, other than bathing (see Lotions, Appendix 1). Chronic or frequently recurrent discharge suggests blockage of the tear drainage system both in children and adults (see Watering, p. 55). A mucocoele of the tear sac causes large amounts of pus to well into the eye, especially after pressure beside the nose.

## Abnormal corneal appearances
(Fig. 5.40)

As the normal cornea is clear it may be difficult to decide how deeply the problem lies without using the slit-lamp. A bright light and perhaps a magnifying lens may help. Associated symptoms, in particular pain or discomfort, are clues to the cause.

### Arcus

The arcus senilis is familiar to everyone though it is poorly named since it is certainly not confined to the old. It may even occur in children and young adults and in younger patients there is a greater likelihood of an associated hyperlipidemia. The arcus begins at the 6 and 12 o'clock positions

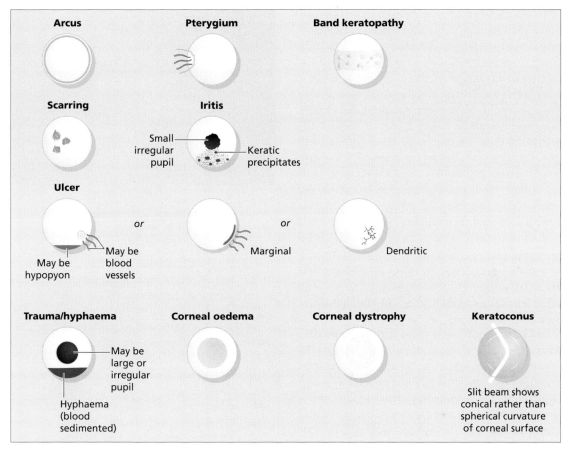

**Fig. 5.40** Abnormal corneal appearances.

and then spreads circumferentially around the peripheral cornea. It is usually bilateral. There is a narrow clear space at the very edge of the cornea (Fig. 5.41).

> Measure plasma lipid levels in the patient:
> • with corneal arcus
> • under 60 years old

## Pterygium

Pterygium is common in those who have spent a significant time in hot arid climates, particularly in Asian subjects. It is usually bilateral but asymmetrical. It is almost invariably non-malignant and rarely a threat to sight. It begins on the medial conjunctiva as a fleshy mass and advances on to the cornea in a wedge shape, pulling with it a leash

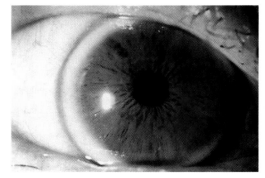

**Fig. 5.41** Arcus of the cornea with fatty deposit in the peripheral cornea and a characteristic thin clear band between the edges of the cornea.

of blood vessels that give it prominence (see Fig. 5.32). The rate of advance across the cornea is usually very slow indeed and removal is rarely indicated on these grounds unless the centre of the cornea is threatened. Sometimes the pterygium may become inflamed, and the blood vessels then enlarge and make it even more obvious. Spontaneous resolution is usual, but if attacks are recurrent then surgery may be reasonable. In general, however, many are referred for pterygium surgery but few are chosen. This is because the surgery itself may scar the cornea and the cosmetic result may then be little better than preoperatively and, more importantly, there is a real risk of recurrence of the pterygium itself and a recurrent pterygium is likely to be more aggressive than the original one. When patients are told these facts, most become happier to put up with what is usually a fairly minor cosmetic blemish.

### Band keratopathy and other corneal deposits

This is the name given to an unusual lesion of the cornea that is confined to the central horizontal zone. It begins peripherally as a grey haze, sometimes with windows of clear cornea within, and is due to the deposition of calcium in the superficial corneal layers. It is usually bilateral and idiopathic in elderly people, but can be associated with hypercalcaemia or chronic intraocular inflammation. Occasionally the deposits can become elevated and make the eye sore, in which case they can be partially dissolved in a laborious operation using the chelating agent EDTA.

It may just be possible to see a pigmentary change, which is usually asymptomatic, in the corneal epithelium of patients on long-term amiodarone therapy. The brown peripheral Kayser–Fleischer ring of copper that occurs in Wilson's disease is vanishingly rare but may be a vital clue to a serious and treatable disorder. It is best seen with a slit-lamp.

### Scarring (Fig. 5.42)

Corneal scarring has a number of causes and of course many of these will produce symptoms in the acute stages. The commonest cause in the UK is recurrent herpes simplex corneal infection, followed by trauma. The scar itself is usually pain-

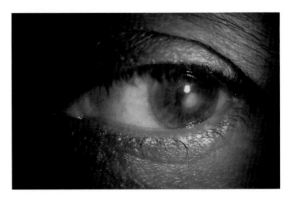

**Fig. 5.42** Opaque corneal scar, usually secondary to previous trauma or infective ulcer. There is also early arcus. (Courtesy of Mr A. Shun-Shin.)

less and only affects vision if it overlies the centre of the cornea. Scarring can vary from minimal to very dense and obvious. Blood vessels in the cornea always signify scarring. Pannus is the name given to a characteristic pattern of vascularized scarring that spreads inward from the edge of the cornea, usually from the top. Old inactive trachoma is the commonest cause and is a frequent incidental finding in patients from parts of the world where trachoma is endemic, particularly in Asians. Prolonged contact lens wear is another cause of pannus, the blood vessels growing into the cornea as a result of hypoxia. Rosacea can also cause pannus, usually of the inferior cornea.

Blood vessels on the cornea are a sign of damage

### Corneal ulcers

A corneal abrasion will leave the cornea clear but stains brightly with fluorescein. An ulcer on the other hand renders a part of the cornea grey or white and this appearance is due to the accumulation of white cells or even frank pus. A sterile inflammatory ulcer of the peripheral cornea is quite common in patients with chronic blepharitis (marginal ulcer) (Fig. 5.40). This has a crescentic shape with a thin band of clear cornea at the edge. This ulcer responds well to combined antibiotic and steroid drops but it is wise to examine these patients with the slit-lamp for confirmation of the diagnosis before steroids are used (see Corneal inflammation and ulceration, p. 73).

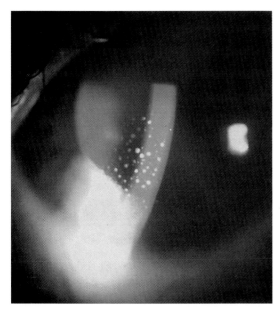

**Fig. 5.43** Precipitates on the lower part of the inner cornea are collections of white cells and indicate iritis. Here they are seen with the slit-lamp, but they may be visible with a torch. Reproduced from Taylor (1992) *Pediatric Ophthalmology* (slide atlas), Blackwell Scientific Publications, Cambridge, MA.

### Iritis

If inflammation in the front chamber (iritis) is particularly acute and severe, aggregates of white blood cells may form on the inner surface of the cornea and can be seen as a series of pale dots or spots (keratic precipitates) whose presence is diagnostic of iritis (Fig. 5.43). If cells sediment in large numbers at the bottom of the chamber they may form a hypopyon or thin white line. Hypopyon is seen with severe corneal ulcers and needs immediate referral (see Iritis, p. 79 and Corneal inflammation and ulceration, p. 73).

> Corneal precipitates indicate iritis

### Hyphaema (Fig. 5.44)

Bleeding within the eye in front of the lens can also settle inferiorly behind the cornea, giving a characteristic appearance known as hyphaema. Its presence usually means the eye has been struck with considerable force and warrants urgent referral for further assessment. (See Chapter 10.)

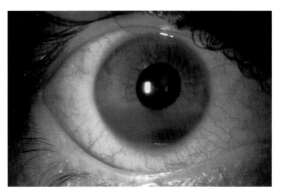

**Fig. 5.44** Hyphaema with blood sedimented at the bottom of the front chamber. This is almost always traumatic.

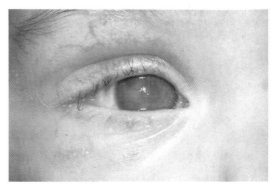

**Fig. 5.45** Cornea hazy with oedema is always significant. Here it is generalized. Reproduced from Taylor (1992) *Pediatric Ophthalmology* (slide atlas), Blackwell Scientific Publications, Cambridge, MA.

### Corneal oedema (Fig. 5.45)

If fluid accumulates within the cornea it becomes opaque and the vision will also fall. A normal cornea subjected to excessive intraocular pressure in acute angle closure glaucoma will respond in this way but corneal oedema is more likely to be seen as part of a chronic eye problem. Surgery such as cataract extraction can be followed months to years later by corneal oedema, although fortunately this is much rarer since the development of microsurgery. Oedema can also occur as part of Fuch's corneal dystrophy. Fluid can accumulate to such an extent that blisters develop under the epithelium and if these rupture the eye becomes very painful. The problem can to some extent be helped by using hypertonic saline eye drops to draw fluid out and by using a large soft contact lens to discourage breakdown of the blisters. Corneal grafting may be needed to restore useful vision. Hazy cornea in a baby or child could rarely signify glaucoma or a metabolic disorder.

### Corneal dystrophy

A variety of corneal dystrophies are distinguished on clinical grounds. Most are inherited in an autosomal dominant manner and become visually disabling in early to middle adult years when opacification affects the central part of both corneas. If the corneal epithelium is involved in the dystrophy episodes of recurrent erosions may punctuate the clinical course (see Pain with an eye cause, p. 50).

### *Keratoconus* (Fig. 5.46)

Keratoconus is an abnormal appearance of shape without opacity, which can be very difficult to detect in the early stages even with a slit-lamp. Keratoconus is the most common corneal dystrophy, and the optician is frequently the first to suggest the diagnosis. Young patients with slowly progressive blurring of vision can be corrected with glasses or contact lenses at first but in some

patients one or both eyes eventually require corneal grafting.

## Lumps around the eye

The eyelids are made up of skin, tarsal plate and meibomian glands, fat, blood vessels and nerves. The lacrimal gland and tear drainage are nearby and the orbital contents lie directly behind. Any of these structures may be responsible for lid swellings.

### Benign lid lumps (Fig. 5.47)

#### *Styes*

These are very common, especially in children. The skin of the lid margins contains the roots of the eyelashes, into which modified sebaceous glands (of Zeiss) empty. These glands may become acutely infected, usually by staphylococci, causing an acute tender, red swelling that points forwards. This is a stye, or 'external hordeolum'. The infection usually subsides spontaneously, sometimes bursting onto the skin. Antibiotic ointment may be given to prevent spread of the infection and hot compresses may help the mini-abscess to burst. Remove the lash. Systemic anti-

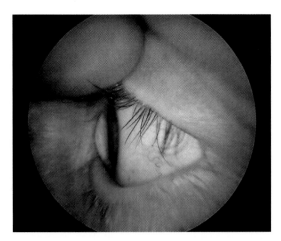

**Fig. 5.46** Conical cornea (keratoconus) causes progressively worsening of vision with pronounced astigmatism. Reproduced from Taylor (1992) *Pediatric Ophthalmology* (slide atlas), Blackwell Scientific Publications, Cambridge, MA.

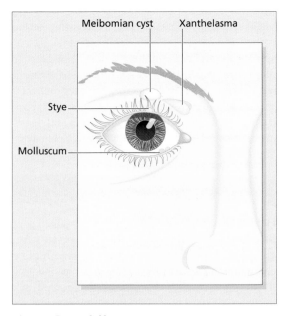

**Fig. 5.47** Benign lid lumps.

biotics or surgical drainage are rarely required. Look for an underlying chronic staphylococcal lid margin infection that may have predisposed the patient. Lash follicle glands may become blocked without getting infected, in which case a very small whitish nodule forms (cyst of Zeiss). Treat this by puncturing with a hypodermic needle and use cautery to the base if it recurs. A very similar swelling which is more translucent can arise from blockage of modified sweat glands in the lid skin. This is called a cyst of Moll (see Fig. 5.38) and is treated in the same way.

*Meibomian cyst* (see Fig. 5.37)
These are very common at all ages. The meibomian glands are modified sebaceous glands, and about 30 of them are buried in each lid. They secrete a fatty material related to sebum onto the lid margin, and this helps prevent tears spilling onto the skin. When a gland orifice becomes blocked, a swelling may slowly appear within the lid. This is also known as a chalazion (pronounced kala'zion) or hailstone. Pull the lid down or evert it and an area of swelling and inflammation is usually visible under the conjunctiva (see Fig. 5.37b). Occasionally the cyst can press on the eye enough to distort the cornea, causing astigmatism and blurred vision. The firm swelling represents a chronic granulomatous reaction in response to the retained oil, and in about one-third of cases resolves spontaneously. In some cases the cyst bursts, usually outwards, outside the lid margin.

The most common lid lump is a meibomian cyst

The surgery (incision and curettage) is simple, though the patient will probably have a post-operative 'black eye' for several days. Anaesthetic drops are given and the lid is infiltrated with lignocaine and adrenaline (epinephrine). The site of the lump can be marked prior to injection if it is small and likely to be obscured by anaesthetic. The lid is then everted and a special circular clamp is tightened around the lump to stop bleeding. The conjunctiva over the swelling is incised. A whitish cheesy material is expressed and the cavity is

cleaned with a small curette. Suturing is unnecessary. Chloromycetin ointment is given immediately, the eye padded for 24 hours and ointment is continued twice a day for 1 week. Those wishing to learn the technique will find further details under Minor surgery around the eyes (p. 186).

Meibomian cysts tend to be multiple and some individuals are prone to them, though fortunately the tendency to develop them often lessens. It is important to remember that cysts are restricted to the tarsal plates and so any swelling right at the medial or lateral extremes of upper or lower lids is not a chalazion, so suspect a malignant tumour. Also, any atypical features of a suspected chalazion, including recurrence at the same site after incision and curettage, should raise the possibility of an adenocarcinoma of the meibomian gland, although this is a very rare lid tumour.

A cyst may become infected and form an abscess, when the lid will quickly swell and become red and tender, obscuring the underlying chalazion. A differential diagnosis is lid, or even orbital, cellulitis (pp. 97–98). The patient may not give a history of a lump in the eyelid. With systemic antibiotics the infection will usually settle and antibiotic ointment with or without hot compresses may prevent local spread and encourage the pus to point. Any remaining lump is best incised and curetted to avoid recurrent infections.

*Lid tumours due to viral infection*
Molluscum contagiosum is a viral infection that is commonest in children (see Fig. 5.13). Numerous waxy elevated and umbilicated nodules congregate around the lid margin, shedding viral particles that may set up a chronic conjunctivitis. The condition resolves spontaneously but this process can be accelerated by gentle cauterization of the nodules. Common viral warts also occur and can be difficult to treat in this site as they may need curettage or excision. For children, this would require a general anaesthetic.

*Angiomas*
The strawberry nevus, or capillary hemangioma (Fig. 5.48), appears at or soon after birth as a small bluish mass in the lids. This increases in size until the age of 6 months or so and then shrinks within

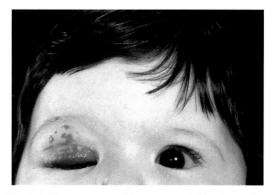

**Fig. 5.48** Haemangioma of the upper eyelid in a 3-month-old child. Reproduced from Taylor (1990) *Pediatric Ophthalmology*, Blackwell Scientific Publications, Cambridge, MA.

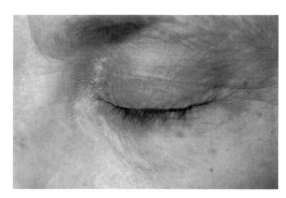

**Fig. 5.49** Fatty deposits in the lids, xanthelasmas, are usually innocent, but the occasional patient has high plasma lipids.

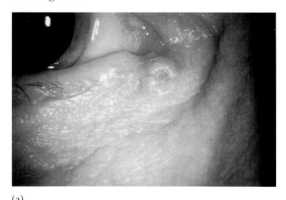

(a)

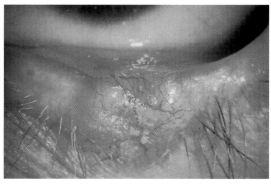

(b)

**Fig. 5.50** (a) An early rodent ulcer (basal cell carcinoma) at the inner lower lid margin. (b) A more advanced rodent ulcer. Note the pearly edge and telangiectasia.

the first 5 years. Anxious parents may bring great pressure to bear for cosmetic treatment. As the eventual scarring is always worse with treatment than with natural shrinkage, for the vast majority observation is best. Parents are sometimes reassured by being shown photographs of typical cases. Occasionally treatment is necessary because the eye is obscured, risking amblyopia.

### Miscellaneous

Xanthelasmas hardly qualify as lumps, but they can be numerous and are slightly elevated (Fig. 5.49). Their association with hyperlipidemia is greatest in young people. Surgery may be done for cosmetic reasons but warn the patient that the lesions may recur. Seborrhoeic keratosis and sebaceous cysts may occur on the eyelids, and

their appearance is similar to that in other parts of the body. Papillomas are the commonest true benign skin tumours around the eyelid. Those with a narrow stalk can be tied tightly with a stout suture. Others are better removed by excision. A good tip here is to follow the lid skin creases (and use them whenever possible) when making the incision (see under Minor surgery around the eyes, p. 190).

## Malignant lid tumours

### Rodent ulcer (Fig. 5.50)

Basal cell carcinoma (BCC, or rodent ulcer) is the commonest primary malignant tumour of the eyelid skin. They arise most often in the inner part of the lower lid, and this is the position in which they are most difficult to treat because they are near the tear duct. Classically, the tumour grows slowly into a pearly nodule with rolled edges and a central crater. The edges often have telangiectatic vessels. Episodes of ulceration, bleeding, loss of lashes or shrinkage may occur. Tumours in this category are not usually difficult to diagnose and they grow slowly, eating into the tissues gradually. Occasionally, the tumour may prefer to spread within the dermis, leaving few clinical signs other than lid thickening, irregularity or distortion. In an elderly person any unexplained chronic lid deformity should be assumed to be a 'rodent' until proved otherwise by biopsy. Rodent ulcers can be treated with radiotherapy or excision, but both become much more difficult for larger tumours, so consider anything suspicious for early biopsy.

> Basal cell carcinoma is the most common eyelid malignancy

> Unexplained chronic lid deformity in an elderly patient is a basal cell carcinoma until proved otherwise

### Squamous cell carcinoma (Fig. 5.51)

Squamous cell carcinoma is the second commonest malignancy of the eyelid skin. It usually grows more quickly than a rodent, and has a varied clinical appearance. Laterally placed tumours metastasize to the pre-auricular lymph nodes, while medially placed tumours spread to the

submandibular nodes. A similar quickly growing nodular or ulcerative lesion, called keratoacanthoma, is benign, yet may easily be confused with squamous cell carcinoma. A keratoacanthoma usually involutes over a period of about 3 months. It is wise to biopsy a suspected keratoacanthoma to help rule out a squamous carcinoma, even though the histological distinction may also be hard to make.

## Lacrimal gland and sac tumours

### Lacrimal gland

The lacrimal gland sits under the upper lid at the outer corner (Fig. 5.52), in a hollow behind the orbital rim and early swelling of the gland may be seen as a fullness here (Fig. 5.53). Pull up the upper lid and look under it, directly at the gland, as the patient looks down and inward (Fig. 5.54). Proptosis may also be present if the lump extends into the orbit behind the eye. Inflammation and lymphoid infiltration account for about half of lacrimal

> • Lacrimal gland swelling appears in the upper outer eyelid
> • Lacrimal sac swelling appears in the lower inner eyelid

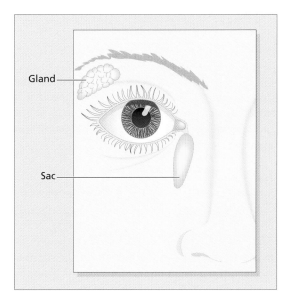

**Fig. 5.52** Lacrimal gland and sac.

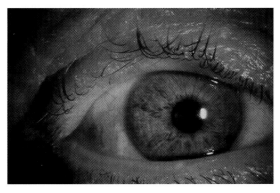

**Fig. 5.51** Squamous cell carcinoma of the upper lid. Rare and easily overlooked. Note the lash loss.

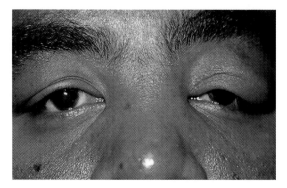

**Fig. 5.53** Swelling of the lacrimal glands, more marked on the left side, with an S-shaped upper lid.

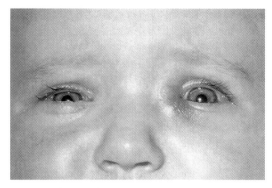

**Fig. 5.55** Infection of the lacrimal sac (dacryocystitis) with localization to the inner angle of the lower lid. Reproduced from Taylor (1992) *Pediatric Ophthalmology* (slide atlas), Blackwell Scientific Publications, Cambridge, MA.

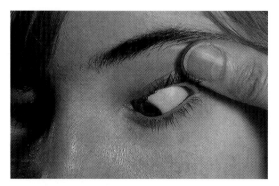

**Fig. 5.54** To examine the lacrimal gland area, pull up the outer lid with the patient looking down and in. The gland may be visible in some patients, especially if enlarged.

gland swellings, the remainder are due to mixed cell tumour or adenocarcinoma. It is best to refer early any patient with a suspected lacrimal gland tumour, particularly if there is pain. Biopsy is avoided, as this may induce recurrence if the tumour proves to be malignant. A suspicious gland is removed entirely.

*Tear sac*
Swelling and redness acutely below the inner canthus is usually due to infection of a previously obstructed tear sac (dacryocystitis) (Fig. 5.55). The infection can progress to lid cellulitis, and the marked lid swelling may then mask the original cause of the problem (see below under Swelling around the eye). Acute infection of the sac usually responds to systemic antibiotics. Occasionally the sac is converted into an abscess cavity and this can

drain spontaneously onto the skin. Incision of a suspected lacrimal sac abscess is best avoided as a fistula may form.

Chronic swelling of the tear sac is almost always associated with a watering eye and is due to a non-tender mucocoele (see Fig. 5.59). Surgery is indicated to deal with the swelling and also to prevent recurrent acute infection. The surgeon should beware that, just occasionally, a swelling at this site may be due to adenocarcinoma of the sac, or to a dermoid cyst or an encephalocoele both of which can herniate from the orbit.

## Swelling around the eye
The tissues around the eye are loose and vascular and particularly liable to swell. The lids can swell within an hour and in severe cases the eye may quickly close. A careful history and examination will allow accurate diagnosis in most cases. Ask especially about trauma, pain, atopy, insect bites, previous lid swelling or pre-existing lid lump or sinusitis. Ask if there is blurring of vision or double vision.

### Acute swelling around the eye
Acute lid swelling has a relatively limited number of causes. Some associated physical findings and likely diagnoses are given in Table 5.33.

*Allergy*
Allergic conjunctivitis can affect the lids, particularly when the patient rubs them vigorously. The

**Table 5.33** Signs and likely diagnoses in acute lid swelling

| Sign | Possible diagnosis |
|---|---|
| Haematoma | Trauma |
| Crepitus | Ethmoid fracture |
| Conjunctival fluid and itching | Atopy |
| Involvement of mouth, larynx, or neck | Angio-oedema |
| Erythema or tenderness | Lid cellulitis |
| Decreased vision, diplopia or disc swelling | Orbital cellulitis |
| Swelling, mostly of lower lid | Lacrimal sac infection |
| Swelling, mostly of upper lid | Infected meibomian cyst or insect bite |

**Table 5.34** Some infective sources for lid cellulitis

Sinuses
   Ethmoid
   Frontal
   Maxillary
Lacrimal sac
   Dacryocystitis
Skin
   Stye
   Meibomian cyst
   Impetigo
   Insect bite
   Herpes simplex

lids will be diffusely swollen without redness or tenderness and conjunctival swelling is likely. There may be an atopic history but allergic conjunctivitis can occur for the first time in adult life. Treatment of the acute episode includes topical vasoconstrictors and systemic antihistamines if severe. Topical sodium cromoglycate (Opticrom) may be indicated for prophylaxis.

> Lid swelling plus lid itching means allergy

### Angio-oedema

This rare dominantly inherited condition can cause alarming periocular swelling within hours of minor trauma, dietary exposure or aspirin ingestion. Its importance lies in the risk to breathing from associated laryngeal swelling and early treatment is needed with antihistamines and systemic steroids. If breathing is already affected give *intramuscular adrenaline (epinephrine) promptly*. The dose for an adult is 0.5–1.0 mg (0.5–1.0 ml of adrenaline solution 1 in 1000 for injection). The number of doses and dosage for children is given in the *British National Formulary*. Refer immediately to a general casualty department in case tracheostomy is needed. The disorder is recurrent and referral to a dermatologist is justified for advice on prophylaxis. Low serum complement levels may be found.

### Lid cellulitis (Fig. 5.56)

Infection can spread around the eyelids from a number of sites, including the air sinuses, lacrimal sac and skin lesions (Table 5.34).

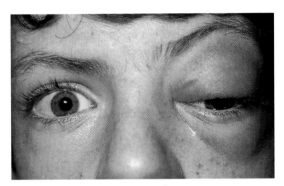

**Fig. 5.56** Swollen eyelids from cellulitis. Important associated features determine whether this is confined to the lids or has spread back to the orbit.

Cellulitis confined to the lid (preseptal cellulitis) is limited by the orbital septum which retards spread of infection backwards into the orbit itself. The skin will be obviously inflamed and tender and an abscess may form. Regional lymphadenopathy in the pre-auricular nodes is common. Lid cellulitis is commonest in children and young adults. It often accompanies or follows an upper respiratory infection and spread in these cases is probably blood- or lymph-borne from the sinuses. Normal sinus X-rays do not exclude the sinuses as the source of infection. Distinction from orbital cellulitis may be difficult (see below), especially if the swollen lids prevent a proper eye examination. If the patient has normal vision, no diplopia or proptosis and normal optic disc then orbital cellulitis is unlikely.

Lid cellulitis is treated with high-dose systemic antibiotics and oral amoxycillin with flucloxacillin is the best initial choice. Up to the age of

7 years the most common causative organism is *Haemophilus influenzae* and amoxycillin should be replaced by cefotaxime or co-amoxiclav. In a child of less than 18 months, or at any age if the patient is generally unwell, parenteral antibiotics are indicated. Referral is not always necessary.

> Refer lid cellulitis if:
> • patient is unwell or has a high fever
> • the eye is protruding
> • lid swelling prevents eye examination
> • previous similar episode
> • vision is blurred or doubled

### *Orbital cellulitis* (Fig. 5.57)

It is important to distinguish this from lid cellulitis because the complication rate for orbital cellulitis is much higher. Complications include cavernous sinus thrombosis and permanent visual loss from optic nerve involvement. Certain features help to establish a diagnosis of orbital cellulitis (Table 5.35).

The causes of orbital cellulitis are similar to those of lid cellulitis but radiological evidence of sinus pathology is more common. The thin medial orbital wall in particular is easily breached by ethmoidal sinusitis and an abscess may then spread into the orbit. Urgent referral of a suspected case of orbital cellulitis is indicated because the patient requires hospitalization and immediate intravenous antibiotics. Also, a CT scan is often indicated to define the extent of infection and the need for surgical intervention if there is a collection of pus in the orbit.

> Orbital cellulitis can cause blindness if treatment is delayed, especially in children

### *Infection of the tear sac (acute dacryocystitis)*

Tears drain into a small duct before passing into the lacrimal sac. A larger channel then drains into the nose below the inferior turbinate bone. Any blockage below the level of the sac will predispose to infection from a 'stagnant pond' effect. A history of chronic eye watering is common. The surface marking of the lacrimal sac is just below and medial to the inner corner of the eye and

**Table 5.35** Distinguishing clinical features of orbital cellulitis

Proptosis
Diplopia
Limitation of eye movements, particularly with pain
Decreased visual acuity
Optic disc swelling

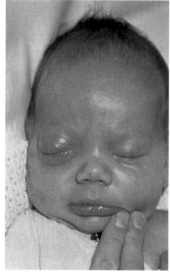

(a)

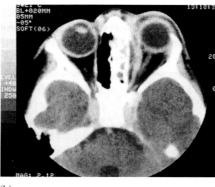

(b)

**Fig. 5.57** (a) Orbital cellulitis in an ill baby aged 3 months, due to *Pneumococcus*. (b) Computed tomography showing orbital involvement (right ethmoid and right orbit on the right side of scan). Reproduced from Taylor (1992) *Pediatric Ophthalmology* (slide atlas), Blackwell Scientific Publications, Cambridge, MA.

swelling begins here. Lower lid cellulitis may follow or the infection may remain localized to the sac and an abscess may form (see Fig. 5.55). Eventually this abscess can burst externally. In the early stages of infection it may be possible to express pus into the eye by pressure on the sac, though it will be tender.

Treatment should be started with an oral penicillin derivative. The responsible organism is most often *Staphylococcus aureus*, though streptococci, including *Streptococcus pneumoniae* are found occasionally. The treatment of first choice is flucloxacillin, 500 mg four times daily for 5 days. Use erythromycin, 250 mg four times daily for 5 days for those hypersensitive to penicillin.

Referral is indicated if an abscess has formed but is not otherwise necessary if the response to treatment is satisfactory. The patient is likely to be left with a watering eye and routine referral may be needed because of this. Acute sac infection may be recurrent and if so a drainage operation is indicated, making a new passage into the nose by a dacryocystorhinostomy (DCR).

### Infected meibomian cyst

Infection within a chalazion can cause lid cellulitis. *Staph. aureus* is usually responsible and the same course of treatment as lacrimal sac infection (above) is suggested. The cause is usually apparent before treatment though sometimes a chalazion is hidden until the lid swelling subsides. If a cyst remains after treatment it should be drained by incision and curettage.

Other skin conditions such as impetigo, erysipelas and herpes simplex or zoster can cause acute lid swelling, as can allergic drug reactions (see Fig. 5.18).

### Chronic swelling around the eye
(Table 5.36)

### Thyroid puffiness

Lid puffiness is occasionally the presenting feature of hyper- or hypothyroidism although associated symptoms and signs are usually present too. It is always worth checking thyroid function if in doubt.

**Table 5.36** Signs and possible diagnoses in chronic swelling round the eye

| Sign | Possible diagnosis |
| --- | --- |
| Bilateral puffiness and dryness | Myxoedema |
| Swelling in upper outer lid | Lacrimal gland tumour or dermoid cyst |
| Firmness or induration | Lymphoma or other infiltrate |
| Swelling in lower inner lid | Mucocoele of lacrimal sac |

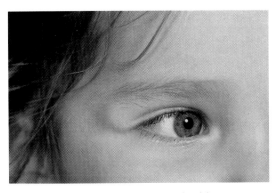

**Fig. 5.58** Dermoid cyst at the outer angle of the upper eyelid. Reproduced from Taylor (1992) *Pediatric Ophthalmology* (slide atlas), Blackwell Scientific Publications, Cambridge, MA.

Remember thyroid eye disease as a cause of lid swelling

### Lacrimal gland tumours

These are evenly divided between malignant and benign. They do not usually cause watering or dryness of the eye but rather proptosis and diplopia because of orbital involvement. Referral is required within weeks.

### Dermoid cyst (Fig. 5.58)

These are benign swellings that can occur around the orbit. They probably arise as inclusion cysts at the time of suture fusion and usually present in childhood or early adult life. They are most common in the upper outer region and can be difficult to distinguish from a lacrimal gland tumour. Also, like lacrimal tumours, they can spread backwards into the orbit.

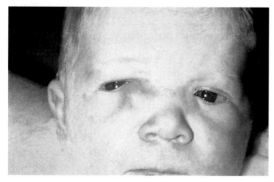

**Fig. 5.59** Mucocoele of the lacrimal sac, a chronic form of inflammation. Reproduced from Taylor (1992) *Pediatric Ophthalmology* (slide atlas), Blackwell Scientific Publications, Cambridge, MA.

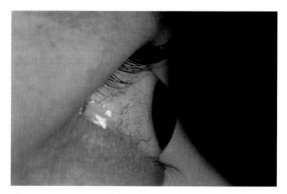

**Fig. 5.60** Protrusion of the eyes (proptosis or exophthalmos), here due to thyroid eye disease.

**Table 5.37**  Causes of proptosis

| | |
|---|---|
| Thyroid associated | Most common overall, particularly in the middle-aged |
| Inflammation | Septic, granuloma |
| Tumour | Bone, lacrimal, optic nerve, secondary, lymphoma |
| Trauma | Blood, arteriovenous fistula |
| Congenital/cystic/ vascular | Minority, but more common in children |

*Mucocoele* (Fig. 5.59)

Swelling of the lacrimal sac occurs when the drainage system is blocked. There may be associated attacks of sac infection. A mucocoele presents as a firm non-tender mass beneath the inner aspect of the lower lid. Pressure on the lump may cause extrusion of mucopus into the eye. Bypass surgery or removal of the lacrimal sac is indicated.

*Lymphoma*

This can arise in the orbit and present as firm swelling in and around the eyelids. The clue is in the firmness of the swelling and any associated lymph node enlargement.

## Proptosis

Proptosis is the appearance of an eye pushed forwards by something behind it (Fig. 5.60), and therefore implies some swelling within the enclosed bony orbit. The appearance is relatively uncommon and there are many possible causes. Investigation is specialized, but the important first step is to recognize the signs and to assess the urgency of referral. The problem may be unilateral or bilateral, and if bilateral is often asymmetrical. Symmetrical proptosis may be the most difficult to recognize in practice.

The eye is displaced forwards and possibly also up or down or to one side. The direction of shift may help in suggesting the origin of the swelling—for instance a lacrimal swelling will often push the eye downwards and also inwards.

The clue to proptosis is usually found in the eyelid position. Forward shift causes the lower lid to fall away from the lower limbus, showing white sclera below, where there is none in the normal eye. The upper lid may be retracted, particularly with thyroid eye disease, but if there is an associated neurological problem with the third nerve or sympathetic nerve affected, there may be ptosis of variable degree. There may be changes of the eye itself, which may be red, or swelling of the lid or conjunctiva. Rarely there may be an ocular bruit, which is interesting to hear, even if only once in a lifetime. There may be abnormal function of the nerves (second, third, fourth and sixth, sympathetic and fifth) or muscles in the orbit which may cause impaired vision (acuity or field), double vision, pupillary changes or sensory loss. These signs must be looked for because positive findings make the referral more urgent.

There are many causes (Table 5.37). In the adult, thyroid eye disease is by far the most common (in

60% of patients aged 20–60 years with proptosis) (see Fig. 5.64). A history of thyroid imbalance is not always clear and the systemic signs of under- or overactivity may also not be obvious, so this can be a pitfall. In children and the elderly, malignant tumours are comparatively more common. Early referral is advised for these age groups and also if at any age the history is short, clearly progressive, painful, involves trauma or includes abnormal neurological signs. A further emergency cause of proptosis, which may occur at any age except the very young, is orbital cellulitis, usually secondary to sinus infection. These patients are usually clearly ill and should be sent to eye casualty without delay as they need antimicrobial treatment and possibly surgical drainage (see above under Orbital cellulitis).

> The most common cause of eye protrusion is thyroid-related disease of the orbit

If the process is more quiet, the patient should still be referred, but not urgently. It may be very helpful if the patient brings a few photographs to give some idea of the rate and pattern of change in the patient's appearance over months or years.

> Refer early if eye protrusion is associated with:
> • sudden onset
> • young or elderly
> • pain
> • cellulitis
> • fall in vision or other neurological sign

The investigation includes scanning by CT or MRI and may involve a biopsy which may be done by an ophthalmic, ENT, neuro- or plastic surgeon depending on the site of the lesion and the expertise of the local surgeons.

## Abnormal eyelid position

Lid position may give clues to important underlying disorders, in particular thyroid dysfunction and neurological problems. There are several traps for the unwary!

It may be difficult to decide *whether or not* the lid position is abnormal and, if the lids are asymmetrical, which *side* is abnormal, whether ptosis or

retraction. Old photographs may be helpful to decide how long the problem has existed, and as a rare bonus may even diagnose a familial ptosis.

### Ptosis

Drooping of the upper lid has many causes (Table 5.38). The lids themselves should be carefully inspected and felt, to detect a lump in the lid or in the lacrimal gland. Enlargement of the lacrimal gland (usually acutely inflamed with mumps or a bacterial infection) makes a characteristic S-shaped ptosis. In elderly patients a fold of lax skin may simulate ptosis. Ask about past trauma to the orbit as a blow-out fracture can displace the eyeball backwards and simulate drooping.

The pupils may help to distinguish a neurological cause, a larger pupil on the droopy side suggesting a third nerve palsy (Fig. 5.61) and a smaller pupil a Horner's syndrome (Fig. 5.62). An acute

**Table 5.38** Causes of ptosis

| |
|---|
| Lid lump or inflammation |
| Neurological |
|     Third nerve palsy |
|     Horner's syndrome |
| Muscular |
|     Myasthenia |
|     Myopathy |
| Congenital |
| Traumatic |

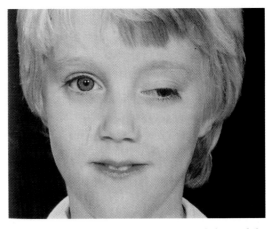

**Fig. 5.61** Third nerve palsy of the left eye with droopy lid, larger pupil and eye deviating down and outwards.

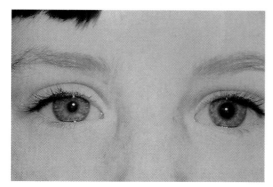

**Fig. 5.62** Horner's syndrome of the right eye, with a smaller pupil and slight droop of the upper lid. Reproduced from Taylor (1992) *Pediatric Ophthalmology* (slide atlas), Blackwell Scientific Publications, Cambridge, MA.

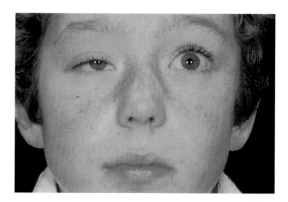

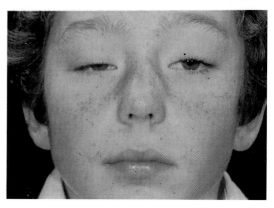

**Fig. 5.63** Myasthenia gravis with variable droop of the upper lids and variable squint. Photographs are taken 10 minutes apart. Reproduced from Taylor (1992) *Pediatric Ophthalmology* (slide atlas), Blackwell Scientific Publications, Cambridge, MA.

ptosis with complete closure is almost always a third nerve palsy. A Horner's droop is always partial and often subtle and may be particularly difficult to detect if bilateral. Double vision may suggest a more widespread problem with extra-ocular muscles, either neurological or muscular in origin, and fatiguing during the day suggests myasthenia in particular (Fig. 5.63). Don't forget that double vision disappears if there is a marked ptosis as one eye can't see, so lift up the lid to do eye movements. Some neurological rarities include myotonic dystrophy and Marcus Gunn jaw winking.

> With a droopy lid, look carefully at the pupils

In children many cases of unilateral or bilateral ptosis of long standing turn out to be congenital and are occasionally familial, so be sure about duration and family history.

Ptosis should not be difficult to distinguish from blepharospasm of the lids which is an active squeezing shut. It is impossible voluntarily to produce true ptosis of the upper lid alone.

### Retraction (Fig. 5.64)
In this case, extra eyeball is visible above (or sometimes below) the limbus. Upper lid retraction is a common sign of thyroid-related eye disease, so look for lid lag in particular. Thyroid retraction is

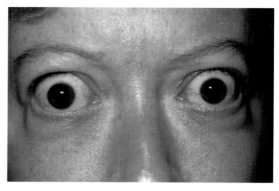

**Fig. 5.64** Protruding eyes with retraction of the upper lids and white showing beneath, due to thyroid eye disease.

usually bilateral but is commonly asymmetrical. Look also for proptosis or protrusion of the eyeball, particularly if there is what looks like lower lid retraction. A much less common cause of retraction, usually bilateral and symmetrical, is a mid-brain problem (sometimes as part of Parinaud's syndrome). Very rarely trauma, tumours or inflammation behind the eye can sclerose and pull back the lids. In aberrant regeneration after a third nerve palsy the upper lid can shoot up in certain positions of gaze, particularly in downgaze, which is disconcerting for the examiner in particular.

Bilateral upper lid retraction in a baby may be due to hydrocephalus.

## Nystagmus

Nystagmus is uncommon but is always significant, so it is important to have an outline idea of types and causes, of which there are many (Table 5.39).

The patient is less likely to notice nystagmus than are relatives, friends or doctor, as the abnormal movements themselves do not give rise to symptoms unless they are so intrusive as to blur vision.

Nystagmus is a repetitive to-and-fro movement usually of both eyes. The name comes from the

Greek for 'nodding off', when the head droops slowly and then jerks back up. Most types of nystagmus are jerky but some are pendular with a wobbling to-and-fro pattern. The movements arise from destabilization of the normal complicated system which keeps the eyes stable while retaining flexibility in fixing and tracking chosen visual targets.

Nystagmus may be seen with the eyes looking straight ahead but is more common and may be more noticeable with the patient looking in different directions, both to the side and up and down. If the pattern is jerky it is conventional to classify the type of nystagmus from the direction of the faster phase, be it right or left, up or down beating. Vertical nystagmus is more likely to be caused by a central nervous system problem.

> Nystagmus is an important sign and should not be ignored

### Types

The type of nystagmus gives some guide to the origin of the problem but a better guide will come from the history. Ask how long the movements have been noticed, particularly in a child. Ask about visual acuity, symptoms which suggest raised intracranial pressure, and about other neurological symptoms particularly balance, vertigo and hearing as well as double vision. Take a drug history, particularly asking about alcohol, sedatives and anticonvulsants.

### Causes

Normal subjects show optokinetic nystagmus in response to a moving target, such as seen in railway passengers watching the passing landscape. It is also normal to have a few beats of nystagmus at the extremes of lateral gaze, but if these are prolonged or persist when backed off from the extreme then they are significant.

Poor vision bilaterally may be associated with nystagmus, particularly if the loss is marked and occurred early in childhood. There is a form of congenital nystagmus which usually dates from childhood which is typically horizontal and often pendular.

**Table 5.39** Least rare causes of nystagmus

*Congenital*—perhaps associated with poor vision from early life

*Intoxication*
Alcohol
Hypnotic
Anticonvulsant

*Eighth nerve damage*
Menière's
Acoustic neuroma
Streptomycin or gentamicin toxicity

*Brainstem*
Stroke
Encephalitis
Tumour
Multiple sclerosis

*Cerebellum*
Stroke
Tumour

Peripheral neurological disorders of the inner ear or vestibular eighth nerve cause nystagmus, often with vertigo, as in Menière's disease or with an acoustic neuroma. It is important to ask about (and perhaps to test) hearing.

Central nervous system problems are another cause. These usually involve the brainstem, including the mid-brain, or the cerebellum. A tumour may need to be excluded. Multiple sclerosis often affects the ocular stabilizing system. Look for ataxia and ask about double vision or oscillopsia (see Sensation of visual movement: oscillopsia, p. 41). Intoxication may be suspected from the patient's past record or drug history.

*Referral*
Most cases will need to be referred for a specialist neuro-ophthalmic opinion, so it is important to spot nystagmus and not to ignore it. The urgency of referral depends more on the duration of the problem and the associated symptoms than on finding a particular pattern of nystagmus. It is in patients with common but vague neurological complaints such as 'giddiness' that the looking for and finding of significant nystagmus may be a vital clue that signals early referral.

## Abnormalities of the pupil

Pupils can be too large or too small. The problem can affect one or both pupils. The response to light and to looking near can be abnormal in one or both eyes. Rarely, the pupil may look white instead of black.

### Equal pupils with an unequal response to light

Firstly, to clear up one popular misconception, in blindness of one eye the pupils will usually be of normal size and equal, as the normally seeing eye dictates the CNS response on both sides. However, the response to bright light shone into each eye separately will be quite different on the two sides: on the normal side the light produces a brisk response (in both pupils, but it is difficult to watch both simultaneously), whereas on the blind side there will be no response (again in both pupils). If vision is reduced on one side, even if the eye is not 'blind' then there will be an asymmetry in re-

sponse to direct light which is most likely to be noticed if the light is swung from one side to the other. The direct response will be unbalanced, as on the deficient side the pupil tends to dilate. (See Input pupillary imbalance, p. 19.)

In patients who are blind from a bioccipital stroke from basilar disease the pupil reactions are normal as the anterior visual pathway remains intact.

### The large pupil
This may be due to:
• third nerve palsy
• Adie's pupil (ciliary ganglionitis)
• iris trauma, ischaemia, pharmacological agents
• mid-brain pathology.

*Third nerve palsy* (see Fig. 5.61)
If the pupil is affected compression is more likely, either from an aneurysm or from an extradural haematoma if there is a history of significant trauma. The fibres running with the third nerve to supply the pupil constrictor come from the parasympathetic system and are located superficially so they are susceptible to external pressure. Look for associated ptosis or limitation of ocular movement on that side.

If there is an acute history with *pain*, referral for investigation is urgent. If the palsy is painless it may still be due to compression but could also be a 'mini stroke' affecting the blood supply to the nerve, as in diabetes.

*Adie's pupil* (Table 5.40 and Fig. 5.65)
This is often discovered by the patient looking into the mirror or it may be noticed by a relative or

**Table 5.40** Features of Adie's pupil

Usually unilateral but sometimes bilateral
Larger than normal early on, later constricts
Reacts poorly to light but better to near
Redilates slowly after constriction (tonic response)
Sensitive to dilute pilocarpine (0.1%), which constricts it
    but not the normal pupil
Discomfort common, but not pain
Ankle jerks diminished in some patients
Benign and not associated with significant neurological
    problem elsewhere

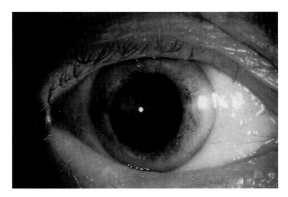

**Fig. 5.65** Large irregular Adie's pupil, which will constrict better to near effort than to light.

friend. In this case there are few accompanying symptoms and referral is not urgent, but those with a training in first aid or neurology may mistake this for a third nerve palsy and cause the patient some concern. Pain is uncommon and never marked. There is never ptosis and eye movements are normal. The patient may notice problems with focusing for near, either because accommodation is poor or because it is tonic (poorly relaxing). The problem usually seems unilateral but subtle signs on the other side may help to confirm the diagnosis. Referral to an ophthalmologist is best as some of the signs are seen best on the slit-lamp. The pupil is dilated, responds poorly to light, better to accommodation and may show a tonic response as it relaxes slowly after constriction in the near position. The response seen on the lamp often shows a spiral twisting of the iris. Absence of ankle jerks makes the diagnosis one of Holmes–Adie syndrome. The aetiology is unclear but may be an inflammation of the parasympathetic ciliary ganglion behind the eye. The diagnosis is confirmed by a supersensitive response to one drop of dilute pilocarpine (0.1%) to each eye. This makes the large pupil constrict to become smaller than the normal pupil (which does not constrict).

### Iris abnormalities

Trauma may rupture the iris sphincter and cause a large pupil which may be irregular. Soon after the injury there may be blood in the front chamber. Iris ischaemia from acute angle closure glaucoma may also paralyse the muscles, making the pupil large, oval and fixed. Dilating agents may have paralysed the pupil sphincter. Drops may be put in accidentally or sometimes deliberately. Any large pupil with a local iris cause will fail to constrict to high strength (4%) pilocarpine drops. In systemic poisoning, for instance with belladonna (deadly nightshade) or other muscarinic agents related to atropine, both pupils will be dilated.

### Mid-brain syndrome

Some patients with mid-brain pathology of various types will have large and poorly reactive pupils, usually bilaterally. Such pupils may react better to near than to light (light–near dissociation).

## The small pupil

Small pupils are common in the elderly. The commonest cause of abnormally small pupils is pharmacological and is related to using opiates, either therapeutically or in addiction, or topical pilocarpine sometimes used to treat glaucoma. A rare but important cause is organophosphorus insecticide poisoning with cholinesterase inhibitors. Pin-point pupils can occur with pontine injury from stroke or trauma. A unilateral small pupil may be part of a Horner's syndrome (see Fig. 5.62)—look for slight ptosis. This should be referred to a neurologist unless it is of longstanding or secondary to a sympathectomy, as it could be caused by a resectable lesion. The classic small Argyll–Robertson pupils of tertiary syphilis are rare but still to be found, though they may be due instead to diabetes. Local iris causes of a small pupil include iritis, either acute or chronic. When dilated such pupils may festoon because of attachments to the lens behind.

## The white pupil (Fig. 5.66)

The commonest cause is a dense cataract with pronounced opacification of the lens proteins. A longstanding detached retina crumpled up behind the lens may look white. A rare but important cause of white pupil in childhood is retinoblastoma. This is a malignant tumour which may arise in both eyes and early detection and treatment is vital. Although a non-specialist is unlikely to see a

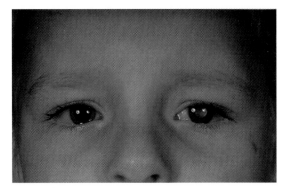

**Fig. 5.66** Child with a white left pupil. This may be due to retinoblastoma and should be referred immediately. (Courtesy of Mr A. Shun-Shin).

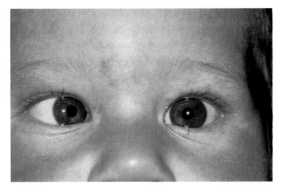

**Fig. 5.67** Right convergent squint in a baby. The left eye is fixing and the left light reflection is central, whereas on the right it is displaced over the iris. Reproduced from Taylor (1992) *Pediatric Ophthalmology* (slide atlas), Blackwell Scientific Publications, Cambridge, MA.

single case in a professional lifetime it is still important to be aware of the possibility. Another childhood cause is fibrosis of the retina after treatment for prematurity.

## Squint

A squint occurs when the two eyes fail to point in the same direction (Fig. 5.67). Patients often complain wrongly of 'squinting' when they really mean screwing up their eyelids.

Squint in childhood is fairly common and is discussed under the section on screening in childhood (see p. 155). Many squinting children continue to squint as adults. They are usually aware of the problem and may give a history of wearing glasses or doing exercises or of patching one eye and they may have had squint surgery. Such patients rarely have double vision as their brain has adapted to ignore one of the images and they often have a 'lazy' or amblyopic eye which has never had good visual acuity. The history may explain many patients who would otherwise present a neurological puzzle. These patients should have an unlimited range of eye movements when each eye is tested separately, with the other eye covered. Adult patients sometimes ask about the possibility of cosmetic surgery for squint and it is reasonable to refer to an ophthalmic surgeon.

Patients who have poor vision in one eye often squint as they have no way of using the two eyes together. Left to its own devices the poorly sighted eye often turns outwards.

Patients who acquire a problem with moving the eyes usually have double vision when they squint. This is discussed in its own section. Such patients often have problems with the third, fourth or sixth cranial nerves but may also have a disorder of the eye muscles themselves, particularly thyroid-related disease. Such patients may need hospital referral either to investigate the cause if the problem is recent or evolving, or to correct the double vision with prisms or muscle surgery if it is more longstanding.

It is worth mentioning that patients who screw up their eyelids may rarely have true blepharospasm. Such patients may benefit from botulinum toxin treatment in a hospital setting.

## Abnormal retinal appearances

This section is designed as a brief checklist for a variety of the more common features that may be seen with a standard direct ophthalmoscope. The use of this instrument and the value of dilating drops are discussed in the section on practical approach (see p. 15). Remember that lesions not involving the fovea will not reduce vision, so these appearances often cause no symptoms.

### Retinal haemorrhages

It is essential to dilate the pupil and have a good look round, including the major branch vessel trunks, the macula within them on the temporal side and the fovea or point of fixation itself. Assess the form and number of haemorrhages. *Flame-shaped* or oval and rather feathery spots (Fig. 5.68)

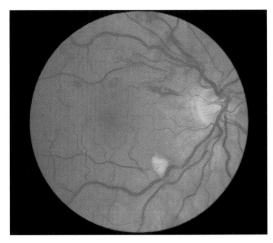

**Fig. 5.68** Flame haemorrhages grouped around the upper branch vessels. Suspect hypertension or hyperviscosity.

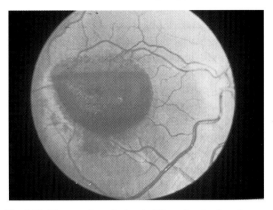

**Fig. 5.70** Haemorrhage in front of the retina is often dense and may sediment into a level. Here it is caused by acute leukaemia.

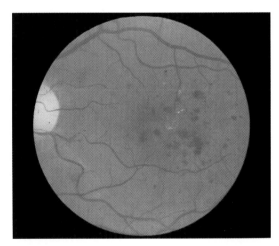

**Fig. 5.69** Blot haemorrhages, here temporal to the fovea and characteristic of diabetes.

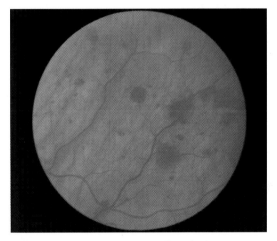

**Fig. 5.71** Large blot haemorrhages, here due to hyperviscosity.

are suggestive of small vessel disorders particularly hypertension or occlusions, perhaps embolic. *Small round dot* areas are suggestive of diabetes and there may also be *larger blot*-type (Fig. 5.69) haemorrhages if there is more advanced diabetic damage. *Larger solid and round* or regular areas (Fig. 5.70) suggest bleeding in front of the retina (behind the vitreous or 'subhyaloid') and may suggest trauma, new vessels or a bleeding disorder perhaps with an underlying haematological problem. *Multiple haemorrhages* with a variety of shapes, if not due to diabetes, raise the possibility of retinal vein occlusion, particularly if unilateral

or in a wedge shape suggesting branch vein occlusion. Alternatively, there may be a haematological disorder or hyperviscosity (Fig. 5.71) (see Haematological disorders, p. 143). Do not forget the possibility of non-accidental injury in children with retinal haemorrhages.

In retinal haemorrhage in a child, consider:
- a blood disorder
- non-accidental injury

**Pale lesions** (Fig. 5.72)

These are a bit tricky to interpret as there is a greater variety:

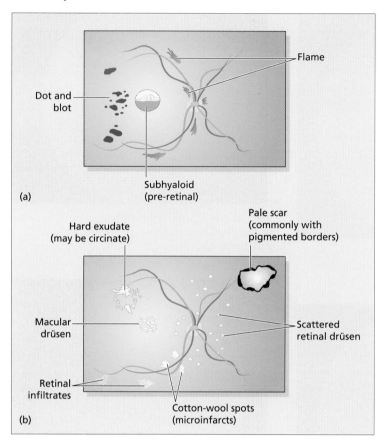

(a)

(b)

**Fig. 5.72** Retinal lesions. (a) Haemorrhages. (b) Pale lesions.

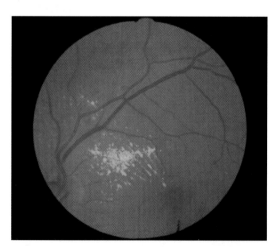

**Fig. 5.73** Shiny, yellowish, hard exudate with streaks towards the fovea, here due to an old branch retinal vein occlusion.

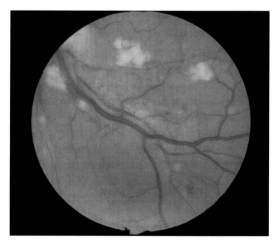

**Fig. 5.74** Pale fluffy patches of cotton-wool spots, indicating vessel closure in accelerated hypertension (here blood pressure was 200/120 mmHg).

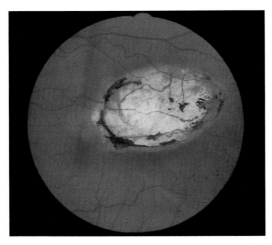

**Fig. 5.75** Punched-out scar of choroid and retina typical of past *Toxoplasma* infection. The pale scar with pigmented areas lies under the retinal vessels.

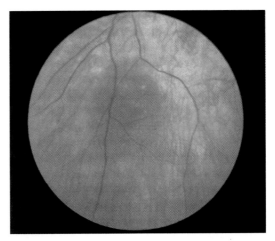

**Fig. 5.77** A pigmented, common, flat naevus is innocent.

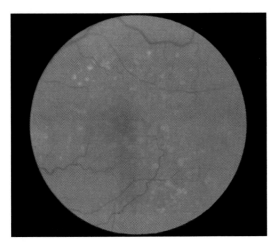

**Fig. 5.76** Drüsen, small scattered pale spots, here especially around the fovea, within the macula.

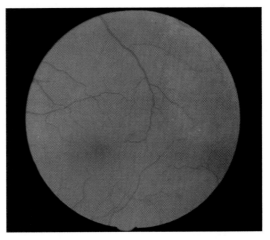

**Fig. 5.78** A pigmented, uncommon, raised malignant melanoma should be referred.

- The commonest is the *hard exudate* which has a dense and shiny appearance due to lipid deposits within macrophages (Fig. 5.73). Hard exudate is most common in diabetes when it may form in a ring ('circinate') around a focal point of leakage within the retina (see Fig. 7.9). It is also found in hypertension if this has been established for several weeks.
- Less dense fluffy areas may be *cotton-wool spots* (Fig. 5.74). These are not exudates but rather

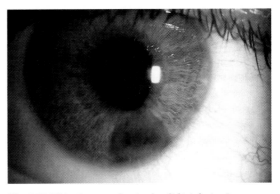

**Fig. 5.79** This pigmented, raised, solid iris lesion is a rare iris malignant melanoma.

sites of swollen nerve fibres due to small vessel ischaemia. They are characteristic of the more severe types of diabetic or hypertensive damage and are always significant and so should be referred.

• Extensive retinal *oedema or ischaemia* as in a retinal artery occlusion may show as areas of diffuse paleness of the fundus but may be difficult to detect with the direct ophthalmoscope (see Fig. 3.4).

• Retinal *infiltrates* are like dense cotton-wool spots but often signify active retinitis, perhaps infective, and may be associated with floaters or cells in the vitreous giving a cloudy view of the retina.

• Old *scars* involving the choroid, as in toxoplasmosis, are not uncommon (Fig. 5.75). They may be large and have well-defined borders. There is often scattered pigment associated with them.

• Degenerative changes, often around the fovea, cause pale *drüsen* of the retina (Fig. 5.76). These have a variety of shapes and textures and a few scattered ones are common and insignificant. In older patients they may be associated with bleeding or scar formation around the fovea (see Age-related macular degeneration, p. 126).

### Pigmented areas

The commonest cause is a flat *benign naevus* (Fig. 5.77) but the lesion that is most easily confused is the less common *malignant melanoma* of the choroid (Fig. 5.78). This causes a dark patch which increases on serial observation and often becomes raised. If the patch is solid looking and clearly raised when first seen, refer immediately. A melanoma may even cause a visible lump to appear within the pupil, darkening the red reflex. If in any doubt, refer. Melanoma of the iris is even less common, causing a pigmented lesion which slowly increases in size, becoming raised and solid looking (Fig. 5.79). Flat iris freckles (naevi) present for many years are much more common, and are benign. Pigment in a *crescent around the optic nerve head* is a variant of normal. Many old choroidal *scars* have pigmented areas. Very dense black spots are likely to be benign *hamartomas* of the pigment epithelial layer, whose only significance is in drawing attention to the rare possibility of associated polyposis coli as an inherited condition.

---

• If in doubt about a pigmented retinal or iris lesion, particularly if solid, raised or enlarging, refer
• It may be a malignant melanoma

# Chapter 6  **Problems with focus, spectacles and contact lenses**

Problems with focus are overwhelmingly the most common sort of eye disorder (Fig. 6.1) and it seems reasonable to give more than the usual explanation in this area, as doctors often feel confused—perhaps less so if they themselves wear glasses and realize their importance at first hand.

## Error of refraction and its measurement

It is the function of the eye to bend light to a focus on the fovea of the retina. If the eye cannot do this there is an error in refraction and vision will be blurred without the help of a spectacle or contact lens. Most people will experience this at some time in their life. To 'refract' means to bend light, but the term is also used to describe the technique of measuring the strength of lens needed. This section describes how the eye should work, what can go wrong and what can be done to correct the error.

### Refraction

When light passes from one medium to another of greater density, it is slowed down. If a beam of light hits a flat surface at right angles, all the particles slow simultaneously so it continues in a straight line. If the beam strikes obliquely, the particles first entering the new medium will be slowed before others which have to travel further. This has the effect of bending, or refracting, the beam. Both the cornea and the lens focus light inwards. As the biggest density difference is between air and cornea, most refraction occurs here. Further refraction by the lens allows the 'fine focusing' onto the retina.

### Accommodation

From close objects, the light diverges as it reaches the eye, and so will need more bending than parallel rays from the distance. When looking close, the eye increases the power of its lens, which becomes fatter, and thus more convex. As the concentric muscle of the ciliary body contracts, the suspensory ligaments of the lens slacken. The lens is able to bulge more and becomes a stronger focusing shape (Fig. 6.2).

### Dioptres

The terminology used for describing lenses is not really complicated. By convention, a 'plus' lens is convex and focuses light inwards whereas a 'minus' lens is concave and turns light outwards. The strength of the lens is measured in dioptres and the higher the dioptre number the stronger the lens, in either a plus or a minus direction (Fig. 6.3). Most average short-sighted people are about minus 2 to 3 dioptres whereas a 'high myope' is about minus 10 or more. The average pair of reading glasses will be about plus 1.5 to 2 dioptres.

## Types of focusing problem

### Presbyopia, or getting older

From the Greek meaning 'old man's eye', this refers to the loss of ability to focus for near that is inevitable with ageing. With time, the protein in the lens degenerates, causing it to harden and lose its elasticity. Contrary to popular belief, it is not the focusing muscles which fail to work. In the early stages, the patient can compensate by holding the book further away so the light is less divergent. Eventually they find that even at arm's length the print is out of focus or too small to see. The solution is to prescribe some convex reading spectacles to do the work in place of their own lens (see Fig. 3.1).

Most people will start to need some help with reading in their mid-forties. At this point they will

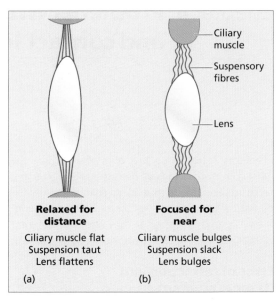

Fig. 6.2 Focusing and the lens.

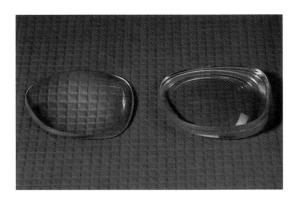

**Fig. 6.3** Spectacle lenses to correct large errors of focus. On the left is a convex +10 lens, thicker in the centre, to correct hypermetropia. On the right is a −10 concave lens, thicker at the edges, to correct myopia.

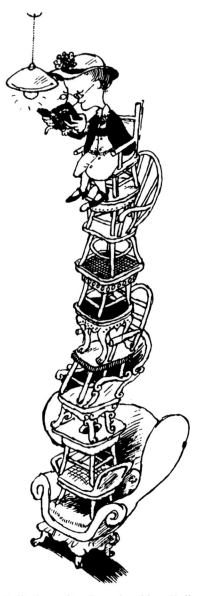

**Fig. 6.1** Difficulty reading. Reproduced from Hoffnung (1962) *Hoffnung's Bookworms* by permission of Gerard Hoffnung © Hoffnung Partnership, London.

still have some focusing ability, and the spectacles need only be about plus 1.00. Eventually the glasses will be doing all the refracting necessary for them to read, and assuming a reading distance of 0.5 metre, the lens will need to be at least plus 2.00. Care must be taken that the lenses give the patient a comfortable working distance of their choice, determined by their activities. Too strong a lens

will make them need to get too close to the object (Fig. 6.4).

Some other factors influence focusing power of the lens, for instance diabetes. It is estimated that one in 20 diabetics presents with blurring of vision due to change in lens shape induced by hydration changes. In many third-world countries the lens ages prematurely, perhaps due to its protein being damaged by severe dehydration. Ultraviolet light may also damage the lens protein.

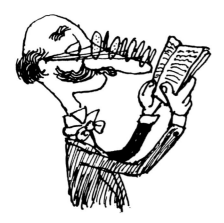

**Fig. 6.4** The presbyope. Reproduced from Hoffnung (1962) *Hoffnung's Bookworms* by permission of Gerard Hoffnung © Hoffnung Partnership, London.

## Myopia, or short-sightedness

This is the next most common problem. The eye's focusing power is too strong for a relatively large eyeball and must be weakened with minus lenses. The eyeball size increases with age in childhood and many adolescents become short-sighted for the first time. They are unable to see the board at school or sit closer to the television to see it clearly. It is worth mentioning here that there is little evidence to support the popular belief that people become myopic by doing too much close work. It is more likely that untreated myopes can see close quite clearly, but the rest of the more distant world passes them by in a blur, so it is perhaps natural for them to become preoccupied with activities involving close work and this is thus the result, not the cause, of their short-sightedness. High myopia is a risk factor for retinal tears and detachment. As the myope ages, he can often correct his presbyopia by removing his glasses for close work, since the taking away of a minus lens is the same as adding a plus!

## Hypermetropia, or long-sightedness

The focusing of some eyes, particularly those of small size, is in effect too weak and must be supplemented with a plus lens. These patients need to focus actively even for distance vision to be clear. In youth, this is not usually a problem as the lens is nicely elastic. As an object comes nearer, even more effort is needed, and it may become a strain to read. Most children are hypermetropic in infancy, but cope well. The danger in childhood is that with more than the usual amount of hypermetropia, a convergent squint (cross eyes) may result from this excessive effort. Such squints are treated by prescribing glasses.

Some eyes remain hypermetropic for life. Such an adult will eat into the reserve of focusing power and will become presbyopic sooner and may complain of 'eye strain' when reading. Later, even distance vision, first television and then driving, will exhaust them and become blurred. Hypermetropic eyes are more likely to develop acute glaucoma (see p. 81).

## Astigmatism

Astigmatism occurs when the cornea has the shape of a rugby ball (USA, football) rather than a football (USA, soccer ball). Such an eye can never produce a clear image at the retina. A small degree of astigmatism is tolerated and most people have up to half a dioptre difference, caused by the weight of the top eyelid on the cornea. Soft contact lenses are not good for correcting astigmatism as they mould to the shape of the cornea. Spectacle lenses to correct astigmatism are shaped to have a different strength in different directions. They must be accurately lined up with the eye. Astigmatism is common after cataract surgery, when the sutures can distort the cornea if tied unevenly. The modern surgical technique of phacoemulsification has reduced this risk considerably, as the incision is tiny and does not usually need to be stitched. Corneal scars may also cause astigmatism. A rare cause is keratoconus ('conical cornea')—see Fig. 5.46.

## The pin hole occluder (Fig. 6.5)

This cuts out the need for refraction by confining the light to a narrow beam which passes straight along the visual axis and so improves vision for a subject with a focusing error. This is not true if there is also cataract or any other problem apart from focusing. It is a very useful part of the examination, and one that is surprisingly often neglected.

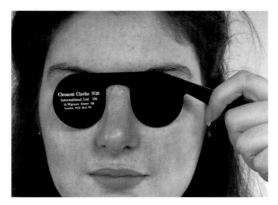

**Fig. 6.5** Pin hole occluder in use. Here, the right eye is covered and the left is viewing a distance chart through one of the holes. The occluder is reversed to measure right vision.

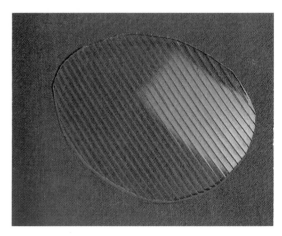

**Fig. 6.6** Fresnel plastic prism to correct double vision (see also Fig. 8.2).

## Prisms

These bend all the light in one direction and may be useful to compensate for double vision. Spectacles can be made to incorporate prisms, either permanently, or as a temporary measure by sticking a flexible plastic Fresnel prism onto an existing spectacle lens (Fig. 6.6).

### Testing for errors of refraction

Known in the trade as 'refraction', this is a means of prescribing glasses suited to the individual patient's needs. Using a retinoscope to watch the reaction to a beam of light reflected from the eye, the refractor can get an objective measurement of the strength of lens needed to correct a focusing error, including astigmatism. Then this is checked by putting trial lenses in front of the eye and checking the patient's response as to how clear the test type is. The lenses are altered until vision is optimal. Small children find it impossible not to focus on the light during the test, so drops may be needed to prevent this. A good refractor can get a very accurate assessment in this way without using test type. Machines are available which will do these measurements automatically, but in the UK the majority of eye tests are still done by optometrists (previously called opticians).

### How to assess spectacle lenses

The type and strength of spectacle lenses can be assessed roughly without special equipment by simply looking at and through the lens. A lens to correct myopia is concave and will be thicker at the edges, where concentric lines often appear, and the lens makes things look smaller. A lens to correct hypermetropia or presbyopia is the reverse. It is thicker in the centre, tends to magnify and may have a 'goldfish bowl' effect at higher strengths. Hold up the glasses and view a straight line through the lens and rotate the lens clockwise and counter-clockwise. If the line also appears to rotate, there is also a correction for astigmatism.

## Professionals qualified in eye care

The optometrist, optician and ophthalmic medical practitioner are all trained professionals who measure patients for glasses and other optical devices. Most of this work is done by 'high street' practitioners, rather than in hospitals. Prior to 1989, they were called either 'ophthalmic' or 'dispensing' opticians, depending on the qualifications and service they offered. Some confusion still exists over this distinction, so some explanation may help in understanding the roles of the various qualified personnel in the provision of eye care outside hospitals.

### Optometrist

Optometrists were formerly called ophthalmic opticians. They are qualified to refract patients and to dispense all forms of spectacles and contact lenses, and advise on the provision of low vision aids. They will have done a 3-year degree course studying the anatomy, physiology and optics of the eye, and will have learned something of its pathology. At the end of this course they will be able to refract and know how to fit glasses and contact lenses, but must spend a further year as a pre-registration student working in practice with a recognized supervisor. Passing their professional exams makes them a Member of the British College of Optometrists (MBCO). Later qualifications may be their Fellowship of the college, or a diploma in contact lens practice (DCLP) issued by that body.

Many, but not all, optometrists will have equipment such as a slit-lamp and visual-field analyser. They are entitled to use topical anaesthetic and dilating drops. A specially trained high street optometrist can therefore help in the screening of patients for glaucoma or diabetic retinopathy. Each optometrist decides the extent of the service to offer and it is well worth getting to know what facilities are available in your locality. The optometrists' register contains a list of all optometrists and their qualifications and is available through the library service. Local lists are held by Health Authorities or PCG/PCTs for their region.

It is a condition of their terms of service that they must refer to a doctor (usually the GP) any patient in whom they find signs of ocular disease. As an increasing number of optometrists check eye pressures, the number of referrals for suspected glaucoma is increasing. The significance of this is discussed in the section on glaucoma screening.

### Dispensing optician

Dispensing opticians hold a less extensive qualification, the Fellowship diploma of the association of British Dispensing Opticians (FBDO), which does not allow them to test patients but only to fit them with glasses made to a prescription issued by an optometrist or ophthalmic medical practitioner.

### Ophthalmic medical practitioner

An ophthalmic medical practitioner (OMP), is a doctor who holds a higher qualification in oph-

**Table 6.1** Entitlement to free annual eye test and voucher

| Free eye test | Voucher entitlement |
|---|---|
| Children under 16 years, students under 19 years | Yes |
| Age over 60 years | No |
| Income Support or Family Credit | Yes |
| Registered partially sighted or blind* | Yes |
| Patients requiring complex lenses | Yes |
| Patients attending an eye hospital | Perhaps |
| Patients with diabetes or glaucoma | No |
| First-degree relatives with glaucoma and aged over 40 years | No |

*Note that many patients registered as blind will have some residual vision and may still need spectacles.

thalmology, and who is registered with the Ophthalmic Qualifications Committee as eligible to provide general ophthalmic services. They must also be registered with the local Health Authority, to be entered on the local ophthalmic list. Many OMPs work on a sessional basis in dispensing opticians, for whom they issue prescriptions. An example of a prescription for the provision of glasses is given in Fig. 6.7.

At present, the cost of an eye test may deter some patients from having an annual check, which limits the role of the optometrist in providing primary preventive care. However, free eye tests are available to patients in certain categories and a voucher system will cover the cost of the glasses too in some cases. The exact regulations are subject to the political policy in force at the time, and can be complex. The booklet HC1 from the Department of Health covers the details, but the main entitlements are listed in Table 6.1.

The Health Authority is the body responsible for funding National Health Service provision in this situation. The vouchers provide a variable contribution towards the cost of the glasses. Many opticians will have a small range of basic spectacles, the cost of which will be wholly or largely covered by such a voucher. More expensive choices must be paid for by the patient.

### Spectacles

Having been issued with such a prescription, the patient is free to take it and have it made up as

NHS Hospital Eye Service                                                                HES (P) 2

## RADCLIFFE INFIRMARY NHS TRUST

Oxford Eye Hospital, Woodstock Road, Oxford OX2 6HE  Telephone (01865) 224740

# PATIENT PRESCRIPTION / STATEMENT

## PRESCRIPTION DETAILS          DATE OF SIGHT TEST

| R I G H T | Sph | Cyl | Axis | Prism | Base | VA | | Sph | Cyl | Axis | Prism | Base | VA | L E F T |
|---|---|---|---|---|---|---|---|---|---|---|---|---|---|---|
| | | | | | | | Dist. | | | | | | | |
| | | | | | | | Near | | | | | | | |

PRACTITIONER'S REPORT

I carried out a sight test today in accordance with the regulations with the following result:

☐ the prescription above was issued

☐ no prescription for spectacles was required

☐ no change was clinically necessary

☐ Tick if complex lenses for voucher purposes

☐ Tick if non-tolerance case

Any other relevant clinical details;

BVD.........mm

PATIENT'S DETAILS

Hospital No. ..................................Mr/Mrs/Miss/Ms

Surname:.............................DOB......./........./.........

Forenames..............................................................

Address...................................................................

..............................................................................

..............................................................................

Prescriber's signature.............................................

### INFORMATION FOR PATIENTS

Read the rest of this form before you get your spectacles. It tells you:
- how to get your spectacles
- about help with the cost of your spectacles

A prescription is valid for 2 years. If you have been given one, keep it in a safe place.

### HOW TO GET YOUR SPECTACLES

If you are under 16 you must take this prescription to a registered optician.

If you are 16 or over you can take this prescription to a registered optician or anyone else who supplies spectacles.

Unregistered suppliers are not allowed to sell prescription spectacles to children or to adults known to be registered blind or partially sighted. Reading glasses may be sold to adults without prescription.

### HELP WITH THE COST OF SPECTACLES

You can get help with the cost of spectacles for any of these five reasons:
- You are under 16.
- You are a full-time student under 19.
- You are getting, or are the partner of somebody who is getting, Income Support or Family Credit.
- You are prescribed complex lenses.
- The DSS decides that you are on a low income.

If you think that you are entitled to help for any of these reasons, please contact the Optometry Department as above.

If you do not already have a certificate HC2 or HC3 for help with NHS charges and if you think that you are entitled to one because you are on a low income, ask for form HC1. For more details, see leaflet HC41.

Refunds are only given by the DSS if a claim is made within 1 month of the date when you obtained your spectacles or contact lenses.

WRI 268 PM1599

**Fig. 6.7** Patient's prescription and voucher form HES (P) 2.

glasses wherever they choose. For most patients, this will be at the same optician as the eye test, but as more low cost dispensing facilities are being established in other shops, the choice is wider. If the patient simply wants reading glasses, these can be bought without testing or a prescription in a variety of outlets, from chemist shop to petrol station. Whilst offering a cheap option which may suit a lot of people very well, the omission of the examination by a qualified practitioner could lead to blindness. Shops cannot sell glasses to those under 16 years of age, or patients on the partially sighted or blind registers.

## Types of spectacle

### Single lenses
Single lenses correct myopia, hypermetropia, presbyopia and astigmatism (see Fig. 6.3). A pair of glasses can be simply assessed by holding them a few inches away from a straight edge and moving them at right angles to it. The edge will appear to move, in the same direction with a minus lens and in the opposite direction with a plus. If a correction for astigmatism is present, rotating the lens will cause the edge to rotate too. A presbyope may choose to have a half-glass, through which to look down when reading and over the top into the distance.

### Combination lenses
These combine lenses of two or more powers in different sections. The most common form is a bi-focal, in which the larger top section of the lens is for distance vision, and a smaller section at the base contains more plus lens for close work (Fig. 6.8). They save the presbyope from having to change glasses when alternating between these two distances. The disadvantage is that the lower section is designed for when the patient is looking down at a book and if instead they look down at the stairs, these will be out of focus. Not all patients will tolerate bifocals.

This idea can be extended to give a third section in the lens, intermediate in position and power between the distance and reading portions. Such tri-focals are chosen by patients who also need to see in the middle distance, such as a musician reading

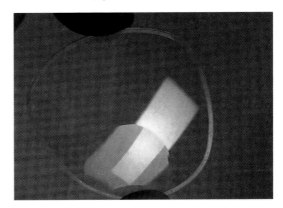

**Fig. 6.8** Bi-focal spectacle lens with distance correction above and reading correction in the 'moon' below.

a score. To avoid the image 'jumping' between the sections of the lens, they may be merged gradually (the principle of the varifocal lens), giving a whole range of working distances, though each part of the lens would have only a narrow band of usefulness.

### Lens materials
Glass, the original material from which lenses were made, may remain the first choice. It is relatively cheap, offers good optical properties, is unlikely to distort under pressure or heat and it resists scratching. The disadvantages are that it is heavy and brittle. Weight is important when the lens has to be thick to correct large errors, especially if the eye's own lens is removed and not replaced (aphakia). Young children may be more likely to fall and break their glasses and certain occupations or pastimes can make the dangers of the glass breaking unacceptably high. Minus lenses, being thinnest in the centre, are more likely to be broken than plus lenses. For high-risk patients, the glass may be specially toughened.

Plastic lenses are an alternative, since they are both lighter and more resilient. On the other hand, they scratch more easily, which can be a nuisance if the spectacles are frequently removed and handled carelessly. Modern resins have overcome some of these problems, but they are also usually more expensive.

Tinting of the lens is possible in both types, and a lens which darkens in response to light (Reactolite type) is now available in plastic. Tinted lenses are usually available only outside the health service unless there is a problem such as dilated pupil or albinism. Tinted lenses cannot harm the eyes but can be dangerous in certain driving conditions. The speed of reaction must be adequate for the rapid fluctuations encountered when driving, for instance through tunnels. Polarizing lenses reduce glare, but can result in distracting patterns appearing on toughened car windscreens. Filters can be incorporated to exclude harmful wavelengths of light in workers exposed to a high intensity of them. A coating can be applied to reduce reflections from the surface of the lenses. Plastic is better than glass in avoiding fogging when the wearer comes inside from the cold.

### The spectacle frames

For most patients, this is simply a matter of personal choice. Nevertheless, it is important that the frames fit well, avoiding undue pressure at the points of contact, yet not allowing them to slip down the nose. This is not only uncomfortable, but alters the effective power of the lens, and may cause distortion. Young children may need flexible wire ends to the side arms, which can hook around their ears and keep the glasses secure.

Certain occupations need side pieces added to the frames to protect the eyes from injury, physical or chemical. Sometimes the frame must be suitable for wear under a helmet or respirator. Patients with severe dryness of the eyes may need frames like goggles which reduce evaporation of the tears. A ptosis prop may be fitted to the top of the frame to hold up a drooping upper lid. Snooker players have made famous their particular requirements in 'frames for frames'! Other sports or occupations may test the optician's skills.

### Intolerance of spectacles

Patients will at times complain that they cannot 'get on' with their new glasses. Usually this is because the brain dislikes the change and must adjust over a period of weeks. If the problem persists, the following should be checked: is the prescription correct; are the correct lenses fitted properly; and do the frames fit adequately? Send

the patient back to the optician if necessary. Intolerance is most common with complex or high power lenses.

### Contact lenses

These sit on the front surface of the cornea, held in place by the surface tension of the tear-film. The shape of the lens plus tears changes the refracting power of the cornea. Most contact lens wearers choose them for cosmetic reasons, or to enable them to pursue a sport or career where glasses are impractical. There are different types of contact lens (Fig. 6.9), each with good and bad points. Nowadays, most are lenses covering the cornea only (Fig. 6.10), unlike the old larger haptic-type lens. Most patients would be well advised to try a rigid but gas-permeable lens in the first instance. It is difficult to predict tolerance but many optometrists offer a free trial fitting.

> Contact lens intolerance may be caused by:
> - allergy
> - dry eye
> - blepharitis

Patients who work in a dusty environment may find this incompatible with lens wear. Patients ask about wearing contact lenses and glasses alternately. If they choose to wear lenses only occasionally then a soft lens may be better tolerated, but if they only wear glasses from time to time a rigid lens can be tried. Vision with glasses is usually less good with intermittent lens wear as the precise corneal shape is unstable from day to day. There is nothing to deter adolescents from trying contact lenses, but remind them that any individual may have a limited period of tolerance of lens wear and they may prefer to 'save' this for later in life: only trying will tell. Disposable lenses used for a month at a time have made it easier for those whose refraction is changing as they grow. Children too young to look after their own lenses or who do not understand the importance of lens care can risk damaging their eyes. On the other hand, responsible children can be surprisingly successful lens wearers if there is a really good indication, perhaps high myopia. The main types available are shown in Table 6.2, together with their advantages and disadvantages.

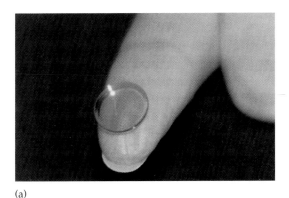

(a)

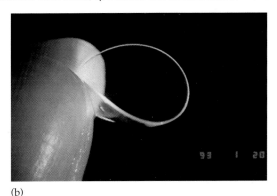

(b)

**Fig. 6.9** Contact lenses: (a) rigid and (b) soft.

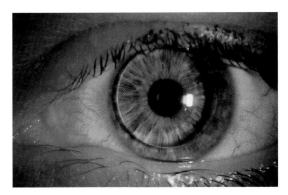

**Fig. 6.10** Rigid contact lens in place on the cornea.

### Extended wear contact lenses

There are soft lenses which are designed to be tolerated for longer than usual and are left in place for several weeks or months before being changed. They are used mostly in the elderly or very young in whom a cataract has been removed without implanting a plastic lens. They carry an increased risk of serious corneal infection. For this reason their use should be discouraged in those patients who may consider them as a 'soft option' compared with the care routine needed for daily wear lenses.

### Disposable contact lenses

These are soft lenses which are advertised as an easy alternative to the chore of the daily wear lenses. Disposable lenses ought to be associated with a lower risk of serious corneal infection but the snag is that to make them commercially feasi-

**Table 6.2** Main types of contact lens: advantages and disadvantages

RIGID GAS-PERMEABLE CONTACT LENS

*Material*
Mixtures of silicone and CAB polymer

*Advantages*
Good vision even with astigmatism
Reasonable oxygen supply
Infection and allergy less likely
Relatively inexpensive

*Disadvantages*
Less comfortable initially
Removed daily
More easily displaced and lost
Poor in dusty environment

SOFT CONTACT LENS

*Material*
Silicone, methylacrylate or vinyl pyrolidone

*Advantages*
Comfortable
Good oxygen supply
Can be worn for longer periods
Safer for contact sports

*Disadvantages*
Vision less good, particularly with astigmatism
More easily damaged and deteriorate more quickly
Risk of infection higher, needing a greater degree of care
Allergy more common
Usually more expensive

ble means that the quality of lens may be poor and also the patient may become rather cavalier in their approach to lens wear. This has resulted in the opposite effect, with reports of increased risk of serious corneal damage associated with disposable lens wear.

### Supervision

It is essential that all contact lens wearers have regular examination by slit-lamp to monitor the effect of the lenses on the cornea, conjunctiva and lids, and that the lenses are checked, since damaged lenses may damage the eye. Hypoxia may cause proliferation of blood vessels at the edge of the cornea. Poorly fitting lenses may produce abrasions, seen with fluorescein. *Beware that fluorescein will stain a soft contact lens*, though this can be leached out over several hours of soaking, or immediately with dilute hydrogen peroxide.

### Lens stuck in the eye

Occasionally, a patient will be unable to remove their own lens. This may be because it has slipped up under the top lid or because they cannot get it off the cornea. A lens that is lodged under the top lid can be most elusive, especially a soft lens. Topical anaesthesia and location with fluorescein may help, and a cotton-wool bud used to wipe under the everted lid to bring down the lens. If unsuccessful, it may be best to refer the patient either to the optician who fitted them or to eye casualty, since a slit-lamp may be needed to locate the lens. If there is any doubt about a lens being retained in the eye, this is the correct course of action, as if left ulceration or infection may follow. In the case of the lens stuck on the cornea, the lens may either be levered off using the lower lid, or a soft lens grasped between index finger and thumb, taking care not to scratch the cornea. Anaesthetic drops may be used with care. Hard lenses can also be removed using a specially designed small suction pad, if you have one.

### Overwear symptoms

Patients who wear their lenses for too many hours in the day or who fall asleep in them can develop symptoms of corneal distress. The appearance and treatment is similar to that of 'arc eye' (see Arc eye, p. 50).

### Criteria for the provision of contact lenses on the NHS

Patients often ask if contact lenses are ever supplied 'on the NHS'. In selected cases this may be possible. These are patients in whom contact lenses will produce much better vision than spectacles, usually those with a high or complex prescription. The conditions that qualify are:
• Hypermetropia or myopia of 10 dioptres or more.
• Anisometropia (difference in refraction of the two eyes) of 4 dioptres or more.
• Aniseikonia (difference in the size or shape of the two images) of about 10% or more.
• Significant corneal irregularity, high astigmatism, keratoconus or scarring.
• Other conditions such as bandage or cosmetic lens.

## Surgery for errors of refraction

Patients may have read about the possibility of having an operation on the cornea or laser treatment to correct focus allowing them to throw away their glasses or contact lenses. The options and problems associated with these are discussed in the section on Refractive surgery on the cornea (p. 182).

# Chapter 7  **Five common eye disorders**

Some of the aspects of *cataract*, *glaucoma*, *macular degeneration*, *squint* and *diabetic retinopathy* are discussed elsewhere. The purpose of this chapter is to highlight their individual features.

## Cataract

The popular idea of a cataract is that it is a 'film' which 'grows over' the eye. In fact, a cataract is any opacity in the normally clear protein of the lens which lies behind the iris (Fig. 7.1). The problem can be likened to white of egg—when fresh this is clear protein, but when damaged (by heat, in the case of the egg) it becomes progressively more opaque. The same thing happens in a cooked fish lens. Worldwide, cataract is the most common cause of poor vision and is estimated to have blinded 20 million people who do not have access to surgery.

- Lens protein is like egg white
- It becomes opaque when damaged

There are few well-defined causes of cataract though many factors may contribute. Age is the most important and dehydration another, particularly in a hot climate. There is little evidence for light-induced damage, though ionizing radiation can produce opacities. Long-term systemic corticosteroid treatment can hasten the process. Congenital rubella or rare metabolic disorders can cause cataract in childhood and diabetics develop opacities earlier than age-matched controls. Trauma to the eye or inflammation inside it may hasten the ageing process.

The patient with cataract complains usually of blurring or 'misting' of vision which is poorly corrected or even made worse with a pin hole. Symptoms are often worse in bright light (especially sunlight) as the opacity both scatters light and is more noticeable with a small pupil if it is central in the lens. The opacity may be visible to a bright light shone onto the pupil but early change can be detected as it causes blurring of the retinal view with the direct ophthalmoscope which cannot be corrected by altering the focusing lenses. With the ophthalmoscope 'backed off' a little and the red reflex brought into focus (together with the pupil margin), the opacity shows as darker spokes, shadows or granular dots against the reflected light, like obscured glass (Fig. 7.2). The pattern is seen better after dilating the pupil.

There are no known preventive measures or medical treatments for cataract. Long-term aspirin has been debated as a retardant, but the results of studies are conflicting. The surgical management has been revolutionized by the development of artificial plastic lens implants, usually inserted into the same position that the natural lens occupied, behind the iris.

Non-specialists often wonder when to refer a patient with lens opacity for surgery. Any patient who is troubled by the symptoms of cataract might be helped by surgery. Younger patients may be particularly bothered by glare from early cataract when driving at night. The elderly are particularly suitable for a lens implant, but this may be feasible in most younger patients. Surgery may be postponed until likely benefit exceeds risk. Children with cataract should be referred early for investigation and consideration for surgery. The aspects of cataract surgery most relevant to the patient are discussed in Chapter 11.

Only refer for cataract surgery if the patient is bothered by the reduced vision

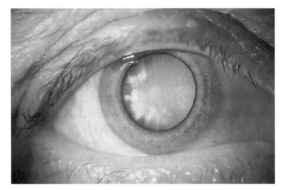

**Fig. 7.1** Cataract, an opacity of the lens, causing haziness in the pupil. (Courtesy of Mr A. Shun-Shin.)

## Glaucoma

This subject is perhaps the commonest cause for concern in the non-specialist responsible for eye care who dreads missing the condition. There is often confusion between chronic and acute glaucoma. The two conditions have in common an eye pressure (like a tyre pressure) which is high enough to damage nerve fibres within the rim of the optic nerve head, but their cause and management are different.

- Chronic glaucoma is painless
- Visual field is lost before vision falls

The major risk factor for chronic glaucoma is age

Other risk factors for glaucoma are:
- first-degree relative has glaucoma
- Afro-Caribbean origin
- myopia
- diabetes

The role of the non-specialist might be summarized thus:
- To *encourage patients to attend for screening* for chronic glaucoma by an optometrist who offers this specific service, certainly over the age of 60, and younger (from the age of 40) if there is a first-degree relative affected by chronic glaucoma. See the section on Glaucoma screening (p. 152), which describes the features of chronic glaucoma and some of the dilemmas in diagnosing it.
- To *recognize pathological cupping of the optic nerve head* (disc) in established chronic glaucoma (Figs

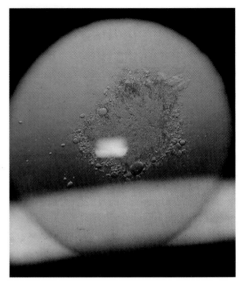

**Fig. 7.2** Lens opacity visible in the centre against the red reflex with the pupil dilated.

7.3 and 7.4). This can be helped by illustrations but the key to confidence is practice in looking at both normal and abnormal discs. It may be possible to attend the local glaucoma clinic for direct experience. If you have difficulty with using the ophthalmoscope, see the section on practical procedures. Cupping of the disc is described in the screening section.
- To have a good index of suspicion for and to *recognize the symptoms of attacks of acute angle closure glaucoma*, which is rare but treatable and speed is necessary in the event. See Acute glaucoma (p. 81) or under Sudden loss of vision (p. 33) for a description.
- To be aware of the rare occurrence of glaucoma in childhood which can present as watering, photophobia or an abnormal eye appearance.
- To have some role in *understanding and supervising the treatment* for chronic glaucoma.

### Treatment of chronic glaucoma

The aim of glaucoma treatment is to prevent optic nerve damage and preserve visual function by lowering the intraocular pressure. This can be achieved by using medication—usually drops, occasionally oral—or by surgery. Traditionally, surgery has been reserved for patients who have

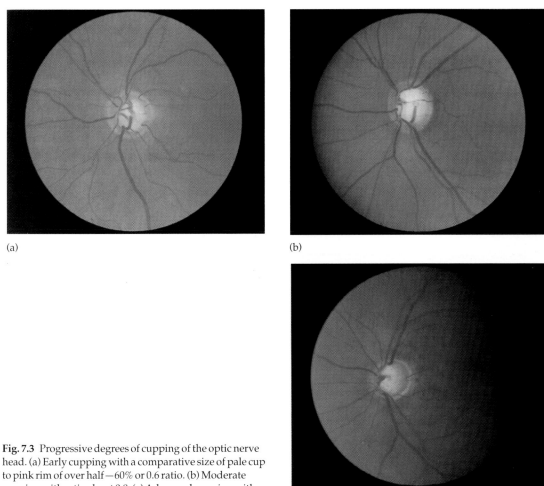

(a)

(b)

(c)

**Fig. 7.3** Progressive degrees of cupping of the optic nerve head. (a) Early cupping with a comparative size of pale cup to pink rim of over half — 60% or 0.6 ratio. (b) Moderate cupping with ratio about 0.8. (c) Advanced cupping with ratio nearly 1.0.

progressed despite medical treatment, but this is not universal practice and from a cost-effective point of view early surgery has much to recommend it. The choice of treatment is particularly important because glaucoma is a chronic condition and the patient will normally require continued care for life.

*Medical treatment of chronic glaucoma*
Although the mainstay of medical treatment remains topical beta-blockers, in recent years new intraocular pressure-lowering drops have become available which are effective, well tolerated with few systemic side-effects, and more convenient as they are used less frequently during the day.

*Beta-blockers*
A range of beta-blockers is available, for example timolol, betaxolol, carteolol and laevobunolol. These all reduce intraocular pressure efficiently by reducing aqueous production. Side-effects are mostly systemic as the dose of the drug in a small drop is surprisingly high (Table 7.1). Use is therefore contraindicated in patients with a slow heart rate, a tendency to wheeze or with heart failure. Beta-blocker drops are used twice daily, preferably at fairly precise 12-hour intervals.

*Pilocarpine*
Pilocarpine lowers intraocular pressure by increasing outflow but its use is limited by difficul-

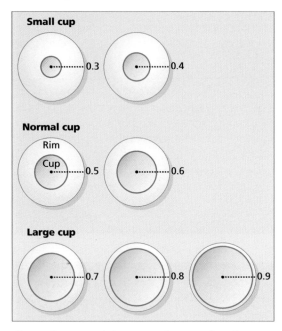

**Fig. 7.4** Progressively larger cup : disc ratios found in glaucoma.

**Table 7.1** Side-effects of glaucoma therapy

| Therapy | Side-effect |
| --- | --- |
| Beta-blocker | Wheezing, bradycardia, heart failure |
| Pilocarpine | Pain, blurred vision |
| Dorzolamide | Bitter taste, conjunctivitis |
| Brimonidine | Dry month, discomfort, allergy |
| Latanoprost | Iris pigmentation |
| Acetazolamide | Malaise, paraesthesia, nausea, anorexia, hypokalaemia, polyuria, renal stone |

ties related to pupil constriction. Headache is common when treatment is started, but often settles after a week or two and it is therefore worth persevering with treatment. Drops must be put in four times daily—a nuisance to the busy and a real problem for those who have to rely on others to put drops in. Newer medications have largely superceded pilocarpine itself, which is available in concentrations of 1%, 2% and 4%.

*Dorzolamide and brinzolamide*
These topical carbonic anhydrase inhibitors reduce aqueous production. They are usually used twice daily and can be used as monotherapy or in addition to a beta-blocker. Dorzolamide and Timoptol are conveniently available together in a single bottle, offering a simplified regime that may help compliance. Systemic side-effects are rare but a transient bitter taste is fairly common, and later emergence of blepharoconjunctivitis may prevent use.

*Brimonidine*
Brimonidine is an $\alpha_2$-adrenergic receptor agonist and a powerful inhibitor of aqueous production,

used twice daily For practical purposes it is as effective as a beta-blocker. It is generally well tolerated but a third of patients complain of a dry mouth. The most common ocular side-effects are burning and stinging, blurred vision and ocular allergy.

*Latanoprost*
Latanoprost is a topical prostaglandin analogue and is the most effective of all glaucoma medications. It is used once daily and increases the outflow of aqueous. It has possible curious ocular side-effects, sometimes resulting in a gradual increase in iris pigmentation or an increase in the number and size of eyelashes.

*Acetazolamide—Diamox*
This is the only oral carbonic anhydrase inhibitor in routine use which gives a rapid and profound reduction in aqueous formation. Its use is limited by side-effects so the drug is best used for short periods of time. Paraesthesiae of the hands and feet are invariable though seldom severe, but worse are malaise, anorexia and light-headedness. Hypokalaemia can be dangerous. The full dose is 250mg four times daily, but a lower dose is often both effective and better tolerated. A sustained release preparation can be used as 500mg twice daily.

**Laser treatment in glaucoma**
Laser trabeculoplasty is a procedure by which small laser burns applied to the trabecular meshwork help aqueous outflow and lower intraocular pressure. Typically, there is a modest fall in pressure which is unfortunately often not maintained

for longer than a year. The technique is mostly used as an alternative to the introduction of a second glaucoma drop or to defer surgery, but it may be preferred as an initial treatment. The treatment is not unpleasant; half the angle is usually treated at one session. A transient rise in intraocular pressure and a mild iritis may follow, so acetazolamide tablets and steroid drops are prescribed for a few days.

> Chronic glaucoma may be treated by:
> - drops
> - pills
> - laser
> - surgery
> - a combination of these

### Surgery in glaucoma

Surgery is usually undertaken when medical treatment is not tolerated or fails to halt the progression of field loss, although in some centres it is carried out on presentation if the disease is plainly severe. The procedure is usually a trabeculectomy (see Chapter 11).

> Chronic glaucoma can progress despite full treatment

### Prognosis

Like other diseases, chronic glaucoma has a wide spectrum of severity. Some patients' glaucoma will be permanently controlled by a single drop regime whereas others show a progressive deterioration with several different agents added together which control the process for a while but the disease then 'escapes'. The timing of surgery can be a difficult decision and the presence of additional problems such as cataract and macular degeneration may modify the treatment plan.

A particular problem is presented by 'low tension' (or 'normal pressure') glaucoma. This is where there is optic disc cupping and typical glaucomatous field loss in the absence of any measured intraocular pressures above the normal range. The condition is likely to be due to poor blood supply of the optic nerve head. It is difficult

by medical means to achieve the low levels of intraocular pressure needed to prevent progressive loss of field, and surgery also cannot be guaranteed to produce these levels so this particular condition has a poor outlook in the long term.

Another therapeutic dilemma is whether to treat the great number of 'ocular hypertensives' now being discovered by optometrists. These people have raised intraocular pressure, but normal disc appearance and full field of vision. Research has so far failed to show that treatment at this stage prevents the subsequent development of glaucoma in some patients. Most ophthalmologists, however, are unhappy to leave intraocular pressures above 30 mmHg untreated, and so treatment may be given.

## Age-related macular degeneration

The human fovea has an extremely high metabolic turnover. Although it is designed to last a lifetime of exposure to bright light levels it is hardly surprising that in an ageing population this part of the retina may show signs of 'wear and tear'.

The symptom of macular degeneration affects mostly central and critical detailed vision which is most commonly noticed first for reading. A visit to the optician cannot correct the problem as it is not an error of focus. A magnifier may help at first, but fine vision tends to deteriorate steadily, though the rate of decline is unpredictable in each patient. Often there is an accelerating problem over many months in one eye, though the other may follow suit. Occasionally the change can be more acute, particularly if the condition sets off leakage of fluid or blood at the central fovea. Unfortunately, it is usually a bilateral problem though it may progress at a different rate in each eye.

> Macular degeneration causes:
> - loss of central vision
> - handicap
> - *not* 'blindness'

There are no certain factors other than age in the development. It seems sensible to avoid very bright light once the early changes are found, but there is no firm evidence that this helps. There has been some interest in whether dietary supple-

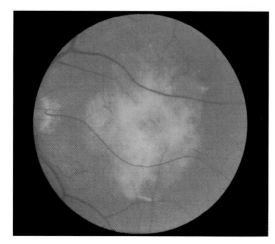

**Fig. 7.5** Age-related macular degeneration with a large pale disciform scar involving the fovea. Detailed vision is irretrievably lost.

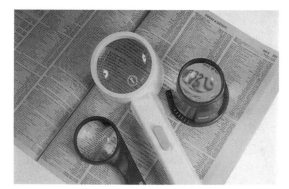

**Fig. 7.6** Various magnifiers may help the patient with poor central vision, and most patients with a macular problem find it possible to read a little, even if the process is laborious.

ments (such as zinc) might be helpful, but the evidence is unclear and supplements are not recommended. Rarely, the condition is familial, especially in younger patients.

The changes to be seen with the direct ophthalmoscope are very variable. The commonest appearance is of retinal drüsen within the macula and particularly grouped around the fovea (see Fig. 5.76). These are pale lesions whose size varies from hard seed-like collections to more soft-looking larger confluent patches (Fig. 7.5). Sometimes there is an increase in pigmentation. Haemorrhage is an ominous sign as it usually signifies the growth of destructive new vessels into the macula from the damaged deeper layers. In some patients the haemorrhage is subtle, in others dramatic. Foveal oedema can also reduce vision but will be difficult to detect with certainty, especially using the ophthalmoscope.

Once vision falls it rarely recovers but for several reasons the patient is best referred for specialist advice. The more acute the history the earlier the referral should be, particularly if there is a clear history of recent onset of distortion of vision close to fixation (see Distortion, p. 43). Established damage can be carefully assessed and the patient given an explanation and estimate of prognosis. Patients will often be told that they will lose central vision but will not go 'blind' in a navigational

sense as they will not lose peripheral vision. The second reason for referral is that a minority of patients may be suitable for laser 'welding' treatment which may stave off damage for a useful length of time, perhaps in the less badly affected eye. Lastly, many patients benefit from a careful assessment for low vision aids and handicapped patients should be registered as partially sighted or blind (see Chapter 12). Most patients with macular degeneration maintain some useful reading ability with the right type of reading aid, though reading is rarely a pleasure for them (Fig. 7.6).

## Squint

A squint is present if the two eyes do not both fix on a single object (see Fig. 5.67) — it does not refer to screwing up the eyelids (which may be what the patient is describing by the expression). Squint is a common condition of childhood, affecting around one in 30 of the UK population under the age of 5 years. It may be present from birth or in the weeks after, or develop later in childhood, often between 3 and 4 years of age. The detection of squint and policies for screening babies and children are discussed in the section on screening (see Chapter 9). The surgical management is discussed in Chapter 11.

Squint affects up to one in 30 of the UK population under the age of 5 years

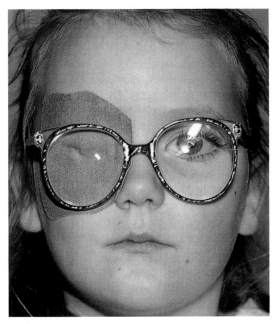

**Fig. 7.7** Squint with glasses and a patch worn over the normal eye. Patching under the glasses gives less opportunity to peep round.

It is untrue that the parents or child will necessarily be aware of the problem and it is true that a squint may be both correctable and, occasionally, an important sign of a serious underlying eye or neurological problem. On the other hand, the squint may be intermittent perhaps lasting for a few minutes at first, so beware of ignoring the parents' observation. If possible, if a squint is suspected or found, try to assess visual acuity in each eye—also described under Screening children, p. 155. Success in detecting a squint depends on several factors including the child's age and personality as well as the observer's skill.

Orthoptists are professionals trained in the screening, assessment and medical treatment of squint and many departments run screening clinics in the community, to which non-specialists may have direct access. If a squint is certain, direct referral to hospital is recommended at any age. If a white pupil is seen, refer urgently as this implies an important internal problem, perhaps even a retinoblastoma tumour.

Various medical measures may be used, depending on the type of squint, under the supervision of a specialist department. These include prescribing spectacles to correct focusing error, patching of the better eye to encourage development of good vision in the squinting eye (Fig. 7.7) and sometimes eye movement exercises. If patching is used, instructions to the parents from the specialist should be clear about the periods and frequency of patching, which may be very important. Normally the better-seeing eye is patched to encourage development of visual acuity in the 'lazy' eye.

Onset of squint due to weakness of the ocular muscles usually causes double vision and restricts full eye movement. This is discussed under Double vision (p. 39).

## Diabetic eye disease

### Change in focus

The commonest visual symptom in diabetics is blurring from a change in focus. About one in 20 diabetics present this way and an informed GP or optometrist is alert to this. The problem arises from change in the hydration and shape of the lens, and is usually reversible with good blood sugar control. When stabilized, the patient may need to visit an optometrist.

### Retinopathy

The most important eye feature in diabetics is retinopathy, which may cause blindness. The problem is potentially treatable at certain key stages and so screening is vital: this is discussed under Diabetic eye screening, p. 145. All doctors in general practice will have diabetic patients, estimated at 40 patients in an average practice of 2000. Of these, perhaps 10 will have retinopathy, which will be serious in three or four. Each practice might have on average one patient blind from diabetes. The incidence will be higher if a significant number of patients are of Asian or Afro-Caribbean descent. It is therefore important that GPs are clear about who is screening the retina and why this is done, as well as checking that this actually occurs or undertaking it themselves. Studies have shown that a GP with motivation, training and a decent ophthalmoscope is able to offer this service, though increasingly optometrists are being trained specifically to provide diabetic retinal screening. It may be worth liaising with the local eye hospital diabetic service to organize a period of training.

> Screening the diabetic retina and referral for laser treatment can prevent blindness

> Retinal screening entails:
> • training
> • practice
> • organization

Diabetes should be suspected in any patient who has microaneurysms, 'dot and blot' retinal haemorrhages or hard exudate (*background retinopathy*) (Fig. 7.8) and the blood pressure should also be checked. The typical pattern of diabetic involvement is the *ring-shaped (circinate) hard exudate* (Fig. 7.9) which forms within or near the macular area enclosed by the major blood vessels, often just temporal to the fovea. Look not only at the nerve head and macula, but specifically at the central fovea (with the patient looking straight into the light) and also in particular nasal to the disc and temporal to the macula (asking the patient to look slightly to right and left to do so). It may be helpful in looking at red lesions to use the red-free (green) filter in the ophthalmoscope.

It is still not clear *why* the retina is affected in diabetes. The problem is undoubtedly in the smaller retinal blood vessels which either leak or close off (or unfortunately in some patients do both). Leakage leads to exudates which may form around the macula and eventually at the fovea itself, with the threat of wrecking detailed vision permanently (Fig. 7.10). This *'exudative maculopathy'* is by far the most common cause of loss of vision in diabetics, especially in the older patients. 'Background' exudates, sited away from the fovea,

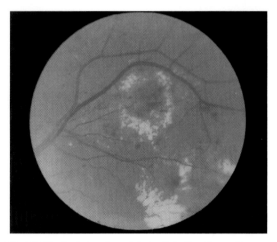

**Fig. 7.9** Circinate hard exudate in diabetic retinopathy, forming a circle around a focus of leakage. Laser welding may help before the fovea is damaged.

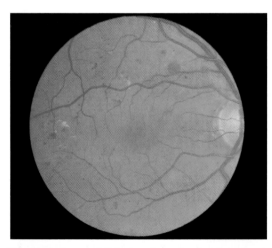

**Fig. 7.8** Background diabetic retinopathy showing a few microaneurysms, blot haemorrhages and hard exudates, but none extensive or near the fovea.

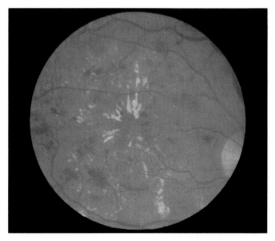

**Fig. 7.10** Established macular change in diabetic retinopathy, with extensive haemorrhage and hard exudate involving the fovea. This is likely to be irretrievable, with poor vision.

may slowly extend towards it and the first sign of trouble may be a slight drop in vision, perhaps with distortion. Laser focally to identified leaking areas may prevent deterioration if done early enough, before the leakage establishes changes at the fovea. The laser scars cause small scotomas in the central field which are not obtrusive to most patients when they use both eyes together. Unfortunately, sometimes foveal leakage is the presenting symptom and is already irreversible.

Significant diabetic damage to the retina causes:
- leakage
- ischaemia
- or both of these

Patients whose blood vessels close off are at risk of forming new vessels on the optic nerve head or elsewhere, in the part of the retina visible with a standard ophthalmoscope after dilating the pupil (Figs 7.11 and 7.12). Attention is drawn to

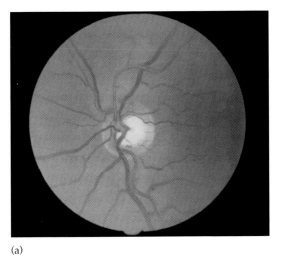

(a)

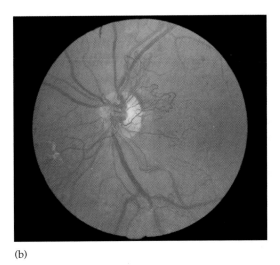

(b)

**Fig. 7.11**  (a) Early disc new vessels in proliferative diabetic retinopathy. These are difficult to see, but small tufts are visible at 6 and 12 o'clock. (b) Extensive new vessels can be seen looping outside the disc margin.

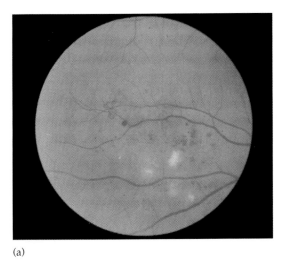

(a)

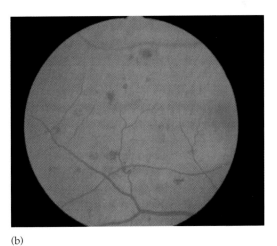

(b)

**Fig. 7.12**  (a) Tuft of peripheral new vessels in proliferative diabetic retinopathy, just above and left of centre. Note several cotton-wool spots, indicating ischaemia. (b) Very early tuft of new vessels, immediately above a loop in the branch vessel below centre.

the important key features of pre-proliferative retinal changes, which are discussed in the screening section, as patients with these features have a 50% chance of developing new vessels within a year.

Any patient with an apparent tuft of frond-like new vessels on the optic nerve head, or elsewhere in the retina, must have prompt specialist retinal assessment. Patients with new vessels are at risk of vitreous haemorrhage which, if repeated, may wreck peripheral as well as central vision. This proliferative response is less common than leakage, accounting for about 5% of all retinopathy, but it is more dangerous and commoner in younger patients. Again, the new vessels are potentially reversible if extensive laser treatment is done before they are too large. It is not clear exactly how laser burning causes reversal of new vessels. Patients who have had the treatment will have defects in peripheral vision which may be most noticeable at night. The treatment itself should not debar a patient from driving unless it is more extensive than usual. Patients in whom treatment has controlled proliferative retinopathy (perhaps in the first year or so) will need continued follow-up to be sure the stabilization is maintained, but most patients who do well in the first instance will have a reasonably good outcome, so they should not feel too demoralized when laser treatment is first planned.

### Fluorescein angiography (Fig. 7.13)

This photographic technique is necessary in some cases of diabetic retinopathy to decide if, and how, diabetic retinal problems should be treated. Leakage or ischaemia can be localized and quantified. The patient sits at a slit-lamp camera and rapid sequence photos are taken after an injection of fluorescein into an arm vein. The procedure is usually complete in a few minutes. Side-effects are quite common but usually minor. Very rarely anaphylaxis occurs and even death has been reported after angiography, so the indications must be secure. The fluorescein causes the patient to look slightly yellow for a few hours afterwards (like a cheap fake suntan), and patients should be warned that their urine will become coloured bright fluorescent yellow also.

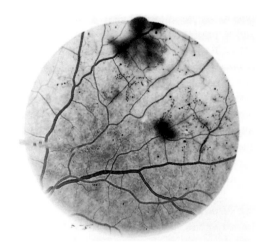

**Fig. 7.13** Fluorescein angiogram in negative form. The retina and vessels in the bottom half are normal. The top half shows bare ischaemic areas and patches of dark leakage from new vessel tufts.

### Laser treatment

Patients are sometimes frightened at the thought of what they perceive to be perhaps dangerous laser treatment. In practice the application of laser burns is usually a straightforward but trying experience. The patient sits at a device similar to a slit-lamp (Fig. 7.14) and is given a fixation target to look at. A contact lens is applied to the eye. They may be reassured to know that the light is only the strength of a normal light bulb which is intensely and briefly focused. The laser energy burns and welds a small spot of retinal tissue at each pulse. The patient will see a bright flash with each burn. Some patients find the burn painful and a minority need an anaesthetic injection behind the eye immediately before treatment. It may be helpful to suggest that the procedure is rather like going to the dentist, and that they must have faith in the operator in just the same way.

Focal laser treatment around the macula usually involves a smaller number of burns (about 20 to 100) but their placing is critical as the operator must not burn the fovea. Patients can be reassured that in practice this very rarely happens. Vision quite often falls slightly for several days or longer immediately after treatment, as a result of macular oedema, but is expected to recover.

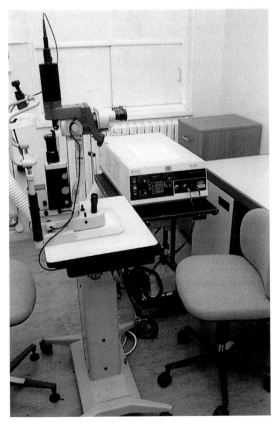

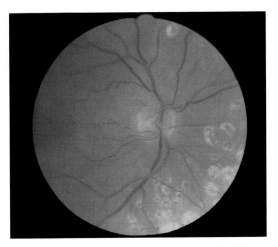

**Fig. 7.15** Treated proliferative diabetic retinopathy. New vessels on the disc have regressed and laser scars are visible inferonasally around the disc in this right eye.

**Table 7.2** Risk factors for diabetic retinopathy

| |
|---|
| Duration of diabetes |
| Age |
| Poor diabetic control |
| Smoking |
| Hypertension |
| Pregnancy |
| Renal impairment |
| Raised serum lipids |

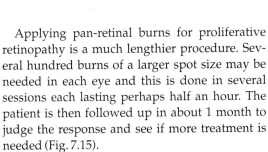

**Fig. 7.14** Laser equipment with adapted slit-lamp.

Applying pan-retinal burns for proliferative retinopathy is a much lengthier procedure. Several hundred burns of a larger spot size may be needed in each eye and this is done in several sessions each lasting perhaps half an hour. The patient is then followed up in about 1 month to judge the response and see if more treatment is needed (Fig. 7.15).

Diabetic retinopathy is a great threat to the patient, of course. They may have to wait on many occasions for long periods in busy hospital clinics perhaps to see an unfamiliar doctor for what is sometimes uncomfortable laser treatment. They emerge from the sessions dilated and dazzled. They meet other patients who have advanced disease and often live dreading the next vitreous haemorrhage with acute loss of vision. Courses of laser treatment may be interrupted until a haem-

orrhage clears. Vision may be impaired immediately after a course of treatment and they must wait and hope that it will improve. They know the problem is almost invariably bilateral and that there is a significant risk of blindness, even if this risk is much reduced by treatment. Patients who only have macular disease without proliferation can be reassured at least that they will not lose the peripheral vision that gives them independence, although for many this is little compensation for the permanent loss of reading vision.

Some patients whose vision does deteriorate will, of course, wonder if the laser treatment was at fault, but it is usually the case that their retinopathy is responsible and they should be encouraged to persist with treatment.

The GP who screens plays a very important role, keeping patients out of hospital clinics until the need for treatment arises (see section on screening). The GP may also need to give explanation and to motivate patients who are being treated, and to liaise with hospital services, including the social worker, if the patient is eligible to be registered as partially sighted or blind (see Chapter 12).

### Risk factors for retinopathy

The major risk factor is duration of diabetes. The estimate is that at 15 years, 80% of diabetics will have background retinopathy. Of these, 5–10% will eventually progress to proliferative changes. Risk factors which may be treatable include diabetic control long term (as reflected in glycosylated haemoglobin levels), hypertension and smoking (Table 7.2). Pregnancy may accelerate ischaemic and proliferative changes and pregnant diabetics with significant background changes should be screened more often than usual, perhaps 2 monthly—dilating drops are safe in pregnancy. Renal disease, including the nephrotic syndrome, anaemia and hypercholesterolaemia increase the risk of leakage, exudate formation and maculopathy.

### Cataract

Cataract occurs at an earlier average age in diabetics. Surgery may need to be done earlier also, so that the retina can be monitored. Most patients are suitable for standard surgical procedures, but there is a higher rate of complications in diabetics, especially of macular oedema. The outcome of surgery must be qualified in patients who may have diabetic macular disease which can be difficult to detect behind a lens opacity.

### Glaucoma

Glaucoma is more common in diabetics. Patients should make sure that a check on intraocular pressure is part of their optician's routine service. Routine eye tests, including pressure measurement, are available without charge for diabetics.

### Neurological disorders

Diabetic patients may develop 'mini strokes', typically painful, involving the motor nerves to the eye muscles (third, fourth or sixth) or the optic nerve itself. Often these improve and may recover within several weeks.

# Chapter 8 **The eye in systemic disorders**

**Thyroid eye disease** (Table 8.1)

It is important to think of thyroid disorders in patients with certain eye problems as the thyroid diagnosis, though fairly common, may not be obvious. The severity of the eye abnormality may not relate to the degree of endocrine imbalance. It seems the link is immunological, though the details of this process are unclear. Quite often the eye and thyroid disorders develop at different times, often years apart. A family history of autoimmunity strengthens the case. It is always worth checking thyroid function, though normality still does not exclude an association.

> Thyroid eye disease can cause:
> - prominence
> - puffiness
> - discomfort
> - double vision
> - redness
> - watering

In thyrotoxicosis the eyes may look *prominent* and staring (Fig. 8.1), a combination of true protrusion because of swelling in the orbital tissues behind the eye and of retraction of the upper eyelids so that white sclera shows above the iris. The appearance may be asymmetrical. The lids are often *puffy*, particularly in the morning. Patients often complain of watering or of *discomfort* and *redness*, usually due to a mild keratitis. Some patients will have *double vision*, often vertical and typically worse in the morning (see Double vision: diplopia, p. 39). Occasionally the eye protrusion is severe enough to put the cornea at risk of ulceration as the eyes may close poorly. Rarely there may be pressure on the optic nerve causing loss of vision and particularly of colour vision. Both these problems need urgent referral. Some patients develop glaucoma.

If thyrotoxicosis springs to mind, look for certain extra features. These are almost always bilateral, though they may only be subtle in one eye and so seem unilateral at first. The conjunctiva is almost always boggy with fluid beneath it and may also be reddened (see Fig. 5.60). There may be 'lid lag' with the upper lid lagging behind the eyeball on rapid downwards gaze, causing a momentary increase in the retraction. In hypothyroidism also there may be puffiness of the lids and double vision from eye muscle involvement.

It is difficult to control minor symptoms and signs. Patients with significant abnormalities may need treatment with immunosuppression or surgery to the lids or muscles. Patients with visual loss need urgent decompression of the orbit. Patients with double vision may benefit from prisms (Fig. 8.2).

## Ophthalmic problems in neurological disorders

### Multiple sclerosis

The commonest problem is optic neuritis which is usually bilateral in established disease. Many patients recover well after the first attacks of acute visual loss but long term most will have some impairment of reading ability and of colour vision. The cardinal sign of a previous attack is pallor of the rim of the optic nerve head (optic atrophy). Patients may become unable to drive. A minority are greatly visually handicapped and are eligible for registration. The difficulty is often confounded by an instability of eye movement, perhaps with double vision, oscillopsia or nystagmus.

> Patients with a first attack of optic neuritis have roughly a 50% risk of developing multiple sclerosis

**Table 8.1** Features of thyroid-related eye disease (not all present in all patients)

Puffiness of lids and conjunctivae, often worse in the
　　morning
Discomfort and redness
Watering
Upper lid
　Retraction
　Lag
Protrusion (with poor closure if severe)
Double vision, often worse in the morning
Visual failure from optic nerve compression (rare but
　　important to treat urgently)

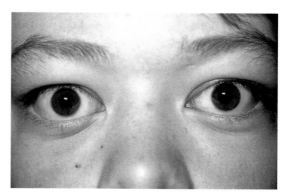

**Fig. 8.1** Thyroid eye disease with puffy eyelids and protruding eyes.

There is no effective management outside the acute attack, which may be shortened in selected patients by systemic corticosteroids, usually given in 'pulsed' intravenous form. Patients should visit a sympathetic optician if they have poor focus. Visual aids are of limited value though some patients may manage to stay in work with the help of a low vision aid, perhaps attached to a computer, so it may be important to try these (see Chapter 12).

## Stroke

The commonest finding is a homonymous hemianopia. Strangely, this is often not recognized by the patient who will never describe the 'halving' of vision one might expect, and may deny any difficulty at all. The lesion is within the visual path behind the chiasm, usually in the radiation as it passes through temporal and parietal areas or in the occipital cortex. Occlusion of the vertebrobasilar circulation may cause bilateral cortical lesions and marked visual disability, though even these patients may find it difficult to describe their difficulty. Visual neglect may simulate a hemianopia and is an equal handicap. Many patients with a defective field have particular difficulty with reading as they lose their place in trying to move from one line to the next. In practical terms there is little that can be done to help, though with time things may improve. Prisms and special spectacles are useless, although the patient should visit the optician as usual to have an up-to-date prescription. Holding a ruler under the line of print may help the occasional patient but is laborious and most abandon it. (See Chapter 12.)

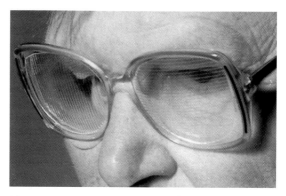

**Fig. 8.2** Fresnel prisms stuck to spectacle lenses to correct horizontal (right eye) and vertical (left eye) double vision in thyroid eye disease.

Patients with a homonymous hemianopia, unless it is very partial, will not be entitled to drive with insurance and they should inform the DVLC of their defect. In equivocal cases it may be worth assessing a formal binocular visual field to see if the patient can achieve the statutory requirement for licensing. At present the recommendation is for a full binocular field within 20 degrees above and below fixation, extending for 120 degrees laterally. Patients with a complete homonymous loss will be barred from driving and may be eligible for partial sight registration.

## Intracranial tumours

A lump inside the head close to the optic nerves, chiasm or radiation may affect visual acuity or visual field. This is why it may be vitally important

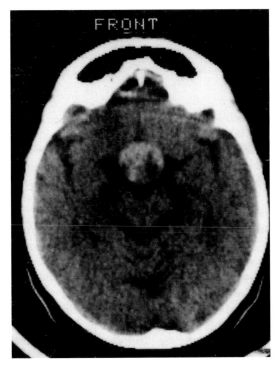

**Fig. 8.3** Computed tomograph showing a bright round midline tumour, arising from the pituitary gland.

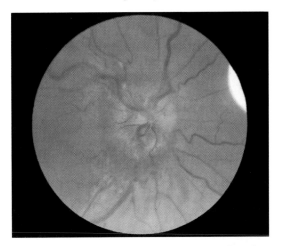

**Fig. 8.4** Papilloedema with optic nerve head swelling due to raised intracranial pressure.

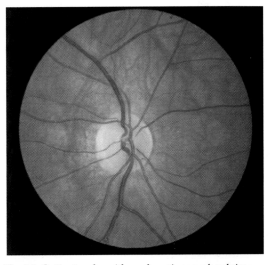

**Fig. 8.5** Optic atrophy with a pale optic nerve head rim, which cannot be distinguished from the cup.

to check both vision and fields in patients with vague but persistent, and perhaps progressive, complaints whether unilateral or bilateral. Headache is not invariable as it is associated with a rise in intracranial pressure which may come on later than the local compressive effects. Brain scanning by CT (Fig. 8.3) or MRI is a reliable investigation which should be done if there is any suspicion of a tumour.

The important signs to look for otherwise are papilloedema or atrophy of one or both optic nerve heads. Papilloedema is swelling caused by congestion from raised intracranial pressure transmitted to the optic nerve sheath (Fig. 8.4). In itself, papilloedema does not usually impair visual acuity though it does increase the size of the blind spot. Optic atrophy (Fig. 8.5) implies death of nerve fibres and will be associated with some impairment of acuity, field or colour vision.

### Benign intracranial hypertension

Patients with papilloedema, raised intracranial pressure but no tumour may have 'benign intracranial hypertension'. (This used to be called pseudotumour cerebri.) This syndrome is usually found in plump young women with persistent headache and menstrual irregularities. The 'stat' regulating CSF pressure seems to be set too high, though the cause is unknown. These patients may respond to diuretics with added Diamox if necessary, but the problem may be very persistent, lasting many years. Some patients may need shunting of CSF or surgery to the optic nerve sheath to control symptoms or to preserve vision. All should have monitoring of visual function and should be under specialist supervision as there is an appreciable risk to vision long term.

### Facial palsy

Patients with weakness of eye closure are at risk of corneal ulceration (see Fig. 5.26) in proportion to the severity of the weakness. Patients with no closure will need taping and perhaps suturing of the eyelid until strength improves. Topical chloramphenicol ointment, at least at night, helps to lubricate and prevent secondary corneal infection.

## Eye problems in joint disorders

Some patients with joint disorders have inflammation of the coats of the eye, such as episcleritis and scleritis. Other conditions are associated with internal inflammation, particularly with iritis. Some are a cause of dryness of the eyes (sicca), so finding eye features may help to diagnose the joint disorder. The eyes themselves may need treatment.

### Rheumatoid arthritis (Fig. 8.6)

Patients with rheumatoid arthritis often have dry eyes, confirmed by Schirmer testing (see p. 11). Dryness may cause discomfort with burning, grittiness or foreign body sensation. In eyes with significant dryness, there will be characteristic staining with fluorescein, best seen with the slit-lamp. The treatment is with tear replacement using artificial tear drops. The type and frequency should be found by trial and success (see Appendix 1). If mucus adheres to the cornea, acetyl cysteine drops may help clear the 'windscreen'. Severe dryness, with loss of mucus production also, may be a serious problem in a minority of rheumatoid patients as there is a threat to the cornea long term and much distress from symptoms. These patients need specialist supervision. The GP can help by supplying regular eye drops and referring the patient to casualty if there is an acute crisis such as corneal ulceration.

> Refer urgently the rheumatoid arthritis patient with a painful or red eye

A significant number of patients develop inflammation of the eyeball, particularly scleritis. This is an ischaemic phenomenon and causes pain and sometimes necrosis of the sclera with the risk of actual perforation of the eye coat in severe cases. These patients may need immunosuppression to preserve vision and can have a poor outcome long term. Refer urgently any rheumatoid patient with a painful eye even if it is not particularly red, or with a red eye, even if not particularly painful.

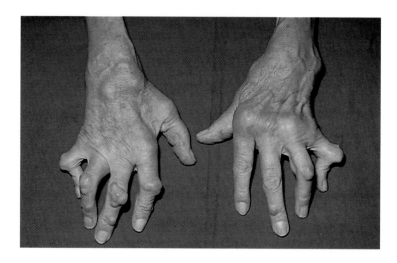

**Fig. 8.6** Patients with rheumatoid arthritis may have a variety of eye problems.

## Ankylosing spondylitis

This occurs in younger patients and causes sacroiliitis or lower back spondylitis. Most patients are HLA B27 positive and there may be a family history. The eye risk is of iritis (anterior uveitis) which is often recurrent. These patients should be referred promptly for slit-lamp assessment and treatment. Most cases respond well to topical agents with no sequelae, but early treatment is least damaging in a recurrent condition. Patients should be encouraged to use their drops carefully and to attend promptly with any relapse. Attacks should be managed with slit-lamp supervision to be sure cells clear from the anterior chamber and that adhesions to the lens do not form. Reliable patients could be supplied with steroid drops (suggest betamethasone 0.1% four times daily) and a dilating drop (such as cyclopentolate 1% bd) to use early in a recurrence, but they should attend for slit-lamp examination as soon as possible in the attack.

> The young man with iritis and a stiff back may have ankylosing spondylitis

## Reiter's syndrome

The eye may figure in the initial attack which precipitates joint problems in susceptible patients, commonly with conjunctivitis which may be chlamydial and possibly sexually acquired. In the subsequent stages of the disorder there may be iritis similar to that seen in ankylosing spondylitis which needs treatment on its own merits (see pp. 79 and 81).

## Sarcoidosis

In patients with joint symptoms and eye involvement sarcoidosis should be considered a possible diagnosis. The acute type is associated with iritis which may be indistinguishable from other aetiologies (Fig. 8.7). The chronic granulomatous phase may be associated with many sites of eye involvement, from eyelids to optic nerve. Particularly suggestive of the diagnosis are small conjunctival granulomatous lumps, dryness and granulomatous iritis or pan uveitis with poor vision. Facial palsy is also suggestive, particularly if bilateral.

## Sjögren's syndrome (sicca syndrome)

This is a joint disorder associated with dryness of the eyes and mouth. The most frequent causes are rheumatoid arthritis, systemic sclerosis, mixed connective tissue disease or sarcoidosis.

## Juvenile arthritis

Children with eye and joint inflammation are a small but important group (Fig. 8.8). Most have juvenile chronic arthritis without rheumatoid factor. The problem is most important in those who develop a low-grade grumbling iritis which is usually without symptoms initially but can lead to blindness if not recognized and treated. Those

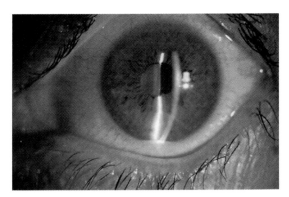

**Fig. 8.7** In sarcoidosis, iritis may be a feature, with or without systemic findings. Note the red eye, and irregular pupil with iris adhesions at 5 o'clock.

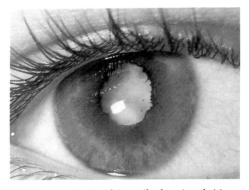

**Fig. 8.8** Young patient with juvenile chronic arthritis — inflammation of the joints and chronic iritis. There is cataract and a festooned pupil. Vision is poor. (Courtesy of Mr A. Shun-Shin.)

most at risk are girls with only one or two joints involved (perhaps just one finger or one knee) who are also antinuclear antibody (ANA) positive. Young patients with only a few joints inflamed should be screened by a specialist so that quiet but damaging iritis may be treated promptly. For this reason, the GP should check that children with joint problems of this sort have regular specialist eye assessment long term.

## Eye problems in skin disorders

Sometimes skin disorders involve the eyelids, and searching for skin pathology elsewhere can help in the eye diagnosis. Vice versa, in some skin disorders a search in the eye may help define the skin diagnosis.

### Allergic reactions

Individuals who have an atopic tendency with an excessive IgE response are prone to atopic eczema and to urticaria. The eyelids may be involved in an acute allergic reaction to an airborne or ingested allergen with marked swelling of the lids on one or both sides. Itching is prominent. The conjunctiva is also often swollen with underlying fluid. The reaction may be an isolated event as seen with ragwort allergy, but is more commonly seasonal as with 'hay fever', or may become chronic if the patient is allergic to a common antigen such as house dust. See Varieties of allergic conjunctivitis, p. 66.

Non-atopic individuals may develop cell-mediated contact dermatitis to a particular allergen. This causes a red itchy scaly reaction in the eyelids which persists as long as the allergen is present (Fig. 8.9). The commoner agents are topical treatments, particularly atropine or neomycin, and the metals in spectacle frames which can include the screws and hinges used in a plastic frame; a reaction to the plastic itself is less common. Some patients are responding to the dichromate in matches or to epoxy resins which are touched onto the eyelids from the fingers. Allergy to eye cosmetics is uncommon though the eyes may be involved in a perfume or hair dye reaction.

### Seborrhoeic eczema

These patients have scaly blepharitis of the eyelid margins which tends to be persistent. They often

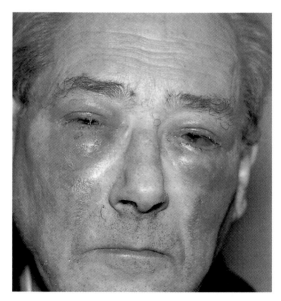

**Fig. 8.9** Contact sensitivity of skin around the eye, usually secondary to eye medication.

have scaling and redness of the eyebrows too. Involvement of the scalp causes scaling and dandruff. Look for similar changes in the ears, chest, back and intertriginous parts. The eye problem may be helped by control of the skin using medicated shampoos containing tar or salicylates.

### Rosacea

This is another important cause of blepharitis which may be persistent and severe. The disorder is also associated with corneal changes which may be severe in some patients (Fig. 8.10). Look for rosaceal changes on the cheeks and nose with redness, papules or pustules. The skin signs may be unobtrusive. Flushing is common. Control of the rosacea with long-term intermittent low dose tetracycline may improve the eyelids; topical treatment does not substitute this effect. Topical steroids to the lids should be avoided because of rebound effects and risk of glaucoma long term.

### Psoriasis

A minority of patients with psoriasis are prone to iritis (Fig. 8.11) which may be recurrent and destructive if not promptly treated. The risk is greater in those with joint involvement, particularly sacroiliitis, who are often also HLA B27

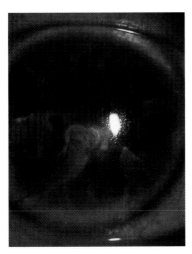

**Fig. 8.10** Rosacea may be associated with corneal ulceration.

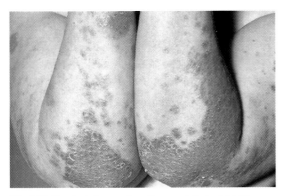

**Fig. 8.11** Psoriasis is occasionally associated with iritis.

positive. Consider also the possibility of ocular side-effects in psoriatics who have had retinoid or ultraviolet treatment (see below).

## Blistering disorders
Certain blistering disorders may involve the eyes. In a minority this may be severe and even result in blindness.

### Stevens–Johnson conjunctivitis
Conjunctival inflammation as part of the acute Stevens–Johnson syndrome with erythema multiforme may progress to scarring and loss of function. This in turn can cause corneal scarring which may be the only major sequel in some patients. Care of the eyes and review by an ophthalmologist

during and after the acute stage is strongly advised.

### Pemphigoid
In some patients skin blistering predominates (bullous pemphigoid) whereas in others eye scarring is the major feature (cicatricial pemphigoid) with conjunctival shrinkage, loss of function and dryness (see Fig. 5.19). Ulceration in the mouth, throat, nose or genitalia are more common in those at risk of eye problems. Biopsy of conjunctival tissue may help in diagnosis. In children the disease may be IgA-mediated. Pemphigoid is distinguished from pemphigus which also causes blisters but does not cause eye scarring.

### Epidermolysis bullosa
This very rare inherited condition causes skin blistering from birth. Some patients have recurrent corneal erosions which are painful and troublesome but rarely cause scarring. See Recurrent corneal erosion, p. 50.

## Alopecia
Loss of eyelashes and eyebrows may occur in the more severe cases of alopecia totalis. Hypothyroidism or atopic eczema may also be a cause. Loss of eyebrows occurs in lepromatous leprosy. Loss of eyelashes may be because the patient pulls them out as a habit tic.

## Infections of the skin involving the eyes
• The eyelids may be involved in primary herpes simplex infections, producing small, usually multiple, blistering lesions on the upper or lower lid associated with marked swelling and redness that mimics cellulitis (see Fig. 5.12). In the case of herpes simplex it is important to examine the eye itself for an associated dendritic corneal ulcer, particularly if the eye is red or painful, or in atopic patients.
• Herpes zoster of the ophthalmic division often involves the upper eyelid and it is important to examine the eye itself carefully for corneal or internal involvement (see Herpes zoster keratitis, p. 76).
• Varicella in children may show lid or conjunctival lesions, occasionally corneal invo-

lvement which causes pain, and in a minority iritis.

• Impetigo may occasionally involve the lids, particularly in atopic patients, when the lesions may be confused with herpes simplex.

• Warts may involve the lids and even the conjunctiva. Molluscum contagiosum produces a characteristic lesion described under lid lumps (see Fig. 5.13).

• Pubic lice sometimes infest the eyelashes, even in children, when there may be a chronic blepharitis. The insects may be seen along the lid margin as small pigmented bodies. Biting produces blood at the eyelid margin. The eggs are adherent to the base of the eyelashes and must be removed with fine forceps, preferably at the slit-lamp to be sure all are eliminated (see Fig. 5.39). Do some discreet detective work amongst the family.

• Insect bites may cause acute swelling of the eyelids which resembles cellulitis but itching usually occurs and the bite site may be visible.

• Many tropical infestations with skin signs may involve the external or internal eye, so refer to a specialist textbook.

## Inherited disorders of the skin with eye features

An exhaustive list would be very long and would include many extreme rarities. Important eye involvement is found in the following conditions which are merely rare:

• Albinism of the skin is associated with defects of iris pigment. This usually causes a pale blue colour rather than 'pink' eyes, but the iris transilluminates with the slit-lamp or ophthalmoscope light set to get a red reflex. Vision is poor because of internal scatter of light and nystagmus is common.

• Pseudoxanthoma elasticum (PXE) is often associated with defects in the elastic supporting tissue (Bruch's membrane) beneath the retina. These show as grey 'lacquer cracks' (also known as angioid streaks) radiating especially from the optic nerve head. They are often associated with macular degeneration and loss of central vision in younger adult patients. This may be accelerated by eye trauma and these patients should mini-

mize the risk by avoiding contact sports and by always wearing a car seat belt.

• The characteristic eye signs in neurofibromatosis type 1 or in tuberous sclerosis or in Fabry's disease rarely interfere with vision but may be important clues to the diagnosis in screening patients (see Screening for genetic abnormalities, p. 159).

• Various angiomatous disorders can affect the eyelids or internal eye. Sturge–Weber with a facial port wine stain may be associated with glaucoma on the same side. Rendu–Osler–Weber disease shows telangiectasia in the conjunctiva inside the lower lid.

## Skin and eye in systemic disorders

• In patients with erythema nodosum look for eye features of acute sarcoidosis, particularly iritis. In patients with skin sarcoid granulomas, there may be lid or conjunctival granulomatous lumps, dryness of the eyes, inflammation inside either eye chamber, or cranial nerve involvement. Sarcoid is a great mimic of many systemic disorders and it is always worth thinking about eye problems as these may help in the diagnosis and the conjunctiva may provide tissue for biopsy.

• Lymphoma may occasionally present or relapse in the eyelids or conjunctiva. The fleshy tissue causes firm swelling and if visible may look like smoked salmon.

• Scleroderma is associated with thickening of the eyelids and dryness of the eyes.

• Dermatomyositis is rare but the diagnosis may be suggested by swelling of the eyelids with a purplish colour, in association with a rash and muscle weakness.

• Lupus erythematosus, either cutaneous or systemic, may cause eye problems. Some patients have lid involvement with chronic blepharitis. Others have recurrent red eyes from episcleritis. Occasionally there may be retinal vascular involvement, particularly vein occlusions.

• Patients with AIDS may develop Kaposi's sarcoma around the eyes or even in the conjunctiva.

## Ocular side-effects of skin therapies

Steroids used topically on the eyelids may spill into the eye and there is a slight risk of inducing glaucoma if used over a long period of time. Patients should not use the more potent steroids in this area anyway; 1% hydrocortisone to the lids should be safe, but betamethasone should only be used intermittently. Systemic steroids over several years may precipitate cataract which can be dealt with surgically if necessary.

Antimalarials are used in some inflammatory skin disorders, in particular in systemic or cutaneous lupus. Chloroquine used long term in the higher dose range can cause macular degeneration with difficulty reading as the usual first symptom. Such patients should be screened and advised before starting treatment (see Screening for drug toxicity, p. 160) and if symptoms arise should stop the drug and be referred promptly for investigation. Hydroxychloroquine appears not to cause retinal toxicity but patients are currently still screened initially.

Retinoids, given for psoriasis and other keratinizing disorders may cause inflammation of the lids and dryness of the eyes and so patients on long-term retinoids should be screened.

Ultraviolet radiation treatment might be expected to cause corneal epithelial loss short term or to cause cataract long term. The eyelids are usually spared in acute phototoxic reactions.

## Eye problems in sexually transmitted disorders

The individual problems are mostly covered elsewhere. Sexually transmitted agents that can cause eye problems include chlamydial conjunctivitis (and Reiter's syndrome), herpes simplex lid or corneal infections, viral warts and molluscum contagiosum of the eyelids. Less common are gonococcal conjunctivitis in the newborn, pubic louse infection of the eyelashes and, in homosexual men, syphilis, which is a rare cause of eye problems in its various stages.

These conditions not only need primary eye treatment but also referral to a GUM clinic for investigation and contact tracing.

In patients with AIDS a new spectrum of problems has emerged. The most serious eye complication is found in AIDS patients with a low CD4 count, who are at risk of developing retinitis due to CMV infection (Fig. 8.12). This can be controlled

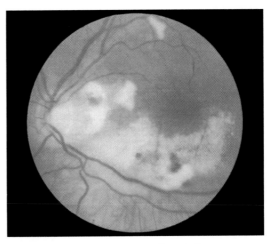

**Fig. 8.12** Late AIDS in a patient with typical cytomegalovirus retinitis. The pale area of retina with haemorrhages (below the fovea) is a characteristic finding. In the USA, this may be termed 'pizza' retinopathy.

with intravenous treatment, but life expectancy is limited in this group, who have a low T-cell count at the onset, unless this can be salvaged with combination therapy against HIV.

## Ophthalmic problems in vascular disorders

The retina has a blood supply which is uniquely visible, so a careful look with the ophthalmoscope can give vital information about the health of small vessels in patients at risk of vascular events. On the other hand, vascular events in the retina or elsewhere in the optic nerves or brain can have devastating effects on visual function.

Risk factors for vascular disease include hypertension, diabetes, hyperlipidaemia, smoking, haematological disorders and systemic inflammatory vasculitis.

### Hypertension

In hypertensive patients the retinal vessel appearance is a good guide as to whether to treat and how urgently. It is customary to classify hypertensive retinal changes, but in practice it is more important to assess certain features individually (Table 8.2). Look for *narrowing or irregularity* of vessels. The retinal branch arteries are usually narrower and more shiny than the veins. Look at a few major

**Table 8.2** Retinal features of hypertension

Vessels, especially arterioles
    Narrowing
    Thickening with silvering or tortuosity
Arteriovenous crossing change
Nipping in of the vein
Haemorrhages
Cotton-wool spots (microinfarcts)
Retinal oedema and disc swelling
Hard exudate, especially after treatment when oedema is
    resolving

*crossing points of arteries and veins to see if there is nipping in or narrowing of the vein* (Fig. 8.13). This signifies significant hypertension or ageing and is a risk factor for retinal vein occlusion. Look also for sheathing, with a narrow cuff of silvery thickening along the edges of the vessels. This is prominent in disorders which have caused leakage into the vessel wall at some time, and implies significant damage either from hypertension or previous branch vessel occlusion.

Examine the retina in hypertension to assess:
• severity
• need for urgent treatment

*Accelerated hypertension* is uncommon in the UK now that blood pressure is widely screened and treated, but remains a very important signal that blood pressure is dangerously high or that there may be an underlying renal disorder. The retinal features are its hallmark, so they are particularly important. Look for small flame-shaped haemorrhages around the major vessel trunks and for fluffy pale cotton-wool spots scattered amongst them, especially between branches of vessels (Fig. 8.14). If the optic nerve margin is blurred the need for treatment is even more urgent. The catch is that vision is often normal in these patients as the fovea is not usually affected and the retinopathy is not noticed unless carefully looked for, preferably after pupil dilatation. As a rough guide, accelerated retinal changes are uncommon unless the diastolic pressure is consistently above 110 mmHg and all patients with pressures above this level should have their fundi examined.

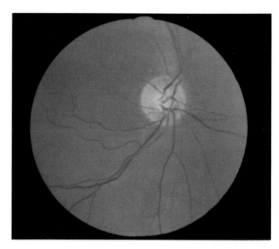

**Fig. 8.13** Narrow and irregular retinal vessels with nipping at arteriovenous crossings, typical of persistent hypertension.

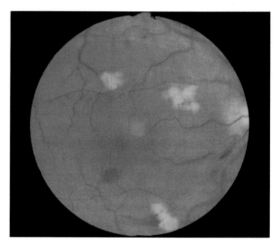

**Fig. 8.14** Pale cotton-wool spots in hypertension are a warning for urgent treatment.

Vision is often normal despite severe hypertensive retinopathy

### Diabetes

Diabetic retinopathy is dealt with under the sections on common eye disorders (p. 127) and screening (p. 145). Any patient with a retinal vascular disorder should have at least urinalysis, if not a formal blood sugar measurement. If diabetes is then suspected, test a fasting level. Cranial nerve palsies causing double vision may be associated with diabetes or hypertension.

## Hyperlipidaemia

Raised fat levels appear to be a risk factor for major vessel disease, particularly in the more pronounced familiar disorders. Eye signs may be an important clue to the diagnosis. Arcus of the cornea (Fig. 8.15) in elderly patients is common with normal lipids, but if the patient with an arcus is under 65 or if there is a family history of early vascular death it is worth checking fasting cholesterol and triglyceride levels with a view to treatment. The same is true of xanthelasmas, the fatty deposits in the skin in or around the eyelids (Fig. 8.16). Raised lipids may be found in patients with retinal vascular occlusions and are worth checking, particularly in younger patients with retinal artery or vein occlusion.

> Eye signs in hyperlipidaemia are:
> - arcus
> - xanthelasma
> - retinal vascular occlusion

## Haematological disorders

The retinal vessels may be affected in blood conditions associated with hyperviscosity (Fig. 8.17) or with a bleeding tendency. The hyperclotting states

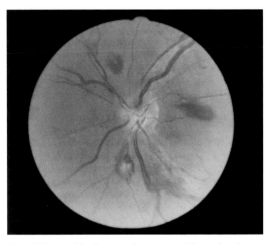

Fig. 8.17  Large blot haemorrhages were bilateral and secondary to myeloma with hyperviscosity.

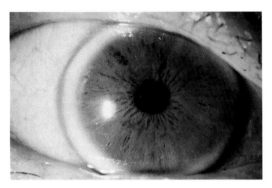

Fig. 8.15  Arcus of the cornea with fatty deposit in the peripheral cornea and a characteristic thin clear band between the edge of the cornea.

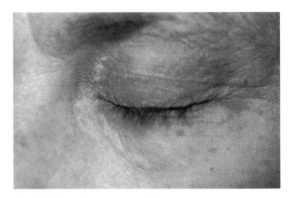

Fig. 8.16  Fatty deposits in the lids, xanthelasmas, are usually innocent, but the occasional patient has high plasma lipids.

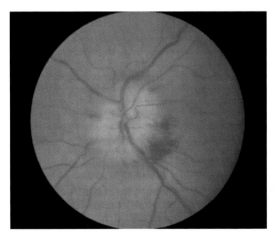

Fig. 8.18  Pale swollen optic nerve head of ischaemia, in this case secondary to giant cell arteritis. Erythrocyte sedimentation rate was 110 mm.

produce sludging and stasis in the small vessels. High red or white cell or platelet counts can cause retinal haemorrhages. Anaemia or a low platelet count make haemorrhages more likely. High plasma proteins as in myeloma or Waldenström's macroglobulinaemia can present with blurring of vision from foveal haemorrhage or oedema: the erythrocyte sedimentation rate (ESR) is usually raised and a plasma protein strip shows the monoclonal band. Patients with sickle cell disease, usually black, may show closure of small vessels in the retina. These patients should be screened by a specialist.

> Suspect a haematological disorder if retinal haemorrhages are bilateral in a patient with normal blood pressure and blood sugar

## Vasculitis

There are many systemic inflammatory conditions of this type which can affect the eye. These include systemic lupus erythematosus, polyarteritis, Wegener's and Behçet's disease. All can affect the external eye with the red eye of episcleritis or the more serious and painful scleritis. Some are associated with inflammation of the internal eye. All can cause retinal haemorrhages or vascular occlusion with a threat to sight.

## Ischaemic optic nerve disease

This problem is *not rare*. The most important type is that seen in elderly patients with giant cell (temporal or cranial) arteritis. This is described under Sudden loss of vision, p. 29. The relevant features are acute and marked loss of vision usually associated with pain in the temples or jaw, a pale swollen optic nerve head (Fig. 8.18), a high ESR and raised CRP.

> Elderly patient with:
> - poor vision
> - pale swollen optic disc
> - plus raised ESR and CRP
> - means giant cell arteritis

Some patients, particularly men who smoke heavily, develop loss of vision in one or both eyes due to optic nerve ischaemia without inflammation. These patients often have a stepwise loss of visual field, sometimes over several years, rather like chronic glaucoma but without the raised ocular pressure and with a pale optic nerve head which is not cupped. Their prognosis for vision is poor although they usually retain some function. All patients with this pattern should also have syphilis serology checked (TPHA or VDRL test).

## Retinal vascular occlusions

The features are described under Sudden loss of vision, pp. 26 and 27. These are small strokes in an important territory, and patients should be screened for risk factors. In arterial disease think of embolic episodes from the carotid or heart. In venous disease remember haematological risk factors and glaucoma.

# Chapter 9 **Screening asymptomatic patients**

## Diabetic eye screening

### Why screen?
• Because even without symptoms significant retinal disease is common, yet treatable at key stages.
• Early detection of sight-threatening changes may mean they can be treated with laser to stop progression.

Diabetes is the most common cause of blindness in the age group 30–64 years and accounts for 10% of those registered blind in the 16–64 age group in the UK. Approximately 4000 new blind registrations each year in the UK are the result of diabetes and yet possibly 60% of these could have been prevented. The prevalence of diabetes is at least 2%, meaning that a GP with an average list size of 2000 will have about 40 diabetic patients. Of these, about 25 will be type II maturity onset and may be well-managed without referral to a specialist hospital clinic, provided their review is regular and thorough and includes regular ophthalmoscopy. This could also apply to many of the type I patients. Incidence of diabetes is increased to up to 9% in those of Asian or Afro-Caribbean descent.

> GPs are in an ideal position to screen for diabetic retinopathy

Some practices run their own diabetic clinic. It has been shown that GPs can be as effective as ophthalmologists at screening for diabetic retinopathy, given some initial training and regular practice. The procedures to be followed are not in themselves difficult (Fig. 9.1). There are no studies of the optimum training period, but the estimate is that about 40 hours would be needed to attend a diabetic eye clinic regularly to learn to use the direct ophthalmoscope with dilated pupils. Some hospital departments organize practical study days specifically for diabetic screening but a longer period of training is usually helpful. Observing and staging the retinal changes is the essence of screening, to differentiate significant patterns and to act on the findings. Training and practice help in distinguishing key features — the most common difficulty is in distinguishing haemorrhages or groups of microaneurysms from pre-proliferative small vessel abnormalities or frank early new vessels. Experience helps in understanding the progression of changes. The retinal pathology is discussed elsewhere (see Diabetic eye disease, p. 127). The intervals suggested for screening are discussed below and the use of the ophthalmoscope under Ophthalmoscopy, p. 15.

### How to screen

> To screen in diabetes:
> • measure visual acuity
> • dilate the pupils
> • assess with the ophthalmoscope

*Measure the visual acuity*
Measure with glasses, if worn, for distance. If the acuity is less than 6/6, test that eye again with the patient looking through a pin hole at the Snellen chart (see p. 11).

*Dilate the pupils*
*Dilatation of the pupils is obligatory for examination of diabetic retinopathy.*

Tropicamide 1% will usually dilate the pupils within 15–20 minutes (Fig. 9.2) and vastly improves the view of the fundus. The commonly held fear, that you might cause an attack of glaucoma (angle closure), is in fact largely unfounded

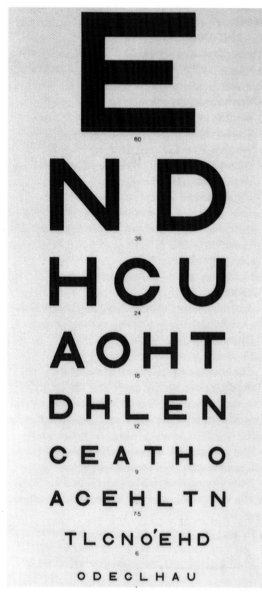

(a)

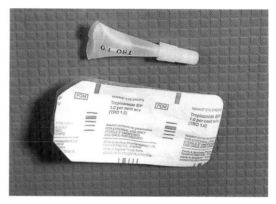

**Fig. 9.2** Drops to dilate the pupil—tropicamide in single-dose disposable minim form.

**Table 9.1** Specimen instruction for patients coming for retinal screening

For a good eye examination, drops will be used. These enlarge the pupil and also blur reading vision for a few hours

Because of glare you will be asked not to drive until you feel safe to do so

In an occasional patient, the drops may cause the eye pressure to rise, usually later the same day

If you have pain in the eye later in the day, telephone the hospital eye casualty department, stating these instructions

if this agent is used. If you would feel reassured, give all the patients you dilate a written warning and instructions about what to do if such an attack occurs (Table 9.1). Even if an attack is brought on by drops, the same would have happened sooner or later anyway. You will blind more diabetics by failing to see retinopathy if you don't dilate than you will by causing glaucoma if you do. Patients with 'ordinary' glaucoma are no more at risk than others, so drops may be used safely. Dilating drops are also safe in pregnancy.

One practical problem is the issue of driving after dilating drops. In law, the doctor may be held responsible for any accident arising because of impaired vision. In practice, it seems more sensible to give the above advice to patients who have no

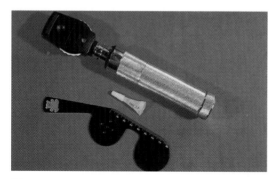

(b)

**Fig. 9.1** (*left*) Basic equipment to examine eyes includes: (a) a Snellen chart for testing vision at 6 metres' distance; (b) a pin hole device, dilating drops and an ophthalmoscope.

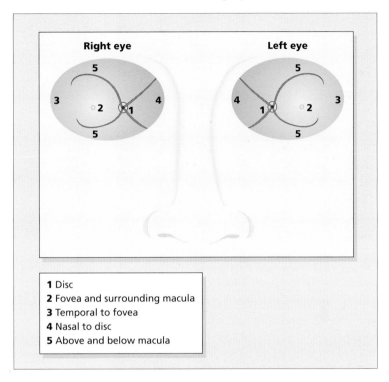

**1** Disc
**2** Fovea and surrounding macula
**3** Temporal to fovea
**4** Nasal to disc
**5** Above and below macula

**Fig. 9.3** Parts of the retina to examine when screening for diabetic retinopathy.

other way of getting to the clinic. Tropicamide is short acting (roughly 2–3 hours) and minimizes the time of dilatation as well as risk of acute glaucoma.

Testing vision and giving drops can be done by a practice nurse in a 'mini clinic' for diabetics, so they see the doctor with pupils already dilated.

> Dilating drops only cause blindness when they are not used in diabetic screening

### Ophthalmoscopic findings
In the following description, *macula* means the area embraced by the major branches of the retinal vessels temporal to the optic disc and *fovea* means the point of fixation (Fig. 9.3) and maximum sensitivity at the centre of the macula (see Glossary). The fovea can only be seen properly after dilating the pupil and should be in view when the patient looks straight into the centre of the opthalmoscope light.

*Basic (or background) retinopathy* (Fig. 9.4)
This characteristically has:

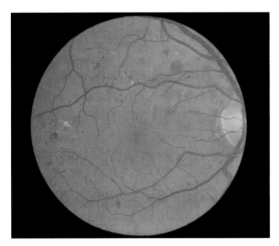

**Fig. 9.4** Background diabetic retinopathy. A few microaneurysms, blot haemorrhages and hard exudates, but none extensive or near the fovea.

• *Microaneurysms*, which form small round red dots scattered about the macula or in adjacent areas.
• *Haemorrhages*, punctate (small or dot), as a result of leakage from small vessels, and flame or

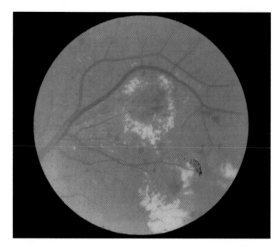

**Fig. 9.5** Circinate hard exudate in diabetic retinopathy, forming a circle around a focus of leakage. Laser welding may help before the fovea is damaged.

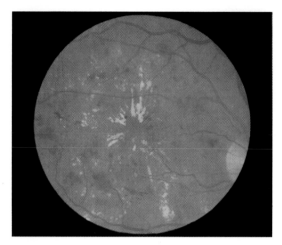

**Fig. 9.6** Established macular change in diabetic retinopathy, with extensive haemorrhage and hard exudate involving the fovea. This is likely to be irretrievable, with poor vision.

blot (larger), spreading according to depth in the retina.

• *Hard exudates*, which look white or yellow with clearly defined edges. These are aggregates of leaked fatty material related to plasma lipids and protein. If they form a partial or complete circle around a leaking focus they are referred to as *circinate* exudates (Fig. 9.5), which are an important hallmark of diabetes. In the background stages exudates are both sparse, and not close to the fovea.

> Background retinopathy exudates are allowed only if sparse and distant from the fovea

### Leakage (or exudative) retinopathy with 'maculopathy' (Fig. 9.6)

This characteristically has:

• *Hard exudates*, which are larger and more numerous than in background retinopathy, particularly *within the macula towards (or even at) the fovea*.
• *Foveal oedema*, which may be difficult to detect with the direct ophthalmoscope.

### Progression of foveal changes to maculopathy

Basic (background) retinopathy has a good prognosis as only 3% of eyes with it will lose useful vision in the following 5 years. It does not therefore need treatment, but must be monitored because

the outlook is much worse if the features of exudative retinopathy appear. Exudate forming within the macula near the fovea can cause the fovea itself to become oedematous, with a drop in visual acuity. Laser treatment to the focus of leakage near the fovea may limit damage if detected early enough, preferably *before the acuity drops below 6/12 Snellen*. If exudates are neglected and actually involve the fovea, the acuity is even worse and at this late stage treatment with laser will not help.

To make matters more complicated, foveal oedema may occur even without visible exudate, particularly if leakage from small vessels is diffuse rather than focal. This change can be difficult to detect with the direct ophthalmoscope but should be suspected if the vision drops and especially if there is distortion (see Distortion, p. 43). In this case fluorescein angiography may be needed to confirm leakage as it may be possible to apply a 'grid' of laser burns within the area of the macula and prevent worsening oedema. For this to be successful, the changes must be detected early. Clues to help in early detection are an otherwise *unexplained fall in visual acuity of two lines on the Snellen chart*, or the appearance of microaneurysms or haemorrhages close to the fovea. Both of these will be picked up with the screening procedure outlined above. It may be wise to suggest as a first

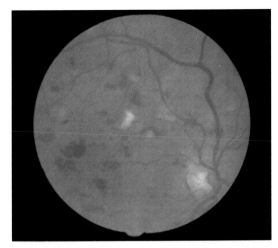

**Fig. 9.7** Ischaemic diabetic retinopathy with multiple cotton-wool spots and many haemorrhages.

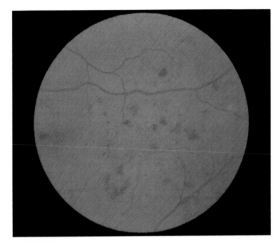

**Fig. 9.8** Pre-proliferative diabetic retinopathy temporal to the fovea, which is on the extreme left. There are multiple haemorrhages and intraretinal microvascular abnormalities would be visible with the ophthalmoscope, especially with a red-free filter.

move a prompt visit to the optician and refer to hospital if the vision cannot be improved beyond 6/9 by changing lenses.

> Macular exudate is the most common cause of loss of vision in diabetics and is more common in maturity onset patients

*Macular changes are the commonest cause of poor vision in diabetics, and occur most often in type II diabetes.* By definition, this problem only affects central vision, sparing the periphery, so that even if detailed vision is lost, the patient may still navigate around familiar environments.

Most patients have predominantly either leakage or ischaemia but some unfortunate patients have both. Unlike maculopathy, the ischaemic and proliferative types of retinopathy can threaten both central and peripheral vision. Laser treatment to control anomalous new blood vessels may preserve central vision at the expense of reduced peripheral field.

### Ischaemic retinopathy

This characteristically has *one or more* of the following features:
- *Widespread blot haemorrhages.*
- *'Cotton-wool' spots*, which look white and fluffy with ill-defined edges (Fig. 9.7). These used to be

called 'soft exudates', but they are not exudates at all. They are rather the result of severe hypoxia or death of nerve cells causing swelling within the axons and are therefore a worrying sign.
- Irregular dilatation and 'beading' of larger veins, perhaps with loops.
- Intraretinal microvascular abnormalities (IRMA) which are clusters of abnormal capillaries at the site of ischaemia (Fig. 9.8). The vessels are dilated, tortuous and form tiny loops. They are often best seen with red-free light using the green filter in the ophthalmoscope. They represent areas likely soon to bud into frank new vessels.

> Pre-proliferative warning signs are:
> - haemorrhages
> - cotton-wool spots
> - changes in larger veins
> - IRMA
> if any feature *is pronounced*

### Pre-proliferative retinopathy

This characteristically has *one or more* features of ischaemic retinopathy but these are *more pronounced*, with multiple haemorrhages, many cotton-wool spots, marked IRMA or widespread changes in the larger veins. These are predictive signs that proliferation is likely to occur. *Refer within a few weeks*, irrespective of whether these features are detected singly or together. Early detection of this stage with early referral and early selection for early treatment is good practice. It is easy for any of these stages to be delayed too long. *Fifty per cent of these patients will develop new vessels within a year.*

### Proliferative retinopathy

This characteristically has *new blood vessels* on the optic nerve head (Fig. 9.9) or in the retina (Fig. 9.10). These vessels begin as small tufts with branching twigs and often with loops. They appear haphazard in direction as they do not supply blood to any particular area of the retina. They are flat at first but, as they grow over weeks or months, may enlarge and move forwards into the central vitreous cavity. They are often best seen with red-free (green) light.

> It is difficult to distinguish:
> - clustered microaneurysms
> - dilated small vessels (intraretinal microvascular abnormalities)
> - early new vessels

*Progression to proliferative retinopathy*
Seventy-five per cent of diabetics will develop some form of retinopathy after 20 years. About

10% of those with mild basic (background) retinopathy will progress to proliferation within 5 years and about 3% would eventually lose useful vision if not treated in the early proliferative stage.

Proliferation refers to the growth of new retinal vessels in response to ischaemia. Once new vessels have formed, they pose a threat to sight from acute vitreous haemorrhage. Before haemorrhage happens, treatment can be given using the laser to destroy the peripheral ischaemic retina which is

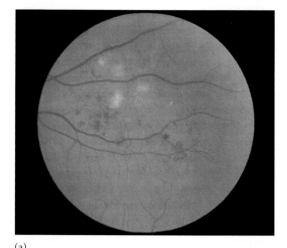

(a)

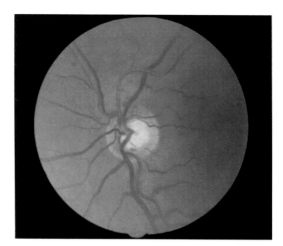

**Fig. 9.9** Early new vessels looping outside the disc margin at 12 o'clock and inside it at 6 o'clock.

(b)

**Fig. 9.10** (a) Tuft of peripheral new vessels in proliferative diabetic retinopathy, just below and right of centre. Note cotton-wool spots, indicating ischaemia. (b) Very early tuft of new vessels, immediately below a loop in the branch vessel above centre.

stimulating the growth of new vessels, rather than directly treating the new vessels themselves. Most vessels will regress within weeks or months with adequate treatment. This treatment preserves central vision at the cost of some loss of peripheral field, which was probably poor anyway as the retina was already ischaemic. Left untreated, the new vessels may cause catastrophic bleeds into the vitreous, which may progress into irreversible fibrosis and risk pulling off the retina as a detachment. Smaller bleeds may clear sufficiently to allow laser later. Occasionally, an operation may remove the blood-stained vitreous (vitrectomy). See under Diabetic eye disease (p. 130) for a description of laser treatment.

As retinal changes almost always occur bilaterally, the prognosis for vision is poor if proliferative retinopathy is not treated. Fifty to 70% of patients with untreated proliferative retinopathy will be blind in that eye within 5 years. Treatment by laser can reduce visual loss by up to 60%.

> Treatment by laser early in proliferative retinopathy can save vision

### A practical screening programme

Table 9.2 shows a suggested scheme for screening the retina in diabetic patients. For this to work, it is obviously important for the patients to be identified and an efficient recall system established. Also, it is important that the notes are organized so that it is easy to see the date of the last screening and the findings. This can be done on a separate sheet, or by stamping the normal notes with boxes for the relevant information. An example is given in Fig. 9.11.

It is suggested that annual screening starts in the younger age group (from puberty to 30 years of age) at 5 years from diagnosis, and in older patients from the time of diagnosis. Pregnant diabetics need to be screened every 2 months. Some optometrists are accredited to offer diabetic retinal screening, sending a report both to the GP and funding body.

Patients with diabetes are entitled to a free annual eye test by an optometrist (optician). In patients over 40 years of age this should include a measurement of the ocular pressures and visual fields as diabetics have a higher incidence of glaucoma. Remember to look for cupping of the optic

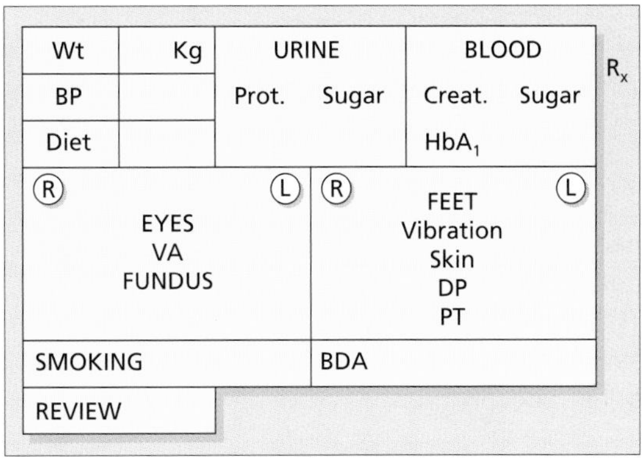

Fig. 9.11 Stamp for recording findings of diabetic screening.

Table 9.2 A practical screening programme for diabetic retinopathy

| Retinopathy type | Prognosis (percentage of untreated eyes blind in 5 years | Action | Suggested treatment | Follow-up interval |
|---|---|---|---|---|
| None | 0.3 | Continue screening | Optimize control | 1 year |
| Background | 3 | Continue screening and return if vision falls | Optimize control | 1 year |
| Maculopathy | | Refer to ophthalmologist | Focal laser | 3–6 months |
| Pre-proliferative | | Refer | | 3 months |
| Proliferative | 60 | Refer | Pan-retinal laser | Monthly until regression |

disc in older patients when screening. Patients at risk of, or who already have, simple glaucoma can have dilating drops without any extra risk of acute rise in pressure.

> • Diabetic patients have an increased risk of glaucoma and cataract
> • They are entitled to free eye testing

### Other factors in diabetic eye care

Optimize blood glucose control as judged best by glycosylated haemoglobin (HbA1) levels. Treat hypertension as an extra risk factor for microvascular disease. As smoking is probably a risk factor for proliferative retinopathy, all diabetic patients should stop smoking. Cataract occurs earlier in diabetes. If vision falls and it is difficult to see the retina because of cataract, then refer for surgical assessment.

> Diabetic patients with retinopathy should not smoke

In advanced cases, perhaps where vitreous haemorrhage prevents treatment to the retina, new vessels may also grow on the iris (rubeosis). This can block off drainage and cause a secondary severe glaucoma. (See also Diabetic eye disease, p. 127, and Chapter 12.)

### Glaucoma screening

Unfortunately, this is a subject which has few clear-cut features, but it is important to get to grips with the problems. The commoner sort of chronic glaucoma still causes patients to become blind. The disorder is painless and gradual. It affects large amounts of visual field before it affects visual acuity at all. It is estimated that the vast majority of nerve fibres (about 90%) will have been lost irretrievably before the onset of symptoms. So, without screening or a high level of awareness among all who care for eyes, the problem will continue, with some patients needing desperate attempts to save remaining vision in the late stages. Successful treatment is possible in most cases of glaucoma, so it follows that early detection is important, before symptoms develop. The GP may be a primary

screener or the link between optometrist and ophthalmologist (or preferably both).

> GPs *can*:
> • encourage screening for glaucoma by optometrists
> • recognize disc cupping
> • explain importance of glaucoma management

*Size of the problem*

In terms of numbers, glaucoma is an important disease. The failures lead to 12% overall of blind registrations in the UK, particularly in the 65 plus age group. The prevalence figures show it to be a common problem: 0.5% in the total population; 1% in the over 45s; 6.6% in the over 75s.

*Risk factors*

Of the risk factors, age and a family history are the most important. Ten per cent of first-degree relatives of someone with the disease are likely to develop glaucoma at some time. Black people, myopes and diabetics are also at an increased risk.

### What is glaucoma?

The hallmark of the disorder is the loss of nerve fibres within the optic disc rim. As the fibres crowd in from the sensory retina they converge on the nerve head (synonymous with 'disc') and turn through a right angle to pass backwards in the nerve itself, forming the pink outer rim at the nerve head. At this point they are vulnerable to pressure. It is believed that in glaucoma the nerve fibres die because pressure on the nerve head reduces the blood supply to the rim. The risk of damage is partly related to the level of intraocular pressure, partly to the health of the vessels. The consequences are loss of fibres, shrinking of the rim as the central cup enlarges (see Figs 7.3 and 7.4), and the appearance of characteristic defects in the visual field. These arch around the central area (arcuate scotoma) (Fig. 9.12) so visual acuity is normal until late. It seems the fibres serving central vision are relatively robust. The whole process is absolutely painless, gradual and irreversible. It cannot be detected except with the skills and equipment to make the right observations. One of these is the optic disc appearance.

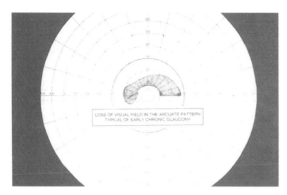

**Fig. 9.12** Arcuate pattern of visual field loss typical of early established glaucoma.

**Table 9.3** Usefulness of features in glaucoma screening

*Raised ocular pressure*
False positives common
Misses low tension glaucoma

*Disc cupping*
Subjective and inaccurate
Requires experience

*Visual field loss*
Equipment necessary
Time-consuming

Diagnosis of chronic glaucoma rests on three features:

**1** Raised intraocular pressure (IOP).
**2** Pathological changes of the optic nerve head (disc cupping).
**3** Characteristic pattern of visual field loss (arcuate scotoma).

A significant group of people have 'low tension glaucoma' with disc and field changes in the absence of raised pressure. This is a group which usually does badly. The converse, raised pressure without disc and field changes is known as 'ocular hypertension', a group which usually does better.

## Screening

Traditionally, glaucoma screening has been carried out on a random basis on those presenting to their optician for an eye test (see Chapter 6). The optic discs were examined, with a rough field test being occasionally performed if the discs were abnormal. Pressure measurement was rare, as few optometrists had much experience of tonometry which involved corneal contact and needed anaesthetic drops. It was quite common for patients who had been regularly refracted to present to the ophthalmologist with symptomatic, usually end-stage, glaucoma in one eye and advanced field loss in the other eye. The situation has changed with the increasingly widespread use of the non-contact tonometer (NCT or 'puff of air', a brief pulse of compressed air) by optometrists. In the belief that raised pressure represents early glaucoma, there is a danger that optometrists may swamp hospital eye departments with referrals.

Let us consider the three diagnostic features in turn, with reference to their usefulness for screening purposes (Table 9.3).

### Intraocular pressure measurement

This can now be done simply and quickly, taking 2 minutes for three readings from each eye, with the non-contact tonometer. The technique has identified large numbers of cases of ocular hypertension, the prevalence of which is estimated at 6.1% of over 40-year-olds or 9.5% of those over 70. This is a very large number of people, and far more than the number with glaucoma. The proportion who will develop glaucoma is estimated variably at between 3.5% and 10% over 5 years. This wide range of risk from various surveys is due to varying criteria for the diagnosis of glaucoma. Despite this, it seems clear that an eye with a pressure at any one time over 30 mmHg is at greater risk. Whether to treat ocular hypertension is a debatable area. An 'only' good eye, glaucoma in the other eye, pressure consistently over 30 mmHg, retinal vein occlusion in either eye, or a family history would all influence the decision towards treatment.

### Optic disc appearance (abnormal cupping)

When looking at the optic nerve head try, in the mind's eye, to draw a line around the outside of the entire disc and also around the boundary between the pink rim and the paler central hollowed cup. Decide whether the rim is a normal pink colour or whether it could be pale. Look to see if the rim is regular in size or if there might be notched areas of focal loss of nerve fibres.

Changes in the appearance of the optic disc in glaucoma include enlargement of the central cup, pallor of the remaining nerve fibre rim and splinter haemorrhages on the disc margin. The size of the cup relative to that of the disc as a whole (cup:disc ratio, see Fig. 7.4) varies in healthy individuals from 0 (no cup) to 0.7 (a large cup) if surrounded by a pink, even rim of nerve tissue. Glaucomatous field loss is much more likely where the cup:disc ratio is over 0.5, but it has been found with much smaller cups. It is therefore impossible to be categorical about what constitutes a 'pathologically' cupped disc. A localized area of thinning of the rim, which may resemble a notch, is highly significant. A difference in cup:disc ratio between the two eyes of 0.2 or more is a risk factor for glaucoma development. Paleness of the rim, either all or in parts, is likely to be significant also as it implies loss of blood supply to the fibres.

Disc assessment is acknowledged to be prone to subjective error. However, in experienced hands such as ophthalmologist, optometrist or GP with training, it can be reasonably reliable. Focusing errors and opacities in the eye media may hamper efforts to assess the disc. Some discs, particularly those of myopes, are impossible to classify. In the screening context, disc assessment suffers from having no clear cut-off point between normal and abnormal, resulting in a potentially large number of false positives amongst suspicious discs without other signs, and a lesser number of false negatives who do indeed have glaucoma without apparent cupping.

### Visual field testing

This detects the functional effect of glaucoma and is therefore the most relevant of the diagnostic criteria. A detectable field defect is usually needed to confirm the diagnosis of glaucoma and will frequently be the basis on which treatment is started. In the past, field testing was time-consuming, insensitive to early changes and required a good deal of concentration on the subject's part. Modern automated static perimetry is quick (4 minutes for two eyes) and sensitive. Many 'high street' optometrists now regularly use a static field screener. As well as picking up glaucoma, including the low tension variety, at a stage when treatment needs to be considered, they have the advantage of revealing interesting non-glaucomatous defects, most of which are likely to be neurological. It is difficult to identify arcuate scotomas with certainty using a red pin but worth a try if the diagnosis is strongly suspected, as finding a field defect increases the urgency of referral.

### Screening programmes

It has been said that screening for glaucoma has undergone spontaneous growth without planning or policy agreement. On the one hand, optometrists are encouraged to refer patients with raised intraocular pressures; on the other, many glaucomatous individuals are not being found. It seems likely that optometrists will continue to be in the best position to screen for glaucoma, as few of the older population most at risk can manage without some sort of optical assistance and optometrists have the necessary skills and equipment. The fee now charged for an eye test, though now only for the under 60s, may present a deterrent to the following-up of glaucoma suspects (such as ocular hypertensives) by optometrists, though patients with a family history of glaucoma are currently exempt from the fee. The availability of spectacles across the counter may offer a cheap alternative, but patients should be aware of the risk of missing serious eye problems in by-passing the optometrist.

Whilst a mass population screening programme for such an important disease as glaucoma might appear to be valuable, its low prevalence in the population at large relative to many life-threatening disorders, together with the inefficiency of pressure and disc assessments as screening criteria without field testing, mean this has never been regarded as an economic proposition. At present the system operates by poorly informed choice and chance, and does not meet the definition of screening.

### How can screening be improved?

If screening is to be more effective and over-referrals reduced, visual field testing must become the test of first choice. Confirmation by

**Table 9.4** Referral of glaucoma suspects

*Early referral*
Ocular pressure greater than 35 mmHg (risk of retinal vein occlusion)
Cupping with field loss (even if pressure less than 35 mmHg)

*Routine referral*
Ocular pressure between 21 and 35 mmHg (on more than one occasion)
Cupping without field loss

tonometry and disc examination are essential. If these are negative, re-examination after 3–6 months would be sensible and hospital referral can then follow if there is still doubt, especially in high-risk groups such as the elderly, diabetics and those with a family history. When assessing priority of referrals for outpatient appointments, the value of having the right information cannot be overstated. A delay of several weeks will not matter for a 'glaucoma suspect' without field loss or with a pressure below 30 mmHg, but if frank glaucoma is suspected an appointment should be made within a few weeks (Table 9.4).

*Role of the GP*
Screening in a general practice setting might be feasible using an automated perimeter operated by a specially trained member of the practice team. For reasons already given, this would be greatly preferable to any attempt to screen on pressure or disc appearance alone. Screening might be confined to a defined older age group or offered to higher risk groups such as diabetics, blacks or those with a family history of glaucoma. The test could be incorporated into existing screening programmes if these groups could be identified. Alternatively, patients identified to be at risk could be referred to the local optometry service for screening. Some groups are exempt from the current fee (see p. 115).

When referring patients on from the optometrist to hospital services it is wise to send the referral form (GOS 18 or 'green form') too. It is important to relay information back to the optometrist after the hospital assessment.

The GP should also understand the features of early and established glaucoma, particularly the optic disc appearances, so that with a high level of awareness these patients will be found more often.

## Screening children

### Why screen?
Learning to see starts at birth and continues until the age of about 4 years. To develop normal vision with the ability to see in depth (binocular vision), each eye must form a clear image. In the brain the two images are merged to give stereoscopic information. If one eye sees better than the other during this time, or if there is a squint and the images would produce double vision, the brain will select the clearer of the two and ignore the other, producing a so-called *lazy eye* (also called *amblyopia*). This can only be avoided by detecting and treating any abnormality, such as a problem with focus, a squint or a defective eye, as soon as possible within the first 4 years. After this age no further learning will take place and the child is doomed to impaired vision in that eye for the rest of life. About 4% of the population has amblyopia. Rare but important conditions may be found such as childhood glaucoma or retinoblastoma.

> Learning to see is a preschool activity

### When to screen?
At the same time as other routine childhood surveillance, at:
- 6 weeks
- 8 months
- 18 months
- 3 years
- preschool to identify any who have not developed normal vision.

### How to screen
With training, patience and practice!

> Screening vision in children needs:
> - a torch from 6 weeks
> - a cover test from 8 months
> - an acuity test from 3 years

Ask a few brief questions:
• Do you think your child sees normally? Have grandparents noticed anything wrong?
• Have you noticed a squint?
• Have the parents or siblings had any trouble with their eyes?
If parents express concern about the eyes they are probably right! Grandparents, with more experience, are most often correct.

Babies who have been on a Special Care Unit, especially if they required high doses of oxygen and are at risk of developing retrolental fibroplasia, will usually have been screened and followed by an ophthalmologist.

Examine the eyes for particular features at various ages.

### At 6 weeks of age
Look for:
• *Ptosis* (eyelid not opening fully).
• *Squint*. Shine a torch and see if it is reflected from the very centre of each pupil. A wide bridge to the nose (epicanthic folds) may give a false impression of a squint (Fig. 9.13). In a squint the reflection is off centre in one eye.

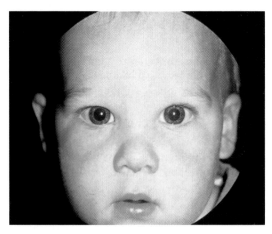

**Fig. 9.13** Epicanthic folds of the inner upper eyelids can mimic a convergent squint, but the light reflections are both central, and there would be no movement on a cover test. Reproduced from Taylor (1992) *Pediatric Ophthalmology* (slide atlas), Blackwell Scientific Publications, Cambridge, MA.

• *Red reflex* using the ophthalmoscope (see Chapter 2). If the pupil is white think of the rare retinoblastoma, though these are even more rare before the second year of life (see below). Other causes are cataract, and fibrosis in premature babies.
• Other abnormal appearances such as: facial asymmetry; different sized eyes; birth mark (strawberry naevus).
• *Photophobia, watering or corneal oedema* suggesting glaucoma, is discussed in the section on the watering eye (see p. 55). Childhood glaucoma is very rare but may be spotted early enough with good screening.

### At 8 months of age
Look for all the above *plus*:
• *Eye movements*, are they full in all directions? Watch as the baby looks round or test by moving an eye-catching object in the field of vision.
• *Cover test to detect squint* (Fig. 9.14). This is difficult to learn without training under the eye of an orthoptist but the test is not complicated, though it must be done with speed. While the baby is looking at an object, cover one eye at a time, using your hand or just your thumb held in their line of vision. If they make a fuss when one eye is covered but not the other, this may mean that one eye is becoming 'lazy' and the other is preferred. Watch at the moment you cover the opposite eye or uncover the eye and notice if it appears to move in or out to look towards the object, suggestive of a squint.

> Mum often does know best in diagnosing a squint (and possibly Grandma knows even better)

### At 18 months of age
Repeat as for 8 months—but it is a bit easier perhaps! Remember now the rare *retinoblastoma*, a malignant retinal tumour. Its prevalence is one per 10 000, so it may not be found even once in a lifetime, but if GPs are unaware of it the chances of delay and ultimate mortality are greater, so no apologies for including it here! It shows as a lump behind or whitening within the pupil. It runs in families, so see the genetic screening section below.

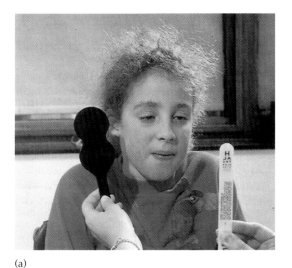

(a)

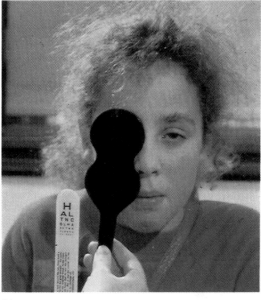

(b)

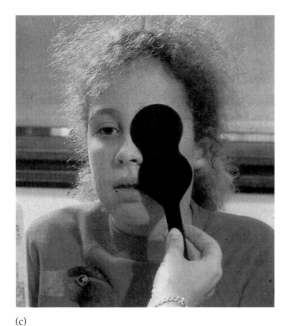

(c)

**Fig. 9.14** Cover test for squint. (a) Shows the right eye is convergent and the left is straight. (b) When the right eye is covered, the left eye does not move but stays straight, as it is already 'fixing'. (c) When the left eye is covered, the right eye is forced to 'fix' and moves out to look straight. This movement confirms that the right eye was squinting inwards. Reproduced from Taylor (1992) *Pediatric Ophthalmology* (slide atlas), Blackwell Scientific Publications, Cambridge, MA.

- Refer promptly any child with whitening of the pupil
- There is usually a serious disorder and it may save a life

*At 3 years of age*
Look for all of the above *plus*:
- *Visual acuity* using a Stycar or Sheridan Gardiner test (Fig. 9.15). Again this is easily learned in an orthoptic department. Each eye is tested in

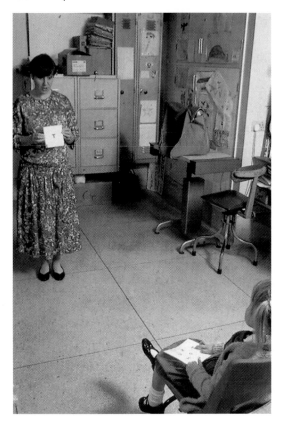

**Fig. 9.15** Testing distance vision in a child using a Sheridan–Gardiner booklet of different sized single letters. The child points to the letter identified each time. Reproduced from Taylor (1992) *Pediatric Ophthalmology* (slide atlas), Blackwell Scientific Publications, Cambridge, MA.

turn, the other being covered with an eyepatch (pirates?). The child sits on parent's lap, the tester stands 6 metres away, and either uses a Snellen chart, or holds up a card with a single letter or shape on it. The child is then asked to identify the symbol by pointing to the matching one on a sheet held by the parent. The size of the symbol presented is reduced as the test proceeds, and from this a semi-objective measure of acuity can be made which corresponds with the Snellen chart, i.e. 6/60 down to 6/5. The child should be able to achieve a vision of 6/6 and if not, should be re-tested soon or referred.

### Pre-school testing

Repeat the 3-year check. It is by this stage probably too late to improve a 'lazy' eye, but parents should be informed and the school can be warned of the child's problem. A squint may need cosmetic surgery. A focusing error will need referral to an optician.

### Later testing (colour vision testing)

Red/green colour 'blindness' is by far the most common defect and is found in 8% of boys and 0.5% of girls. There is little evidence that this causes any learning difficulties but is significant when deciding on certain careers. Some occupations require normal colour vision and it is helpful to be aware of this. These include certain jobs within the armed forces or the fire service, work involving colour-coded wiring such as electrician, and some jobs in fashion or industry involving colour choosing or matching. Some would advocate the screening of all boys on entry to secondary education, at least. The Ishihara test is an easy and sensitive means of doing this (see Fig. 3.29a).

### Sharing with other professionals

Various professionals are involved in childhood screening and it is essential that they work as a team. Policies and practices vary between different localities as to who does what, but the personnel involved may include the following.

*Health visitors* are perhaps the key workers as they have a statutory duty to provide childhood surveillance which should include vision testing. They will have been trained, probably by an orthoptist, to test vision in babies (using coloured objects) and older children (using a test like the Stycar or Sheridan–Gardiner). In addition they will know how to do a cover test and to examine further for squint.

*School nurses* are trained to test visual acuity using a Snellen chart in older children and may be confident to do a cover test. Not all authorities use the school nurse in this way, however.

*Child health clinic doctors and GPs* should be able to do all the above tests and also to use the ophthalmoscope. It is usually the responsibility of the doctor to do the 6-week check, at which the eyes should be examined. If, as a result of screening at any age, you are unsure whether or not the child has a problem, there are two things you can do:

• *Repeat the examination after a short interval.* The tests are not easy, and you may get better co-operation the second time. Confer with the health visitor at this stage.

• *Get a second opinion.* Often the health visitor has done the initial screening, except for the 6-week check, and the GP may be the 'second opinion' but, if there is still doubt, ask for the child to be screened by the orthoptist from the local eye department. Orthoptic departments often offer screening at community clinics. Some orthoptists visit health centres on a regular basis for this purpose and will accept referrals directly from the health visitor. Otherwise they will see children at the hospital. The orthoptist will then decide whether or not the child needs follow-up and treatment by themselves or with an ophthalmologist. Of course, if you are sure that a problem exists, refer directly to the ophthalmologist, stating your diagnosis.

> 'Two are better than one' applies to eyes and also to opinions if you are unsure about a child's eyes

## Why bother to screen all children? (A contentious issue)

Some authorities on community health bodies doubt the value of routine screening for visual disability on the basis that it is not cost-effective and that parents will always notice if their child is not seeing properly, and will seek help. They would recommend that only children with a strong family history are routinely screened at 18 months and 3.5 years, and that all other children are left to have a check when they first attend school. In contrast, many workers in this field find considerable benefit in the early detection of problems which need to be explained or corrected. Several areas of screening and prevention could have the same cost-effective arguments applied and there is no logic in excluding visual screening from the examination of children who are already being seen in a surveillance programme. Also, it is only by the regular practice of the skills of examining the eyes that primary care workers can become expert and confident. This is providing that they have been taught correctly in the first instance; maybe training is the key to effective and economical screening.

## Screening for genetic abnormalities

The ophthalmologist may work as part of a screening team which may include a clinical geneticist and a paediatrician. The principle of screening is to detect the presence of a particular feature in members of families at risk of specific inherited disorders. The family members may then be counselled about the outcome for themselves and the predicted outcome for their children, and may be offered appropriate treatment.

> Eye screening in selected patients at risk may help detect important dominant life-threatening conditions:
> • Marfan's syndrome
> • neurofibromatosis
> • Von Hippel–Lindau disease
> • retinoblastoma

Marfan's syndrome is a relatively common dominant disorder. The features may include abnormalities of eye size or of lens position. Slit-lamp examination with dilated pupils will detect lens dislocation or instability even in toddlers. Younger children are screened for squint, refractive error or abnormality of the red reflex, and are re-screened later by slit-lamp. Most children will co-operate with the slit-lamp by the age of 3 years. Correction of refractive problems with glasses will improve vision and may prevent amblyopia in younger children.

Neurofibromatosis type 1 (Von Recklinghausen's disease) is quite a common dominant gene. Affected individuals have a 95% chance of having small Lisch nodules on the iris, best seen with the slit-lamp by an experienced observer. Other eye or visual problems can occur and may be correctable.

Retinoblastoma is a disorder with a dominantly inherited component. Although rare, screening is important as the condition poses a threat to life which increases in each successive generation. The early lesions are found by screening the fundi. Later, the mass may be visible within the pupil and may cause it to look white. Treatment can be given at any stage, the earlier the better. (See also under Screening children, above.)

## Screening for drug toxicity

It is uncommon for drugs used in therapeutic doses to have serious side-effects on the eye. It is only worth screening all patients taking a drug if the effect is reasonably common, potentially serious, reversible if detected early, and if the symptoms of early toxicity might go unnoticed. The tests chosen for screening must detect the problem reliably enough, so that there are few false negatives, and early enough that stopping the drug reverses the effect. They should ideally also be inexpensive and fairly quick to complete.

### Corticosteroids

Systemic corticosteroids are among the commonest drugs to have side-effects, but in practice it is not worth screening all patients regularly. The drugs cause cataract, and affected patients will present usually with a fall in vision, especially for reading. Often the drug cannot be stopped, and although the change in the lens is irreversible the problem can be tackled surgically. The risks of lens extraction are no higher in this group, most of whom are suitable for an intraocular lens implant. It is not worth screening because this adds nothing to the outcome; wait for the patient to present.

### Antimalarials

Antimalarial drugs of the chloroquine group are known to have toxic effects on the retina, in particular the macula. Affected patients notice impairment of fine vision, especially when reading, and may have disturbance of Amsler grids or colour vision. The affected retina shows an increase in pigmentation in the early stages, progressing to a 'bull's eye' appearance later. Toxicity is well-documented, although uncommon, in patients who have taken chloroquine itself regularly and daily for rheumatological problems such as rheumatoid arthritis or lupus erythematosus. In practice toxicity is not seen in patients taking chloroquine in the usual dose for malaria prophylaxis, even after many years, unless they have abused the drug (as a readily available alternative to aspirin in the tropics). Hydroxychloroquine could potentially produce similar toxicity, but so far regular screening has produced very few cases in the world literature.

Screening for patients on antimalarials should begin with a baseline assessment in a hospital setting. This would include visual acuity, inspection of the macula and perhaps macular photographs, and some test of macular threshold sensitivity that is reliable, reproducible and easily repeated. In practice the Amsler is rather too crude for reliable testing and a Dicon threshold screen is better. The patients are counselled about the low risk of toxicity and asked to report any change in reading function that cannot be corrected by their own optometrist.

### Ethambutol

Another drug for which screening is necessary is ethambutol, usually prescribed for treatment of tuberculosis. This can cause optic neuropathy which is reversible if the drug is stopped early enough. Baseline assessment includes visual acuity and colour vision testing, usually by the hundred-hues method, with inspection of the optic nerve head. Re-testing should be every 3 months, but the patient is warned to report any subjective change as soon as it occurs as the effect can progress rapidly. Toxicity is uncommon at the usual dose of 15 mg/kg daily, but there are patients whose optic nerves seem particularly sensitive to the drug.

Screening visual function is necessary for:
- long-term chloroquine
- short-term ethambutol

## Other drugs

At present routine screening is not undertaken for other drugs, unless for pharmaceutical companies when a new drug comes on the market. This was the case with amiodarone, which causes corneal deposits. Screening established that the deposits rarely caused symptoms and led to no significant toxicity long term, so screening is not now necessary.

# Chapter 10 **Trauma**

Damage to the eye and structures around it can vary from the trivial and transitory, such as a sub-tarsal foreign body, to the severe and permanent such as a penetrating injury by glass. This chapter will consider the importance of the clinical history in assessing risks to the eye itself, the symptoms and signs of eye damage and the immediate management of various injuries. Only selected injuries need referral and the patient with a painful eye will be very grateful for primary care (see Fluorescein staining the cornea, p. 8 and Irrigation, p. 170). If referred to hospital, the patient should not drive (as the eye may be padded), should avoid rubbing the eye and should not attempt to remove foreign material, unless this is easily done.

## Importance of the clinical history

The circumstances in which the eye was injured give important clues to the likely site and severity of damage (Table 10.1).

### Risk of foreign body within the eye

If a foreign body sensation develops during the use of powered machinery such as a drill or sander the possibility arises that a tiny piece of metal could have penetrated the eye. An intraocular foreign body is very rare except in power-tool or hammer and chisel injuries. If the head of a chisel is not kept well-filed slivers of metal are forced to the edge during repeated hammering and eventually one of these breaks off at high speed and may penetrate the eye with remarkable ease (Fig. 10.1). It is important to remember that this can happen with few clinical signs and symptoms. Remember to ask about circumstances in any patient with a metal corneal foreign body. Unfortunately, there may be medicolegal implications in failing to refer patients with these specific accidents. Slivers of

flying glass are likely to cause corneal abrasion but penetration is less likely, though detection of a glass foreign body is particularly difficult.

### Risk of significant blunt trauma

This is most common with high-speed missiles which are large enough to reach the eye itself rather than damage the bone around (Fig. 10.2). They include squash balls, golf balls and champagne corks. Examine the front chamber and pupil carefully for internal bleeding or iris damage.

### Risk of penetrating eye injury

Injuries to the eye are sometimes divided into blunt (eye wall intact) and open (eye wall breached). The clinical history gives major clues to the likely category. The blow from a squash ball will rarely puncture the eye but a head-on car crash without seat belt protection, when the head plunges through the windscreen, is likely to cause an open eye injury. Ophthalmic surgeons tend always to wear their seat belts, from bitter experience. Beware also some gardening or agricultural injuries, as thorns may be involved. Garden canes can produce very unpleasant corneal abrasions and the risk of penetration. In children beware when an injury involves pencils or if the account of the circumstances of the injury is unclear.

> Preventive ophthalmology: encourage your patients to use goggles with power tools and, in gardening, ping pong balls to cover cane tops

### Risk of chemical injury

Eye injury may be caused by chemicals, either particulate, liquid or gas. These are usually minor but there are exceptions which merit particular em-

**Table 10.1** Features suggesting risk of significant eye
injury

*A particular history*
Hammer and chisel
Missile, especially golf ball, squash ball or cork
Certain chemicals, especially ammonia, alkali and acid
Gardening or agricultural setting
Pencils, especially in children

*Rough guides to the severity of injury*
Severity of pain
Level of vision

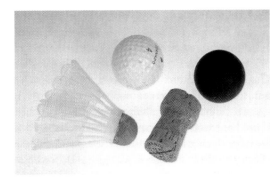

(a)

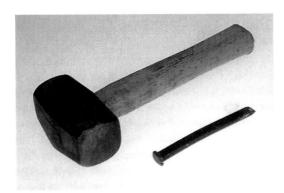

**Fig. 10.1** Hammer and metal chisel—beware of the danger
of an intraocular iron foreign body from the head of the
chisel (see also Fig. 10.5).

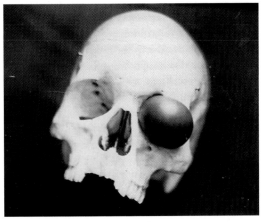

(b)

**Fig. 10.2** Missiles hazardous to the eye, travelling at high
speed and small enough to pass bone.

phasis. Alkaline substances penetrate the cornea
rapidly and trigger a severe toxic reaction that
can lead to permanent scarring of the cornea. Hazardous substances include household ammonia,
bleach, dishwasher cleaner, plaster used for walls
and cement (Fig. 10.3). In any case of chemical
eye injury the history should include the delay
between injury and irrigating the eye since this
is crucial in determining prognosis for vision. See
below for advice about immediate irrigation with
tapwater.

Beware eye injury with:
• ammonia
• alkali, acid
• bleach, lavatory cleaner
• plaster, mortar, cement, lime

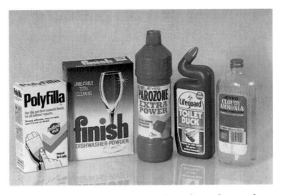

**Fig. 10.3** Some household chemicals are hazardous to the
eye, including plaster, dishwasher granules, bleach, acid
lavatory cleaner and ammonia.

## Warning signs in eye trauma

### Foreign body sensation: look carefully

The eye, and particularly the cornea, is extremely sensitive to foreign bodies and scratches but cannot distinguish between them. In other words a patient may be convinced that something is in the eye when this is no longer the case. A sudden grittiness or foreign body sensation which persists for hours or even days is characteristic of a foreign body stuck on the undersurface of the upper eyelid or on the cornea. Under the upper lid small particles can become firmly embedded with scratching of the cornea during each blink. The pattern of fluorescein staining on the cornea, seen best with the slit-lamp, is highly characteristic, with many little vertical lines. Everting the upper lid (see p. 9) usually reveals the offending piece of grit. A foreign body can also lodge on the cornea itself and, if it contains iron, rust will diffuse into the surrounding cornea within a matter of hours. Glass is difficult to detect but can be located using fluorescein at the slit-lamp.

> The acutely painful red eye warrants:
> • fluorescein staining of the cornea
> • inspection of the everted upper lid

### Black eye: usually straightforward

The eye is very well protected from most blunt injuries because of the bony orbital rim. When blood vessels are damaged a black eye develops. The bruising can assume dramatic proportions because of the normal laxity of the very vascular tissues, but damage to the eye beneath is uncommon. Rarely, blunt injury can result in bleeding behind the eye or orbital haematoma. The eye may then be shifted forwards, the eye muscles may be affected causing double vision and compression of the optic nerve by haematoma may cause vision to fall. The optic disc may be swollen.

### Hyphaema: bleeding within the front chamber is always significant

With sufficient force a blood vessel within the eye may rupture. Squash balls are a classic cause of this injury as their size and flexibility allow them to transmit energy directly to the eye. The commonest site for vessel rupture is in the iris when the blood will spread into the front chamber and vision will fall to a variable extent. Examination may show a blood clot on the iris and the iris itself, particularly the pupil margin, will appear hazy because of turbid blood within the aqueous fluid. After a few hours the red cells tend to settle under the influence of gravity and a characteristic red crescent forms at the bottom of the chamber (see Fig. 5.44). As the blood settles the vision improves but movement of the eye can stir up the blood and result in blurring of vision again. This is like shaking a glass dome of a Christmas snow scene so that the flakes swirl about.

### Dilated pupil: a sign of significant trauma not to be mistaken

Blunt injury to the eye can cause temporary paralysis of the pupil sphincter and a dilated pupil. This does not significantly interfere with vision, though it may cause glare, and it usually wears off within a week or so. There are often other signs of trauma, particularly hyphaema. Recognition of this cause of a dilated pupil is particularly important since it avoids a mistaken diagnosis of partial third nerve palsy. Iris injury is much more likely when the trauma is directly to the eye (Fig. 10.4) and when there is no ptosis, diplopia or limitation of eye movements to suggest a neurological cause.

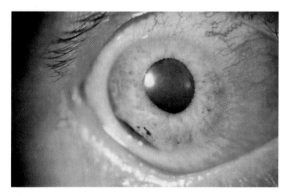

**Fig. 10.4** Traumatic iris tear at the periphery at 7 o'clock, causing a dilated irregular pupil. (Courtesy of Mr A. Shun-Shin.)

Iris trauma causing a dilated pupil is easily mistaken for a third nerve palsy unless the slit-lamp is used

Conjunctival haemorrhage plus laceration means suspected foreign body inside the eye

## Subconjunctival haemorrhage: beware sometimes

Such a haemorrhage with a history of trauma indicates that the eye has been hit with a moderate force, enough to rupture blood vessels on the surface of the eye. The haemorrhage resolves over 1 or 2 weeks and causes no long-term damage. There are two circumstances in which the presence of a haemorrhage should be viewed with suspicion.

• A haemorrhage with an overlying conjunctival defect (use fluorescein and cobalt blue light to check) may indicate the site of penetration of the eye and perhaps an intraocular foreign body (Fig. 10.5). Always take seriously a conjunctival haemorrhage in a child, particularly if a pencil or a fall may be involved.

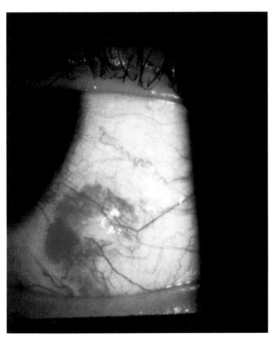

**Fig. 10.5** Entry site for a small foreign body marked by a conjunctival haemorrhage. The conjunctival wound would stain with fluorescein.

• A haemorrhage whose back border cannot be seen may indicate that the bleeding comes from the orbit or that there is an orbital fracture. Although uncommon, this is serious because of the risk of optic nerve compression (see Black eye, above).

## Crackling of the skin: indicates traumatic emphysema

Traumatic emphysema indicates a fracture involving the sinuses. The orbital pressure rises as the eye is forced backwards and part of the bony orbital wall ruptures. This is most common in the ethmoid sinus medially as the bone is exquisitely thin here. Air may not track into the orbit and lids until the patient blows their nose, when marked periorbital swelling may happen and will probably precipitate the patient into your waiting room. Refer for clinical and radiological assessment.

Sudden lid swelling after nose blowing means a sinus fracture

## Vitreous haemorrhage: always significant

A sudden onset of floaters at the time of injury or shortly afterwards indicates damage to the vitreous which is only caused by severe eye injuries. When an eye is struck hard the distortion may cause the vitreous to pull away from its attachment to the retina. Traumatic detachment causes floaters if bleeding occurs into the vitreous and does affect vision to a variable degree. Whether or not there is blood in the vitreous, trauma may cause retinal tears with the risk of subsequent retinal detachment. This usually takes days or weeks to develop and retinal detachment is only an acute feature of the most severe eye injuries.

## Retinal oedema: may be hard to detect

Retinal oedema may cause poor vision after blunt eye injury due to reversible damage caused by sudden pressure or a shearing movement in the overlying vitreous (Fig. 10.6). The oedema shows

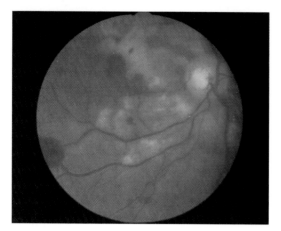

**Fig. 10.6** Commotio of the retina, with pale oedema and haemorrhages, from a blunt injury.

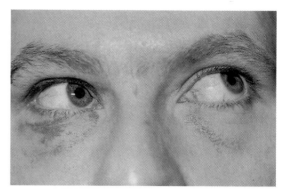

**Fig. 10.7** Fracture of the right orbital floor ('blow-out') with poor elevation of the right eye.

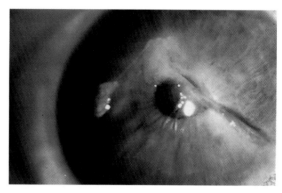

**Fig. 10.8** A perforated eye with a full-thickness laceration of the cornea, caused by glass.

as an area of pallor with irregular margins that can be hard to see with the direct ophthalmoscope. It subsides within several days usually with return of normal vision and no long-term damage.

### Double vision

Double vision is a symptom only, of course, when both eyes are open. It is therefore important to raise the upper lid even if it is very swollen to assess damage, test vision and ask about diplopia. For most patients the cause of double vision is not apparent and recovery is complete within 24 hours, otherwise an orbital fracture should be considered (Fig. 10.7). Look for limitation of upward movement of the eye because the inferior rectus muscle may be trapped in the fracture site. Rarely is diplopia attributable to a cranial nerve palsy, when a history of major head trauma is usually apparent.

### Is the eyeball intact?

Do make an attempt to examine the eye itself. Swelling around the injured eye may make examination difficult. Gentle pressure is safe (see Fig. 2.11), but excessive pressure on the lids to open the eye can itself cause further prolapse of ocular contents and this should be avoided, so it is best not to make strenuous efforts to open an injured eye. Put on a pad instead (see Appendix 3) and refer. The eye wall is usually only broken by laceration but is occasionally forced to split by being hit very hard. In either case intraocular pressure is reduced to zero, so the eye feels very soft and may collapse, and vision is severely affected. Evidence of other eye damage will certainly be clear, such as periorbital bruising, extensive subconjunctival haemorrhage, corneal abrasion or hyphaema. If the perforation has occurred in front of the iris, the iris will plug the gap (Fig. 10.8 and see Fig. 10.11). Pigmented iris tissue may be apparent on the surface of the eye and the pupil will be distorted. If clear vitreous jelly prolapses through a wound further back, damage is extreme and prognosis poor.

- Try to examine the eye with lid swelling, *but*
- Do not use undue force to separate the eyelids — refer instead

A badly distorted pupil indicates penetrating eye injury

## Lid lacerations: should be repaired carefully

These are common and rarely associated with eye damage. A minor injury can seem severe because of bleeding and an early priority is to clean the lids gently to see the site and severity of the laceration. Of course it is also critically important to examine the eye itself. Beware lacerations involving the inner parts of the lid margin when there is a risk of damage to the lacrimal drainage system and injuries here may not be suitable for simple suturing. Also, if there are areas of skin loss associated with lid lacerations, as in some dog bites, there is a risk that late scarring will result in permanent distortion of the eyelids.

Laceration of the inner eyelid needs expert repair

## Loss of vision — summarizing the causes

• A central corneal foreign body or abrasion: stain with fluorescein.
• Bleeding in the front chamber: look at the iris pupil and chamber.
• A dilated pupil: ask about glare.
• Vitreous haemorrhage and retinal oedema: look with the ophthalmoscope.

After injury, reduced vision without an obvious cause may be due to:
• bleeding within the eye
• retinal oedema
• optic nerve damage

## Management plan for the injured eye

Minor eye injuries can generally be managed without the need for referral but it is very important that the patient's symptoms can be fully explained by the physical findings. Any discrepancy should lead to referral. In particular, this will help to avoid the unlikely disaster of missing an intraocular foreign body which may give few symptoms and signs in the acute stages.

## Subtarsal foreign body

Always ask how the foreign body got there, and beware hammer and chisel events. Remove by everting the upper eyelid and wiping with a cotton bud. Lid eversion (see Upper eyelid eversion, p. 9) is simple and painless and should be a routine procedure when a patient complains of a foreign body sensation. Topical anaesthetic is usually not necessary and the patient is often considerably more comfortable within seconds. There is usually no need to pad but some chloramphenicol ointment may reassure the doctor.

## Lost contact lens

Reassure the patient that these can always be found and removed. If in doubt give fluorescein which will pool round a hard lens and stain a soft lens to help locate it. If the lens is not seen, evert the top lid. The lens can be gently nudged round the conjunctival sac with a cotton bud and can be removed as it tilts (hard) or crumples (soft) with your fingers or forceps. If a hard lens has broken (uncommon), it would be wise to refer if discomfort persists and check that the pieces fit to a whole lens. Look for corneal fluorescein stain and treat for abrasion.

## Corneal abrasion (see Fig. 2.7)

A large abrasion may heal completely within 48 hours. These patients are often in considerable pain and immediate primary care is helpful. A drop of topical anaesthetic will relieve their misery and make examination of the eye much easier. Apply a pad pressed firmly over the closed eyelid since an eye that opens under a pad is liable to further injury (Fig. 10.9). If the abrasion is small the patient is allowed to remove the pad after 24 hours and report back only if the eye still feels painful. For a large abrasion it is best to see the patient in 24 hours and assess the need for further padding by restaining. If there are other signs such as haemorrhage, refer.

• A simple corneal abrasion heals in 48 hours
• Persistent symptoms suggest a foreign body or corneal ulcer

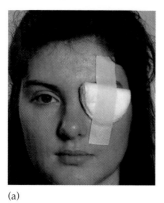 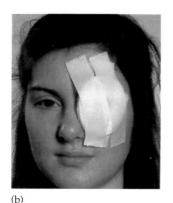

(a)    (b)

**Fig. 10.9** Padding the eye to heal a corneal abrasion, using (a) one or (b) two pads.

> A drop of local anaesthetic makes examination of the painful injured eye much easier

### Corneal foreign body (Fig. 10.10)

Corneal foreign body removal is best undertaken with a bright light and magnification and with the patient lying down. Give anaesthetic drops. Use a hypodermic needle (gauge 27) held with the point tangential to the corneal surface to lift off the foreign body. Remind yourself that the cornea is much tougher than is generally supposed, and heals rapidly. Apply chloramphenicol eye ointment and a pad (Fig. 10.9, and see also Appendix 3). Any foreign body not easily removed in this way should be referred. Don't make many attempts at removal particularly in the central cornea because this may itself damage the cornea and cause long-term scarring. Beware particularly

of the iron particle that has been present for a day or so because rust will have diffused into the surrounding cornea. Remove the particle itself if you can and refer for slit-lamp examination and removal of rust.

> • Iron on the cornea rusts quickly
> • Refer early if near the centre

### Black eyes and other blunt injuries

The patient with a black eye can be a difficult management problem because although nearly all black eyes are 'simple' without underlying eye damage, it is hard at the initial consultation to be confident of this because the swollen lids may make eye examination difficult. If the eye can be opened and is seen to be uninflamed with good vision and a clear red reflex it is reasonable to wait 24 hours and reassess. If initial eye examination is impossible or abnormal, or if there are problems at later reassessment, referral is justified. An eye which also has a subconjunctival haemorrhage should be referred if there is a history of power-tool or hammer and chisel use. Lid emphysema warrants referral because of the need for orbital X-rays though these fractures are usually not themselves serious and need only a short course of systemic antibiotics.

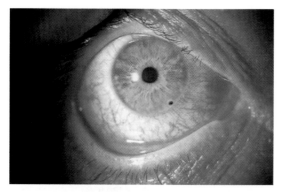

**Fig. 10.10** Corneal foreign body: a small black speck at 5 o'clock. Note the eye is most red just adjacent to it. (Courtesy of Mr A. Shun-Shin.)

### Double vision

Refer the patient with an urgency dependent on associated injuries. If the orbital floor fractures, the infraorbital nerve and inferior rectus muscle are most at risk. Examine for anaesthesia of the skin below the lower eyelid and diplopia on upgaze. Surgery may be necessary, but not as an emergency.

## Internal blood: hyphaema and vitreous haemorrhage

Blood in the front chamber of the eye (see Fig. 5.44) is an indication for immediate referral. Do not dilate the pupil. A careful search needs to be made in due course for other damage such as a retinal tear. The blood itself usually reabsorbs in a few days without permanent damage but there is a small risk of recurrent bleeding in the first 48 hours which may be much more severe. If the injured eye does not see normally or if there are multiple floaters, look with the ophthalmoscope at the red reflex and retina. Refer if there is vitreous haemorrhage or unexplained loss of vision.

## The damaged eye that appears to be perforated

An eye that is severely damaged, especially if there are clear signs of perforation such as leaking clear fluid or continued bleeding from under the lid, should not be disturbed beyond the minimun needed to confirm the injury. Usually there will be considerable periorbital bruising or lacerations and a clue to the nature of the eye injury when the lid is lifted. Instead of the normal resistance felt, the eye may feel soft beneath the lids. Other features of severe injury may be obvious such as hyphaema, corneal laceration (Fig. 10.11) or iris prolapse. Apply a gentle pad. Immediate referral is needed for these cases. No treatment should be given unless a substantial referral delay is expected in which case systemic antibiotics may be started. The patient should be told to starve ready for surgery. Their tetanus immunity should be boosted if necessary.

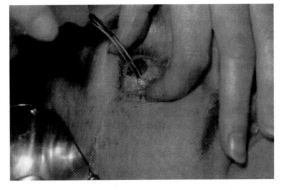

**Fig. 10.12** Irrigating the eye using a beaker, with the patient lying down.

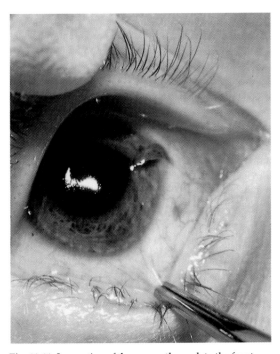

**Fig. 10.11** Laceration of the cornea through to the front chamber, with a plug of pigmented iris and a distorted pupil.

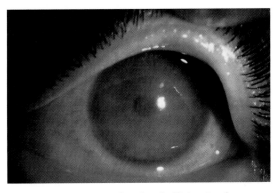

**Fig. 10.13** Hazy cornea after chemical injury is a danger sign of significant damage.

## Chemical injuries

Chemical eye injuries are common but rarely severe enough to warrant referral. In general, damage from chemicals occurs in the first few minutes after injury. Anxious patients will often come for advice many hours after minor chemical exposure. If the eye is white with normal vision and no corneal staining with fluorescein then the patient can be reassured that no harm has been done. Look particularly at the lower cornea and conjunctiva as injuries are commonly confined here because the eye has already begun to close and turn upwards as a reflex.

### Irrigation

Immediate irrigation of the eye is extremely important and may save vision if carried out within minutes of injury. It is still important even after hours if not carried out thoroughly at the time of injury. Particulate matter such as cement can remain for long periods and cause persistently high tear pH. There should be no delay in irrigation and tapwater is perfectly adequate. If possible, give a local anaesthetic drop first, lie the patient down and pour water steadily into the eye while the patient blinks (Fig. 10.12), trying to catch it in a bowl held against the face. It is better to have a wet patient than to delay irrigation. Continue for a minute or so, up to 10 minutes, and err on the side of overdoing it particularly when the chemical is alkali, plaster or cement. It is important to evert the lids at some stage during the irrigation to dislodge all but the most stubborn subtarsal particles with a cotton bud. This is kinder after topical anaesthetic.

Stain the cornea with fluorescein after irrigation and refer cases where staining is obvious. Otherwise, 24 hours of topical antibiotics and a recheck should be adequate treatment. If there is haziness of the cornea (Fig. 10.13) or blanching of the conjunctival vessels then refer. **But irrigate first— refer second.**

In chemical eye injury:
- irrigate immediately with a lot of water
- better to use tapwater than to delay
- better a wet patient than a damaged eye

## Superglue

A classic injury is accidental inoculation of superglue into the eye, sometimes because the patient uses chloromycetin ointment and makes an unfortunate mistake in picking up the wrong tube! Fortunately in most cases the eye closes quickly and apart from temporary bonding together of the eyelids no harm is done, as the lids separate spontaneously overnight and the eye is usually unharmed. Most patients would be reassured by a hospital visit.

# Chapter 11 **Eye surgery**

This section will give an outline of when surgery is appropriate, what the undertaking will imply for the patient, a brief account of the procedure and a guide to after-care and complications.

## Cataract surgery

With modern surgical techniques it is not necessary to wait for a cataract to 'ripen' as surgery may be done at any stage without undue risk. The decision to operate is based on the degree of visual disability. This may mean that a young person with 6/9 acuity and glare from a unilateral cataract may be suitable for surgery while an 80-year-old who is content with 6/36 vision and bilateral cataracts may not. The mere presence of a cataract is not an indication for its removal. To some extent it is the patient who must decide whether the level of vision has fallen enough to make surgery worth while. After all, the patient will sign the consent form, and despite what many people think, a cataract operation is not risk free.

> In deciding on cataract removal, think:
> - how much can the patient see out
> - *not* how little can the doctor see in

Almost all adult patients are now suitable for intraocular plastic lens implantation which has the major advantage of restoring sight quickly without the need for heavy glasses or a contact lens.

### Day-case cataract surgery

This has become very common, both because patients prefer it and because it is cheaper. Patients for day-case cataract surgery should usually be suitable for local anaesthesia and have uncomplicated cataracts. They should also be able to arrange their own transport for the frequent trips to the hospital that will be required, and for the trip home after surgery they should avoid public transport. A typical programme would involve three separate visits for pre-operative assessment, the operation and the first postoperative day. Thereafter the follow-up is identical to that of inpatients. A suitable day-case patient will also have someone able to help with the daily chores in the early days and to put in the eye drops necessary postoperatively.

### Local anaesthesia for cataract surgery

This is becoming increasingly common and lends itself particularly well to day-case surgery, and the predominantly elderly often have relative contraindications to general anaesthesia anyway (Fig. 11.1). Local anaesthesia is preferred for many patients because it carries little risk to their general health and the patient recovers and goes home more quickly. Most patients who have local for their first eye choose to have local again for their second. Some patients hate the thought of being awake during an eye operation and a general anaesthetic may be necessary. Other patients unsuitable for local include the confused, unco-operative or deaf (who might move during the operation) and a patient who does not speak the same language as the surgeon. Many surgeons would also request a general if the patient has only one seeing eye, as complications are minimized.

> Most patients who have local anaesthetic for their first eye operation, request it again for their second

> Local anaesthetic injection prevents the patient from seeing the operation

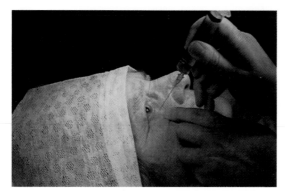

**Fig. 11.1** Local anaesthetic, given to selected patients before eye surgery, such as cataract extraction.

Local anaesthesia requires one or more injections around but not within the eye, which sting for some seconds. Afterwards the eye should be immobile, the lids incapable of squeezing and the eye insensitive to the bright light of the operating microscope. The injections will also blur and dim the vision, and patients need not worry that they will see the operation 'before their eyes' so to speak, though it is true to say that sensations of movement and bright flashes/patterns of colour are commonly experienced. The eye will be numb and the vision blurry for some hours afterwards, there may be some lid and subconjunctival bruising, and an eye patch will therefore be necessary for some time. Because of this some surgeons now advocate surgery with local anaesthetic eye drops alone (so called topical anaesthesia), though this practice is not yet widespread. Occasionally there is some bleeding at the time of giving the local around the eye in the path of the needle (retrobulbar haemorrhage) and this makes it unsafe to operate. The eye itself is not in danger though the patient may be alarmed to discover a black eye when returning to the ward. The patient is allowed home the following day and readmitted in about a month's time for surgery under general or a different type of local anaesthesia.

### The operation (Fig. 11.2)
The cataract operation itself usually lasts about 20–30 minutes and most patients tolerate the whole procedure very well, with minimal discomfort or none. Small incision surgery using a technique known as phaco-emulsification—or 'phaco' for short—is rapidly becoming the treatment of choice for the majority of patients. In comparison, extracapsular surgery involves a larger incision and is reserved for a small minority of cataracts, such as those which are very dense and are not amenable to the phaco technique (Fig. 11.3). The great advantage of phaco is that suturing is often unnecessary as the cataract is ultrasonically fragmented and sucked out through an incision which need be no larger than 3 mm! Of course this also means that the replacement intraocular lens must be folded up prior to insertion and technological developments have produced a wide range of foldable lenses (Fig. 11.4).

During cataract surgery, great care is taken to preserve the capsule or original covering of the lens. The intact back capsule in particular prevents vitreous jelly from protruding into the operative site, and so maintains normal anatomy and reduces the risk of retinal detachment. Once the new lens is in place, a judgement is made whether the wound is watertight or requires a stitch, and then the eye is padded for a few hours. If the patient has poor vision in the other eye, padding can be omitted and a clear eye shield used instead (Fig. 11.5).

### Postoperative care
Visual recovery is rapid, particularly after phaco-emulsification surgery, and many patients are pleased to find that their distance vision is clearer and brighter immediately the pad is removed. Further improvement usually occurs over the next few weeks, and a visit to the optometrist is usually recommended at 4 weeks.

After day-case surgery the eye is usually examined the following day, though there is now a trend toward 'same day' dressings. This saves the patient the return visit which reduces the advantages of day-case treatment. After the initial check, a further review is at about 2 weeks. An antibiotic and steroid eye drop combination is normally prescribed for a month after surgery.

With small incision surgery the restrictions on postoperative activities have eased considerably, and the patient can be told that most day-to-day

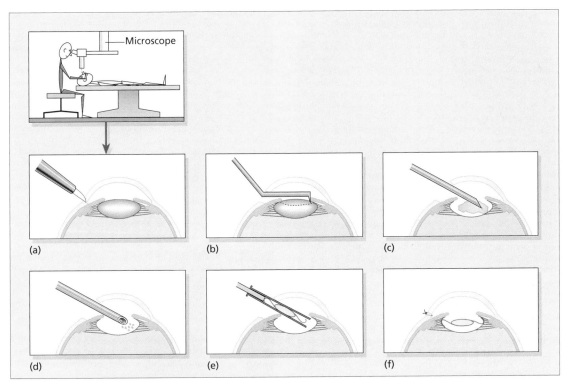

**Fig. 11.2** Phaco-emulsification surgery with lens implantation. (a) A small (3 mm) incision is made close to the edge of the cornea. (b) A bent needle punctures the front capsule of the lens in circular fashion, and a circle of lens capsule is removed. (c) The central hard nucleus is removed by an ultrasonic device which emulsifies the nucleus and sucks it out. (d) The remaining soft cortical lens matter is removed with a suction/infusion device. (e) The foldable intraocular lens implant is 'injected' into place behind the iris. (f) The lens lies within the capsule, stabilizing its position. The cornea sometimes needs a single stitch.

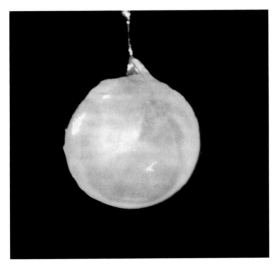

**Fig. 11.3** A cataract which has been removed at surgery — the opaque lens. (Courtesy of Mr A. Shun-Shin.)

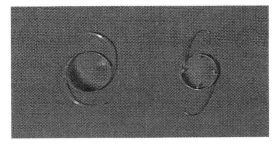

**Fig. 11.4** The plastic lens implant, inserted in place of the cataract. The legs stabilize the implant in the same position, behind the iris.

activities are perfectly safe immediately. The only real risk is a physical blow to the eye, so anything which increases this risk should be avoided for a month or so. Driving should be fine after the 2-week check if this gives the all clear, though a seat

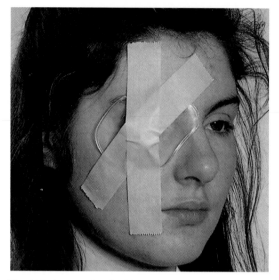

**Fig. 11.5** A protective shield may be worn at night after surgery to the internal eye.

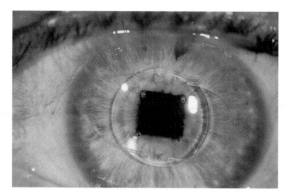

**Fig. 11.6** Unusual lens implant, clipped to the iris and causing a square pupil. Beware—do not use dilating drops.

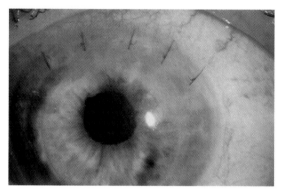

**Fig. 11.7** Five sutures in the upper cornea after traditional cataract surgery. These are often left *in situ* indefinitely.

belt must be worn without fail. Any amount of 'using the eye' is perfectly acceptable while waiting for new glasses.

Many patients are keen to be put on the waiting list for second eye surgery as soon as possible. If not, the patient can be discharged from hospital follow-up at the 2-week visit, unless there is a further problem such as glaucoma or diabetes.

> 'Using' the eye to see after a cataract operation will harm neither it nor the other eye

## Complications

The main operative complication is rupture of the back capsule of the lens. This allows vitreous jelly into the front part of the eye and increases the risk of retinal detachment. The jelly must all be removed with a specialized suction/cutter and placement of the new lens will be more difficult because of loss of the capsular support so that an iris-clip lens may be necessary (Fig. 11.6).

Much rarer, but also much more serious, is postoperative infection within the eye, endophthalmitis. This comes on a few days after surgery, and causes blurring and pain. It requires intensive antibiotic treatment and carries a risk of blindness. This underlines the need for patients to sign

a consent form and to understand that despite many technical advances a cataract operation cannot be risk free.

With the advent of small incision phaco surgery, corneal sutures are needed less frequently (Fig. 11.7), but when they are used they can break months or years later, resulting in one end of the suture sticking up proud of the cornea and causing a lot of discomfort. A good light and magnification will aid in spotting the problem, and a visit to the Eye Unit will probably be needed for the suture to be removed at the slit-lamp.

A further complication which may occur months, or even years, after surgery is clouding of the back capsule that supports the lens implant. Patients will often think that the cataract has returned. Fortunately a hole can easily be made in the thickened membrane using the YAG, or cut-

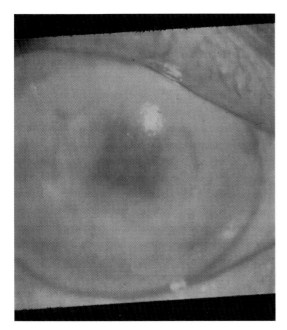

**Fig. 11.8** Corneal oedema may be a late complication after cataract surgery.

ting, laser in the outpatient department. It is a particularly satisfying form of treatment because it is quite painless and vision improves very quickly. There is little risk of the membrane ever causing trouble again.

> Laser cannot be used to treat cataract, but may be useful after the operation to clear the remaining capsule

Another delayed complication, nowadays rare, is corneal oedema, which can reduce vision dramatically (Fig. 11.8). This responds poorly to medical treatment and may be an indication for corneal grafting (see below).

## Glaucoma surgery

Surgery is needed for selected patients with chronic 'simple' glaucoma, not to improve vision, but to avoid further deterioration. All patients with acute angle closure glaucoma are treated, either by laser or conventional surgery.

## Chronic 'simple' glaucoma

When a patient is on maximum medical therapy and the intraocular pressure is still too high and/or the visual field is deteriorating, surgery is needed. The simplest procedure involves making holes with the argon laser in the anterior chamber drainage angle to try to open up a new drainage path—this is called argon laser trabeculoplasty and is quick and easy to perform at the slit-lamp as an outpatient procedure. However, the response is somewhat variable, and any beneficial effect may wear off within a year or so.

Trabeculectomy is the commonest operation, which can be done under local or general anaesthetic, but not usually as a day case. A hospital stay of 2 or 3 days is planned, and the vision can be quite blurred for a few weeks after that. A small hole is made in the sclera very close to the corneal junction, and then this is partially reclosed to allow fluid from the eye to escape through a lower resistance path (Fig. 11.9). If successful, a blister-like appearance, or bleb, develops under the upper lid which shows that fluid is successfully accumulating under the conjunctiva. The bleb appearance is thus an expected finding after trabeculectomy and the patient should be reassured. Unfortunately, postoperative scarring can close over the hole, so increasingly an antimetabolite such as 5-fluorouracil or mitomycin C is used, applied topically at the time of surgery to minimize postoperative scarring, or injected around the trabeculectomy postoperatively if the bleb is thought to be failing.

### Acute (angle closure) glaucoma

Patients with this condition are admitted to hospital urgently and treated medically with systemic acetazolamide and/or pilocarpine eye drops (see Acute glaucoma, p. 33). Once the intraocular pressure has come down and the corneal oedema resolved, a laser iridotomy or a surgical peripheral iridectomy is needed, usually to both eyes. Either of these procedures will prevent further attacks of acute glaucoma by allowing the aqueous fluid produced behind the iris a short circuit exit into the trabecular meshwork (Fig. 11.10). Laser is easier and quicker, and is usually tried first. If it fails, or if the patient is unable to sit still at the laser, then a surgical iridectomy is better.

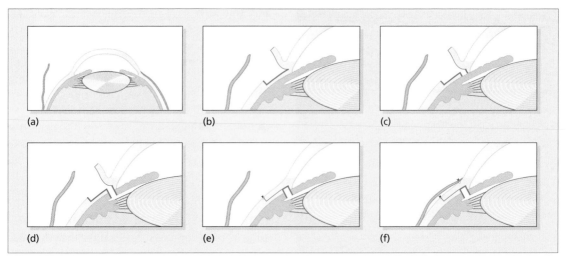

**Fig. 11.9** Trabeculectomy for chronic glaucoma. (a) The conjunctiva is dissected off the eye. (b) A partial-thickness scleral 'flap' is made ('trapdoor'). (c) A much smaller, full-thickness hole is then cut into the front of the eye. (d) A peripheral iridectomy is made. (e) The scleral 'trapdoor' is loosely stitched back into place. (f) The conjunctiva is stitched back into place.

## Retinal detachment surgery

Most patients with a retinal detachment should have surgery within days of diagnosis because the detachment can deteriorate quickly and lost vision may not be restored if surgery is delayed. Patients will find themselves being admitted from the casualty department and planned for surgery the same evening or the following day. Exceptions to this include a detachment obviously of long-standing and those which are complicated, requiring further investigation or subspecialist referral.

### Timing of surgery

A detachment results from a tear or tears in the retina (Fig. 11.11) which is usually peripheral and beyond the range of the direct ophthalmoscope. The tear allows the retina to lift off its bed and collapse into the eye. Gravity helps this if the detachment is in the upper part of the retina (see Fig. 3.9). Fluid accumulates between the retina and its base as the detachment progresses and this is encouraged by eye movements and vitreous detachment. The process can take weeks to progress to total detachment and in the early stages when only the peripheral retina is 'off' the patient may not be aware of any visual defect and may ignore symptoms such as flashing lights and floaters. As the detachment spreads it eventually causes the macula to come off when vision will fall dramatically (Fig. 11.12). The macula deteriorates quickly when deprived of its source of oxygen in the underlying choroid and recovery of vision depends directly on the speed with which surgery is carried out once the macula is off.

### The operation (Fig. 11.13)

A general anaesthetic is usually given and the operation can take several hours. The patient is warned beforehand that the other eye will be carefully examined at the time of surgery and any weak areas in the retina will be treated with cryotherapy or laser (see below). This may make the eye sore but will not affect vision. The operated eye will be much more sore.

The main principles of retinal detachment surgery are:
• Carefully examine the retina of both eyes to detect all retinal tears.
• Apply forces to move back the detached retina into contact with the retinal pigment epithelium base.
• Cause an inflammatory reaction around any retinal break so that scarring will prevent fluid getting under it again.

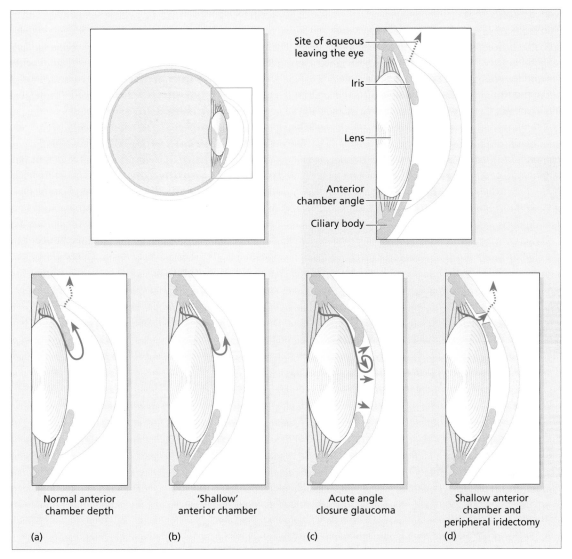

Site of aqueous leaving the eye

Iris

Lens

Anterior chamber angle

Ciliary body

Normal anterior chamber depth

(a)

'Shallow' anterior chamber

(b)

Acute angle closure glaucoma

(c)

Shallow anterior chamber and peripheral iridectomy

(d)

**Fig. 11.10** Peripheral iridectomy for acute glaucoma. (a) Normal drainage. In a shallow anterior chamber, the peripheral iris rests too close to the aqueous drainage channels (b). If the iris blocks off the drainage, acute angle closure glaucoma develops (c). This cannot happen in the presence of a peripheral iridectomy (d).

There are two ways to achieve the second aim. Either the outside of the eye can be pressed inward to meet the detached retina, or a bubble of gas can be placed inside the eye to push the retina outward. In many cases both techniques are used. Vitrectomy surgery is becoming increasingly popular because it allows a much larger bubble to be inserted, and also because it is done with an operating microscope and the magnification available allows better recognition of small retinal breaks.

Scleral buckling together with a gas bubble which may be combined with removal of the vitreous—vitrectomy—is the most common operation, usually under general anaesthesia. From the patient's perspective it may be useful to describe the buckle and the bubble as the two ends of a clamp, between which the retina is sandwiched and pressed back into place with slow-set 'gluing' with laser or freezing (cryotherapy). After a week or two the clamp is released as the bubble spontaneously reabsorbs and by then the glue has set and the retina should stay in place.

At the time of surgery the non-affected eye is also carefully examined because sometimes the retina will show that a tear might form, or a tear may already be present without frank detachment. In either case, because the retina is not detached, all that is needed is some 'gluing' with cryotherapy or laser in the damaged area to cause a scar which will prevent fluid getting under the retina and detaching it.

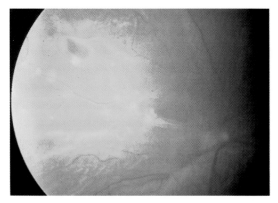

**Fig. 11.11** Detached retina with fluid collected below the optic nerve head on the lower left. An oval tear is visible at 10 o'clock to the disc and a pink retinal hole further to the right.

## Postoperative care

Postoperative care has come a long way from the old days of 2 weeks prolonged strict bed rest with the head immobile between sandbags. For the first week or so the patient will probably be asked to adopt a head-down position much of the day to help the bubble press backwards. Once the bubble disperses the patient is usually aware that side vision has been restored, but recovery of central vision can take months and is rarely complete. Depending on the ease with which the patient adapts to positioning, a return home is likely within 2 or 3 days.

## Complications

The main complication is failure to reattach the retina, occurring in about 20% of cases, even in the

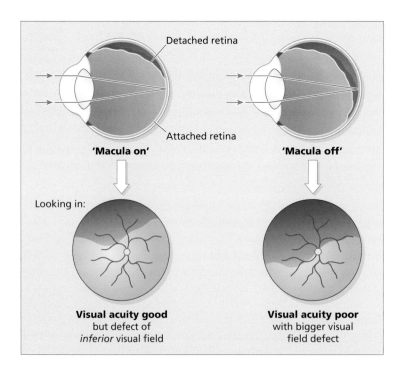

**Fig. 11.12** Vision and retinal detachment.

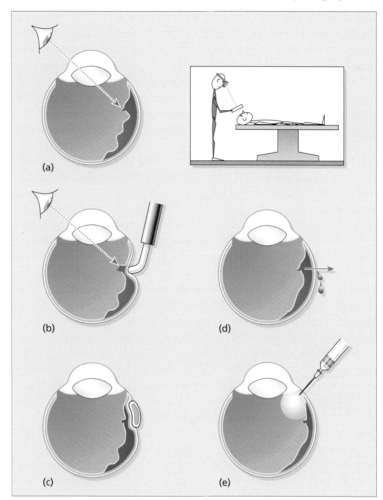

**Fig. 11.13** Retinal detachment surgery. (a) The retinal hole(s) or tear(s) are found. (b) A cryoprobe is used to initiate an inflammatory reaction involving the retina and choroid around the break. (c) A scleral buckle (silicone sponge or rubber) is stitched onto the eye to indent it and keep the retina pressed against the choroid. (d) If the retina is widely detached, it is sometimes necessary to puncture the eye with a small needle so the fluid under the retina can drain out. This allows the cryotherapy probe to freeze the retina. (e) Sometimes a bubble of gas is injected into the eye to help keep the retina pressed against the choroid. The patient will be asked to adopt an abnormal head posture for some days.

best surgical hands. Some retinas are poor material to begin with, and tear very easily. If the retina has been folded up for some time it may be very difficult to smooth out and flatten back into place successfully, so be guarded in suggesting outcome. With further surgery the anatomical success rate goes up to well over 90%, and in these difficult cases intraocular liquid silicone oil may be used. The use of scleral buckles alters the shape of the eye, causing astigmatism by twisting and sometimes myopia by lengthening, so a change in glasses is often necessary to get best vision. The scleral buckle can cause chronic discomfort, or may extrude through the conjunctiva, in which case removal will be necessary even though there

is a small risk of recurrent retinal detachment. Occasionally, despite repeated operations, it proves impossible to re-attach the retina, because scar tissue forms on the surface converting it from a thin and supple membrane into a thickened and more rigid sheet of tissue which resists being pressed back into place. This process is called proliferative vitreo-retinopathy or PVR.

## Squint surgery

Squint surgery for children is usually cosmetic, while in adults it may either be to improve appearance or to overcome double vision. Squint in early childhood does not usually cause diplopia because the brain suppresses one of the images, but this ability is lost in adulthood. An orthoptist is usually involved in the decision to operate, and management after surgery will also often be monitored by the orthoptist.

The main priority in childhood squint is visual development and avoidance of amblyopia, often with patching, and sometimes also with glasses. Surgery can be done at any time if parents' concern about the appearance is great, especially if the child is becoming self conscious, but patching and glasses may still be needed for some time postoperatively. A popular time for surgery is in the fifth year, before or soon after starting school, to avoid the particularly unkind teasing that other children can give the squinting child. In older children who have lost the ability to suppress doubling, surgery may be needed as eye strain may be followed by diplopia, particularly when reading or studying if the child does not take a break. Some squinting adults may ask about cosmetic surgery, sometimes rather shyly at a time when they are looking for a partner, so it is wise to be sensitive to their request and it is worth referring for assessment.

A childhood squint that persists into adult life can deteriorate, whether or not operated upon, because the 'squinting' eye has a tendency to drift further and further outwards. Surgery should help, though the eye may wander again.

### The operation (Fig. 11.14)
General anaesthesia is usual, though in selected cases a local anaesthetic may be preferable. There are two ways an eye can be straightened, and sometimes both are needed if the angle is large. Either the muscle that works in the direction of the squint is loosened (recessed), or the twinned muscle being stretched can be shortened and strengthened (resected). For recession, the muscle tendon is detached from the eye close to its insertion, and reattached to the eyeball a measured distance further back. For resection, the tendon is again divided, but this time the muscle is shortened by a measured amount before being re-attached to the eye at the original place. The same principles hold for vertical squint surgery, though this tends to be more complicated; the two directions may be combined in one operation.

The amount the muscles are moved is very tiny—a matter of millimetres—and it is often difficult to get the eyes perfectly straight. Some surgeons now use adjustable sutures which are loosened or tightened a fraction until the double vision is gone, with the patient awake after the operation. This can be done at the bedside under local anaesthetic. The technique is particularly useful in patients with thyroid eye disease. It is not as unpleasant as it sounds, though it is not suitable for children.

Many squint operations are now done on a day-case basis. An operated eye will be red and a bit sore because of stitches on the surface, but this only lasts a few days. Antibiotic drops are prescribed for about 2 weeks, during which time swimming should be avoided. Then an orthoptic check is carried out. Children tolerate the surgery very well, and eye patching is not necessary afterwards.

Sometimes an injection of botulinum toxin into one of the eye muscles can substitute for surgery, or may be helpful in assessing the need for surgery. The injection can easily be done under topical anaesthetic and is not as dangerous as it sounds.

## Corneal graft surgery
Corneal grafting to improve vision is usually done as a planned operation; occasionally an urgent graft may be needed to repair a badly damaged or perforated cornea. Herpetic corneal scarring and keratoconus (see p. 92) are the two most common indications. Until relatively recently it was not possible to maintain donated corneas in a viable state for more than 48 hours, so corneal grafting always had to be carried out at short notice. Now it is possible to keep a donated cornea in culture medium for up to a month, which means that surgery can be planned well in advance. Corneal material is obtained from the United Kingdom Transplant Service, who will be asked to provide donor material for a given date when a patient is due to be admitted for surgery.

General anaesthesia is often preferred but is not essential. The operation takes an hour or two, and can be combined with cataract surgery if necessary. Usually the entire thickness of the cornea is removed in the form of a disc and replaced with a

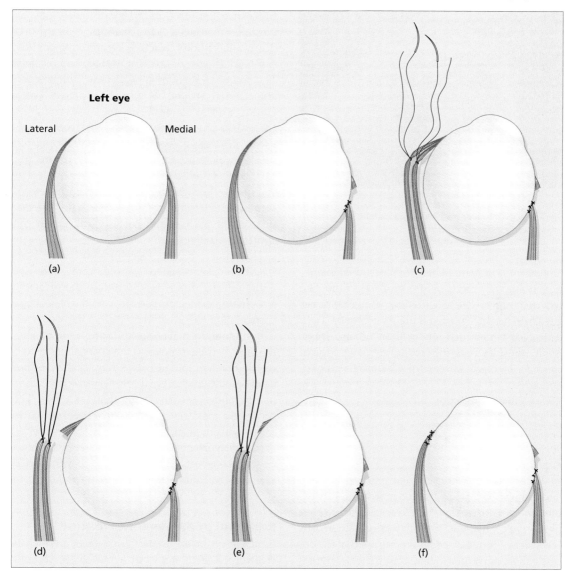

**Fig. 11.14** 'Recess/resect' squint surgery. (a) Representation of inward deviation of eye (convergent squint). (b) The medial rectus muscle insertion is cut, and the muscle reattached at a measured distance further back (typically 5 mm). (c) The lateral rectus muscle is ligated a measured distance back from its insertion (typically 5 mm). (d) The lateral rectus muscle is cut in front of the stitch and the muscle stump is cut off. (e) The shortened muscle can now be reattached to the eyeball. (f) Because the medial rectus has been weakened and the lateral rectus tightened, the eye is straightened.

donor corneal 'button' about 8 mm in diameter stitched in place, an operation called penetrating keratoplasty (Fig. 11.15). Sometimes only the superficial cornea is replaced—a lamellar keratoplasty—which has the advantage of low risk of rejection.

Grafted patients require close follow-up in the early stages, and may well be in hospital for a few days postoperatively to start eye drops and to check for wound leaks or early graft rejection. Multiple outpatient visits will be needed, and the patient will be encouraged to report urgently with

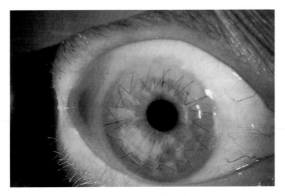

**Fig. 11.15** Sutures of a corneal graft with a zig-zag pattern. These may be removed once the wound has healed if they cause astigmatism or irritation.

any increase in pain, redness or blurring of vision, which are warning signs for graft rejection. The risk of rejection lessens with time, though it never goes to zero, thus grafted patients use steroid eye drops for very much longer than others. Treatment of graft rejection with intensive topical steroids is often successful if started quickly enough.

Corneal graft rejection may cause:

- aching pain
- photophobia
- redness
- fall in vision.

Visual recovery after corneal grafting is slow, and it may take up to a year or more. The sutures inevitably cause some uneven pulling which twists the cornea into irregular astigmatism, but the stitches cannot be removed immediately because the wound takes a long time to heal. There is likely to be some residual astigmatism even if all the sutures are eventually removed, and most patients will need glasses or a contact lens to get best vision. The patient can become despondent during the time of waiting and may imagine the graft has been a failure. Of course if astigmatism is not present new glasses can be prescribed early.

### Corneal refractive procedures

Patients may have heard of these latest developments in the popular press and may ask about their availability. Some years ago it became possible to lessen myopia by making a series of cuts in the cornea, known as radial keratotomy—now an outdated treatment. A much simpler laser procedure called photorefractive keratotomy, or PRK, can treat greater degrees of myopia more safely. The laser, of 'Excimer' type, is now widely available, though in the UK only on a private basis. Under topical anaesthesia the laser removes corneal tissue to modify corneal curvature. Usually the curvature is lessened to correct myopia, but it is now possible to increase the curvature and treat low degrees of long sightedness. Understandably, the surface of the eye is very sore for sometime afterwards, and occasionally the patient is left with a faint corneal scar which can spoil the visual result.

The most recent development has been 'LASIK'—laser-assisted *in situ* keratomileusis. Although the title is long winded, the principle is actually quite simple. To avoid the surface corneal damage inflicted by PRK, a flap of cornea is first hinged up, like decapitating a boiled egg, the laser is then applied to the corneal tissue and the flap is then folded back—remarkably, it does not need stitching. Visual recovery is quicker, less painful and eventually better than with PRK. The prospects for very short-sighted people to do away with their glasses have never been better, though at a price of course—no surgery is without risk, and the best advice for someone who is used to glasses or contact lenses is still, by and large, to stick with them!

### Removal of an eye (enucleation)

Enucleation means removal of an eye which is clearly a drastic step, but a malignant tumour may be present, or the eye may be blind and also painful. The removal of a blind eye that is disfigured may also be justified on cosmetic grounds. Finally, a severely damaged eye may be removed early after injury to avoid a very rare complication known as sympathetic ophthalmia.

General anaesthesia is needed. The muscles are detached and the optic nerve is cut. An orbital implant is often placed to occupy the space, the muscles are stitched to give this a degree of movement, and the conjunctiva is carefully sewn over the front to prevent the implant working through to the surface. The conjunctiva forms a smooth

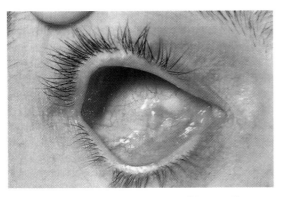

**Fig. 11.16** Eye socket after enucleation of the eye. This is fitted with an artificial eye.

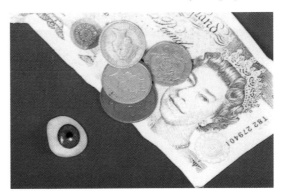

**Fig. 11.18** The patient with an artificial eye may use it 'to keep an eye on' money overnight if they prefer not to sleep with it *in situ*.

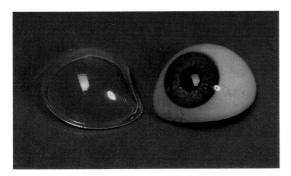

**Fig. 11.17** A glass shell helps to conform the new eye socket, and the patient is then fitted with a personalized artificial eye, made of plastic and moulded to the socket.

pink healthy pouch or socket, looking like the inside of the mouth (Fig. 11.16). A glass shell placed over the conjunctiva maintains the normal eyelid position while the patient waits to have an artificial eye fitted (Fig. 11.17). The patient is taught how to put the shell in and take it out on a daily basis because it should be cleaned to avoid infection. It may take a few days for the patient to become confident with this technique, after which he is allowed home. About a month later an artificial eye is fitted, similar in shape to the glass shell and like a hard plastic hemi-dome rather than a sphere, with iris detail hand painted on it to match the other eye.

The eye should be thought of rather like dentures are, and many patients prefer to remove and clean their prosthesis at the same time as their dentures. One patient remarked that he would put his false eye next to his money beside the bed, to 'keep an eye on it' (Fig. 11.18)! The prosthesis needs to be polished if it becomes unsightly or if the socket becomes sticky. Treat stickiness as conjunctivitis. If the patient looks cosmetically poor, refer back to the artificial eye service for advice. Following eye removal and successful fitting of an artificial eye, no ophthalmic follow-up is needed, though the patient will keep in touch with the prosthetist from the Artificial Eye Service. Complications include extrusion of the implant and later orbital shrinkage so that further oculoplastic surgery may be needed.

## Postoperative eye drops

Most eye operations are followed by a course of eye drops, usually antibiotic or steroid or a combination of the two. Cataract patients for instance will usually be given a combined antibiotic + steroid preparation four times a day for the first 2 weeks, then perhaps twice daily for another 2 weeks. After corneal grafting the treatment regime is much more intense, often involving hourly or 2 hourly steroid drops in the first week to avoid rejection. Squint surgery on the other hand may only require an antibiotic drop, four times a day for 2 weeks.

Important practical points to remember are:
• Postoperative eye drops are important.
• Re-prescribe promptly if requested in the first 2 weeks.

- Use drops four times daily if correct dosage is unknown—this can do no harm.

Postoperative drops commonly prescribed include the following.

### Antibiotics, such as chloramphenicol

Prescribed after most eye operations. One drop four times daily is adequate, which can be increased to a drop every hour if infection is present.

### Corticosteroid

Used to shorten postoperative inflammation and to minimize scarring. Not usually prescribed without an antibiotic. Numerous combinations exist. Most common are Betnesol N (betamethasone and neomycin) and Maxitrol (dexamethasone and neomycin). The commonest dosage is four times daily.

### Dilating

Prescribed for patient comfort and/or to keep the pupil dilated for examination. Intraocular surgery can cause a degree of iritis with resultant photophobia for which twice daily atropine works well. It is used most often after retinal detachment surgery; most cataract surgery patients do not need postoperative dilating drops.

### Pressure lowering

It is quite common for the eye pressure to rise in the first few days after intraocular surgery, for which a beta-blocker such as timolol can be used, with Diamox tablets if necessary. The Diamox is stopped quickly as the pressure falls, but the timolol may well continue for a few weeks.

## Minor surgery around the eyes

Minor operations around the eye are those that can be done under local anaesthetic, using few instruments, need only low-power magnification (if any) and do not expose the patient to risk. For some operations, the skills can be learnt just with brief training, and any doctor with reasonable dexterity who is interested could do them in their own surgery. Others are better done in an eye unit. No clear boundary separates the two. What follows lists the equipment necessary. Training should be available by contacting the local oph-

thalmologist and arranging to attend a minor surgery list. This book does not aim to be a manual of surgery, but explains the indications for, and briefly describes, the operations with the likely outcome and follow-up where appropriate.

Three procedures which are ideally suitable for GPs to learn are removal of ingrowing eyelashes, syringeing tear ducts and drainage of a meibomian cyst. They are common problems which are rewarding to treat, both for the patient and the doctor, and the techniques are not hazardous.

> Three minor procedures the GP might offer:
> - remove an ingrowing eyelash
> - syringe a tear duct
> - incise and drain a meibomian cyst

Patients attending for minor surgery, except for syringeing, should be warned that they are likely to have a patch on the eye afterwards, and should not drive home.

> If an eye patch is on, driving is off

The minor operations need to be done with the patient lying down and with a bright anglepoise-type light.

### Ingrowing eyelashes (trichiasis)

Eyelashes may grow in the wrong direction and scratch the cornea even without the lid turning in. With a good pair of flat-ended forceps and a loupe, these can easily be pulled out, giving instant relief to the patient, who is usually most grateful for this simple service. *Every general practice should offer this service*, at least. It is safe, simple and effective. If the problem is recurrent, and many are, the patient can be referred for electrolysis to the hair follicle. This fiddly job is best done under good magnification and illumination, so an operating microscope is ideal. An injection of lignocaine is needed in most cases. A fine electrode is inserted beside the offending lash, and its root is destroyed by cautery.

### Syringeing the tear ducts (Fig. 11.19)

This is appropriate for patients with apparently normal eyes which 'water', with tears spilling

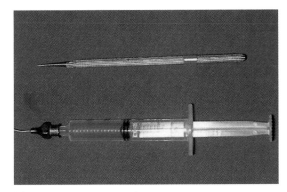

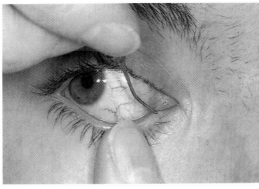

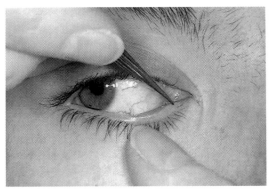

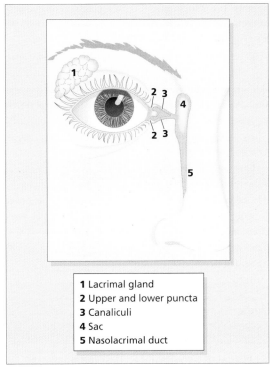

**1** Lacrimal gland
**2** Upper and lower puncta
**3** Canaliculi
**4** Sac
**5** Nasolacrimal duct

**Fig. 11.20** Tear production and drainage, based on an illustration by Lizzie Ambler.

**Fig. 11.19** Dilating the lacrimal punctum and syringeing the duct for a patient with a watering eye. (a) Equipment. (b) Dilatation. (c) Syringeing.

down the cheek (Fig. 11.20). Syringeing the tear drainage might clear an obstruction. The cannula is passed along parallel to the lid margin, towards the nose.

*Instruments*
• Nettleship's dilator with a good straight point.
• Fine metal cannula.
• Two millilitre syringe.
• Normal saline.

*Anaesthesia*
• Benoxinate drops, or equivalent, to the eye surface.

*Magnification*
• A binocular loupe may help.

*Procedure*
• Put in a few drops of anaesthetic.
• Dilate the lower punctum, pushing firmly but not roughly once sure the tip is in the duct.
• Insert the cannula gently into the tear canal.
• Inject saline, which should pass into the tear sac and down the duct into the patient's nose. The saline may reflux through the top punctum, which

means the blockage is further down the duct, otherwise the saline cannot go anywhere, except to squirt back out of the lower punctum.

When syringeing fails to stop the watering, the patient will need to be assessed by a surgeon. As the operation to make a new canal or duct is a delicate procedure, usually done under general anaesthesia, and with variable success, many older patients prefer to continue carrying a handkerchief instead.

Do not try to syringe babies with watery eyes, who usually get better if you wait long enough. Those which persist beyond 12 months may need a probing, when the syringeing goes slightly further, and the cannula is passed down the duct. This requires day-case admission with a general anaesthetic such as ketamine.

> Be wary, very occasionally:
> • tear duct block is due to a tumour
> • a meibomian cyst may be really a dermoid cyst

### Removal of a meibomian cyst (chalazion)
(Fig. 11.21)
After an initial acute inflammation, these lumps may remain uncomfortable and ugly, and the patient asks for their removal. They are incised and curetted from the conjunctival side of the lid.

*Instruments*
• Chalazion clamp.
• Small curette.
• Scalpel (15 blade).

*Anaesthesia*
• Oxybuprocaine hydrochloride (benoxinate) drops or equivalent to the eye, and
• 2% lignocaine with adrenaline (epinephrine) injected into the lid.

*Magnification*
• None essential, but presbyopes should wear their reading glasses!

*Procedure*
• Give the anaesthesia (Fig. 11.22).
• The clamp (Fig. 11.23) is applied to the lid to encircle the lump.

• The lid is everted and the cyst incised vertically and curetted, taking care to avoid the lid margins and tear canal.
• The eye is padded for 4 hours, after which chloramphenicol ointment is applied three times a day for 3 days.
• The patient can return to most normal activities the next day, except for contact lens wear which must wait for 72 hours. This cyst should not recur, but other new ones may form in the future.

**Caution! Make sure a 'chalazion' in the top lid near the outer margin is not really a dermoid cyst emerging from deep in the orbit!** (See Chronic swelling around the eye, p. 99, Fig. 5.58.)

### Retropunctal cauterization (Fig. 11.24)
If the patient resembles a bloodhound, the watering may be due to the lower punctum falling away from the eyeball so that the tears cannot enter the normal drainage. By causing a scar inside the lid, just below the canal, the punctum will be drawn back into place as the scar tissue shrinks.

*Instruments*
• Hand-held cautery (Fig. 11.25).

*Anaesthesia*
• Oxybuprocaine hydrochloride (benoxinate) drops or equivalent to the eye, and
• 2% lignocaine with adrenaline (epinephrine) injected into the lower lid.

*Magnification*
• Loupes may help.

*Procedure*
• After giving the anaesthetics, the lower lid is everted and, taking care to avoid the lower canal by going below and lateral to it, four or five cautery burns are made through the conjunctiva into the lower lid. How long to apply the cautery varies with different instruments, but as a rule use enough to produce whitening of the tissues to twice the radius of the cautery point. In practice, this should take about 5 seconds with the battery-operated cauterizer. One side-effect is the burning smell, so warn the patient not to be alarmed.

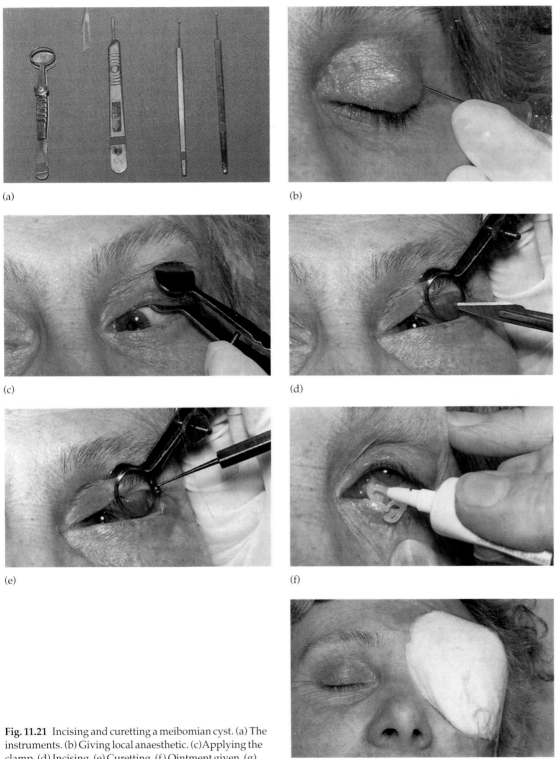

**Fig. 11.21** Incising and curetting a meibomian cyst. (a) The instruments. (b) Giving local anaesthetic. (c) Applying the clamp. (d) Incising. (e) Curetting. (f) Ointment given. (g) Firm double pad applied.

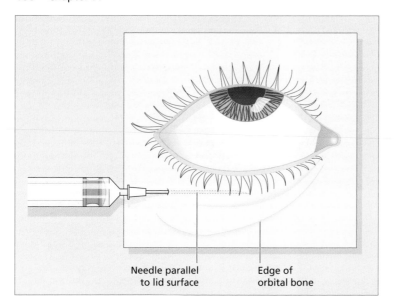

**Fig. 11.22** Injecting anaesthetic into the lower eyelid.

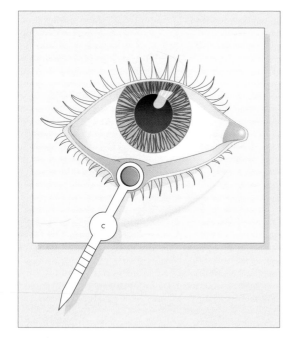

**Fig. 11.23** Chalazion clamp applied.

• Chloramphenicol ointment is applied and the eye is padded for 4 hours. The eye is sore for less than a week, for which time topical antibiotics can be continued twice daily.

### 'Three snip' operation (Fig. 11.26)
If the eye waters because the lower punctum is too small, a bigger hole must be made. Such patients benefit from dilatation and syringeing but watering soon returns.

*Instruments*
• A pair of very fine pointed spring scissors.
• Nettleship's punctum dilator.

*Anaesthesia*
• As for retropunctal cautery (p. 186).

*Magnification*
• Loupes.

*Procedure*
• Give the anaesthetics.
• Dilate the lower punctum.
• Insert one blade of the scissors and make the three snips on the conjunctival surface: one at right angles, one parallel to the lid margin, and the third across the base of the triangle of tissue made by the first two.
• Chloramphenicol ointment is applied and the eye padded for 4 hours.
• The eye is sore for about 5 days during which time continue ointment at night.

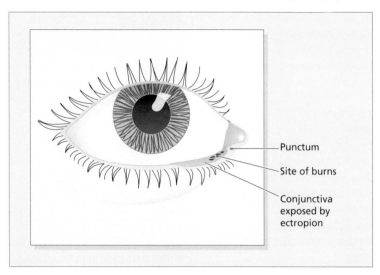

Fig. 11.24 Retropunctal
cauterization.

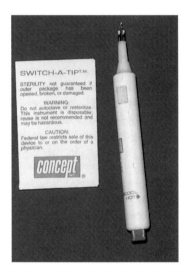

Fig. 11.25 Equipment for cauterization behind the lacrimal punctum.

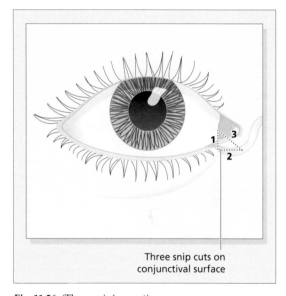

Fig. 11.26 'Three snip' operation.

## Tarsorrhaphy

This is an operation to keep the eyelids closed by sewing them together, either totally, or more usually just on the lateral side. This is to protect the cornea when blinking is poor or eye closure is lost (e.g. Bell's palsy or thyroid eye disease), or perhaps the cornea has lost sensation, with a risk of ulceration.

A strip of lid margin is removed from the corresponding edges of both lids to create raw surfaces which are then stitched together. The sutures are tied over rubber tubing to stop them cutting in to the skin, as they have to be tight enough to allow the two lids to heal together, and they are left in for at least 2 weeks. This minor operation can be undone at any time in the future if the protection is no longer needed.

More recently, 'superglue' has been used instead, which will stick the lids together for short periods. Longer term (2–3 months) coverage of the cornea just using the top eyelid can now be achieved using botulinum toxin. This causes a ptosis which gradually wears off over 8–12 weeks, when a further injection can be given if needed.

## Entropion

An entropion is where the edge of the eyelid is turned inwards, so that the eyelashes rub on the cornea. In western countries this is usually part of an ageing change and affects just the lower lid. In patients from some third-world countries, the entropion may be due to scarring of the conjunctiva from chronic infection with trachoma, when the top lid is most affected. In either case, not only is it painful to have eyelashes scratching the cornea, but this may cause scarring and blindness. Surgery is needed to treat entropion, though some patients manage to relieve the symptoms by pulling down on the lower lid with tape stuck vertically downwards from just below the lid margin to the cheek.

A variety of operations exists, determined by the type of entropion and the surgeon's preference. All can be done under local anaesthetic, infiltrated into the lids. The commonest operation on the lower lid is when a 'tuck' is taken in the outside of the lid by cutting out a full-thickness wedge and sewing the edges of the wound together, thus tightening the outer lid margin. This heals well within 2 weeks, and is not as uncomfortable as it sounds. A useful alternative, especially for the infirm or immobile patient, is to use a suturing technique. This involves inserting three double-ended 6-00 catgut sutures in to the lower lid. The needle passes from the lower fornix, through the lid, emerging just below the lashes. As each pair is then tied, the lid turns out. The sutures are left to dissolve, and the track of scar tissue creates the tension needed to maintain the lid position. More complicated procedures are needed for upper lid entropion. Even the simpler operation needs care in sewing the lid back together without causing a notch in the margin, which would disturb the tear-film. A period of training would be necessary for anyone thinking of doing this operation.

## Ectropion

This describes a lower eyelid which sags away from the eyeball, like a bloodhound. As with entropion, it is most common in elderly patients with lax skin, but paralysis of facial muscles may be the cause, such as a Bell's palsy, or leprosy in endemic areas. The effect either way is that tears spill down the cheek and the exposed conjunctiva of the lid becomes inflamed, so surgery becomes appropriate. A vicious circle can develop as the patient dabs the eye and so drags the lower lid further down. The operation is like that for entropion, to tighten the lid by excising a wedge, but in this case from the inside. Some ectropions are secondary to chronic skin conditions of the face such as eczema, rosacea or scleroderma, in which case this underlying cause must be treated to prevent recurrence.

## Conjunctival cysts (see Fig. 5.35)

Patients may complain that such cysts look unsightly, or that the eye irritates. This is due to the cyst lifting the lid clear of the cornea, causing a dry patch. Using an anaesthetic eye drop, it is easy to burst the cyst with a needle, but they often recur. In that case they can be cut out, sewing the conjunctiva back together with a dissolvable suture, but even this may cause another inclusion cyst to form. For excision, a bleb of lignocaine is put under the conjunctiva first.

## Pterygium (see Fig. 5.32)

A pterygium is a fleshy 'growth' which can creep onto the cornea, usually from the medial side. They cause much alarm, but are seldom a problem, and they are benign. Like a conjunctival cyst, they may cause drying of the adjacent cornea, which is irritating but responds to lubricating drops or ointment. Patients fear that they will grow right across the eye and blind them, but this is almost always unfounded. Only those which are clearly rapidly growing should be removed, as they tend to recur even after the most careful shaving from the cornea. This should only be done by an experienced surgeon using an operating microscope, so it is not a minor operation.

# Chapter 12 **Management of visual handicap**

Learning that poor sight is not going to improve is a painful moment in anyone's life. The nature of the problem, its prognosis, and details of any ongoing treatment will have been explained in the clinic, and arrangements made for low visual aid assessment. It is at this time very helpful if a specialist medical social worker is available, who will have the expertise and time to listen to the patient's worries, help to put things into perspective and, if necessary, to interpret medical information. Letting people know how others in the same situation have coped makes the difficulties more bearable. S/he can also advise on making the best use of remaining vision to get organized in anticipation of possible further deterioration. Most of us would benefit from more methodical habits.

Visual handicap, arising as it does from a variety of disease processes, is not a homogeneous entity. The field of vision, as well as the visual acuity, affects the individual's capacity to function in a world designed for the sighted. People's needs differ, too. What is intolerable to the lonely retired academic will probably not worry the busy housewife with a supportive family. Many patients with poor vision worry particularly about keeping up standards of appearance, either personal or domestic, when they can no longer tell if things are clean or dirty.

## Loss of central vision
This is usually due to macular disease, most often age-related macular degeneration, the commonest cause of blind registration in those over 65. The gradually progressive 'dry' sort generally, though not always, causes smaller areas of retinal degeneration than the sudden 'disciform' type, which means that a variable area of relatively sensitive retina around the fovea may be available to be exploited by the use of magnifying aids. Macular degeneration, by definition, does not affect peripheral vision, something in which the ophthalmologist, as well as the patient, can take comfort when discussing the matter. Diabetic maculopathy is another common cause of poor central vision, mainly in older type II diabetics, and tends to cause a rather patchy central loss. It may, of course, be accompanied by proliferative retinopathy which carries a threat to all vision.

Practical problems may arise with 'near vision' tasks. The following is a selection with which most difficulty is found:
- reading letters and newspapers
- sewing
- seeing prices in shops
- signing things
- eating meals
- telling the time
- pouring liquids
- cutting finger and toe nails.

Driving, which needs around 6/9 Snellen acuity binocularly, will have been abandoned by the time these activities give trouble. Other 'distance' difficulties are seeing the numbers on buses, and, very frequently mentioned by patients, and obviously very important, recognizing friends and acquaintances in the street. It's surprising how little understanding can be shown. Fortunately, mobility is less of a problem as peripheral vision is preserved.

## Loss of visual field alone
The degree of handicap will depend on the nature and extent of the visual field deficit. Surprisingly, bumping into things is rarely complained of before the field approaches the proverbial tunnel. By this time, locating such everyday things as one's plate of food or the clock are major hurdles. Driving is precluded by homonymous or bitem-

poral hemianopias, and any other condition giving a smaller binocular field than the statutory 120 degrees in the horizontal and 20 degrees above and below fixation (Fig. 12.1). Advanced glaucoma, retinitis pigmentosa and, occasionally, extensive pan-retinal photocoagulation for proliferative diabetic retinopathy can all lead to this amount of loss of field. Reading is difficult with a homonymous hemianopia, especially one to the right, and with a very constricted field from glaucoma. It is often hard for people in this situation to grasp that their reading will not be facilitated by 'stronger' glasses. Try to explain that it is not a focusing problem but rather something wrong with the 'computer'.

## Loss of both acuity and field

Handicap here varies from mild, as in the case of early cataracts, to severe, as following bilateral vitreous haemorrhages due to proliferative diabetic retinopathy (fortunately now comparatively rare as a result of laser treatment). With cataract, practical difficulties may be greater than the Snellen acuity would imply. In bright conditions, glare can considerably reduce vision. Commonly, profound loss of central and peripheral field of vision is due to a combination of diagnoses, such as glaucoma plus macular degeneration or cataract.

## Other visual handicaps

### Colour vision defects
These are mostly of importance in choosing a

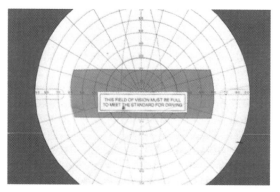

**Fig. 12.1** The field of vision (with both eyes open) needed for driving is shown in pink.

career. Eight per cent of the male population has congenitally imperfect colour vision, almost always of the 'red/green' variety. Inheritance is of sex-linked recessive type, unaffected female carriers passing the gene to 50% of their sons. Bright colours can usually be matched but problems arise with pastels or dark colours. The Ishihara colour vision test will pick out all colour anomalies. Further testing is needed to determine the relevance of the particular defect to the occupation under consideration. Some occupations such as the railways (train crew), the fire services and the Royal National Lifeboat Institution require normality on Ishihara testing, whereas others perform their own, less exacting testing (the Civil Aviation Authority, the Royal Navy). Colour vision defects are not a bar to driving, despite traffic lights.

A specialist medical social worker provides great support to those newly registered as blind or partially sighted

Disease confined to the macula should not affect mobility

### Night blindness
This is most often due to retinitis pigmentosa and usually dates from early in life (see p. 45). Affected individuals regard it as normal not to be able to see in the dark! The condition can preclude driving and various careers including the fire services.

### Loss of vision in one eye
Adaptation to using one eye alone takes longer in the old than in the young. It is not in itself a reason for Partially Sighted Registration or a bar to ordinary driving, assuming there is normal vision and field in the remaining eye. However, professional and vocational (formerly Heavy Goods Vehicle and Public Service Vehicle) driving is precluded. Monocularity will also exclude a number of other careers.

### Low vision aids
Many people, finding that their reading glasses are not 'strong enough' will buy a magnifier for

themselves and start resorting to large print books. If these are insufficient for their needs, referral to the local eye department's low vision clinic may be useful. Unfortunately, provision of these clinics nationwide is patchy. A few opticians provide a low vision service, but this has to be paid for by the patient. Generally, it is easier to provide magnification for near than for distance (Fig. 12.2). High 'plus', strong convex lenses resembling reading glasses are the most popular, giving a wider field of view and leaving the hands free, as well as looking more 'normal'. Visual acuities of less than 3/60 are unlikely to be helped by optical aids. A lot of motivation is needed to persevere with low visual aids if the vision is very poor, as increasing the magnification means reducing both the distance at which the work is in focus and the field of view. It cannot be overemphasized that a strong, focused light like an anglepoise, directed at the reading material from behind the reader, can help dramatically (see Fig. 6.1).

For those in work, but experiencing problems because of their sight, a variety of aids can be provided by the Employment Services agency, ranging from a dictaphone to closed circuit television, following assessment at an approved centre. The same agency is also able to arrange work assessment for those having to change their work because of loss of sight.

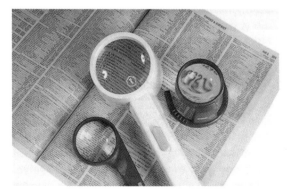

**Fig. 12.2** Various magnifiers may help the patient with poor central vision, and most patients with a macular problem find it possible to read a little, even if the process is laborious.

## Registration as blind or partially sighted

This can be initiated by the poorly sighted themselves, their relatives, GP, health visitors and social workers, but in most cases the suggestion is likely to come from a doctor in the eye clinic, on noticing that a patient's vision has deteriorated to the appropriate level (Table 12.1). Ideally, the pros and cons of registration should be discussed by the patient with an experienced social worker before going ahead. Registration, which is entirely voluntary, is by form BD8, filled in by a consultant ophthalmologist. Copies go to the patient, their GP, the social services department for their area and the Office of Population and Censuses.

After registration, a social worker (sometimes a specialist) will visit the registered person at home, assess what assistance can usefully be offered and provide practical help with daily living skills, mobility training and modification of the home environment. The greatest benefit is to be had by improving lighting. People can be surprisingly reluctant to abandon their 40 watt bulbs! Braille in particular is quite difficult to learn and not an advantage to many people nowadays.

**Table 12.1** Registration of visual handicap

*Initiated by*
Patient, relative
GP, health visitor, social worker
Hospital ophthalmic service

*Completion of form BD8 by consultant ophthalmologist*

*Rehabilitation officer*
Daily living skills
Mobility training
Home modification
Braille and touch-typing

*Benefits and concessions*
Tax allowance
Free sight test and low vision assessment
Rail, bus and parking concessions
Disability living allowance for over age 65
Disability working allowance for under age 65

*Voluntary agencies*
Clubs and holidays
Royal National Institute for the Blind
Guide Dogs for the Blind
'In Touch' help line
Self-help groups

**Table 12.2** Guidelines for registration

*As partially sighted*
6/18–6/60 binocular, depending on visual field

*As blind*
Worse than 3/60 with a full visual field
Better than 3/60 with a restricted visual field

## Requirements for blind registration
(Table 12.2)

Although certification is defined as appropriate if a person is 'so blind that they cannot do any work for which eyesight is essential', guidelines are laid down (fortunately!):

• Visual acuity below 3/60 in the better eye (i.e. patient must stand at 3 metres to be able to read the top letter on the 6-metre chart).
• Visual acuity above 3/60 with a very contracted field of vision, especially in the lower field.

## Requirements for partially sighted registration

There is no legal definition of partial sight, but the following guidelines have been laid down:

• Visual acuity between 3/60 and 6/60 with full field in the better eye.
• Visual acuity up to 6/24 with moderate field loss.
• Visual acuity of 6/18 or even better with gross field defect such as hemianopia or retinitis pigmentosa.

Note that a patient with one blind eye is not eligible as the good eye exceeds the requirements.

> There is no 'blind pension'

## Benefits and concessions for registered blind and partially sighted people

Contrary to popular belief, there is no 'blind pension'. The following list gives some of the more important benefits. The help of an experienced welfare rights worker would be an essential to guide anyone, not just the visually handicapped, through the forest of forms that is required to claim benefits.

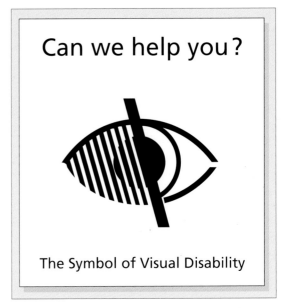

**Fig. 12.3** Partially Sighted Society symbol of visual disability.

• Special personal income tax allowance (blind only).
• Some exemptions from deductions from Income Support (blind only).
• Parking concessions (blind only).
• A tiny discount on the television licence (blind only).
• Free NHS sight test and low vision aids through the hospital eye service.
• Railcards and bus passes.

A Disability Living Allowance for care and/or mobility may be available for the blind person under the age of 65, including children. Allowances are not usually given to those over 65 whose only handicap is poor vision, but those both blind and deaf would qualify. The Disability Working Allowance is a means-tested benefit for those in low-paid employment, designed to 'top-up' their income. Both blind and partially sighted should qualify.

**Voluntary help** (Fig. 12.3)

Voluntary organizations run clubs, where activities can use skills that give satisfaction to the individual. These clubs tend to cater mostly for an elderly clientele and younger visually handicapped people are less well provided for. Holidays may be organized. Local voluntary groups are also, increasingly, taking on the provision of high-quality information.

The Royal National Institute for the Blind (RNIB) provides a large number of services, including information on benefits, braille and cassette libraries, as well as running its famous 'Talking Book' service. This last is available to anyone with near vision of N12 or less. Social services departments may help with the subscription.

Guide Dogs for the Blind can be approached directly by interested people but remember that not all blind people can manage or wish to care for a dog. Assessment for suitability can be arranged with the charity. They impose no age limit. Self-help groups exist for many ocular conditions. The weekly BBC Radio 4 programme (*In Touch*) makes good listening for anyone, but especially those for whom it is intended.

## Visual handicap in children

Visually handicapped children are a very mixed group, the size of which cannot be accurately determined because of the difficulties inherent in measuring visual function in children. Also, as many as 50% of poorly sighted children may have multiple handicaps, especially mental handicap, which make the poor vision comparatively unobtrusive. Up to 25% of visually handicapped children may not have an established diagnosis.

Criteria for blind and partially sighted registration of older children is the same as for adults. Unless obviously blind, registration of young children as partially sighted is encouraged. The 1989 Children Act, now in force, requires local authorities to provide such help as is necessary for any child to grow up as normally as possible, with an obligation to assess needs and provide services to meet these needs.

**Table 12.3** Help for visually handicapped children

Pre-school peripatetic teacher
Low vision aid assessment and optical aids
Specialist resource teacher in school
Special schools
Self-help groups
Disability Living Allowance

The primary purpose of the registration of children is for the identification of their need for special help with education (Table 12.3). This should start as early as possible, with a peripatetic teacher visiting the home, recommending toys and pointing out ways that parents can show their poorly sighted child all the things that other children absorb effortlessly. If necessary, the RNIB can put parents in touch with qualified specialist teachers. Later on, if the child is able to attend an ordinary school, a specialist resource teacher should be available to back-up the class teacher. Special supplies and equipment must also be provided. Low vision assessment is started as early as possible and appropriate glasses and magnifiers provided. Some blind children will need to attend a special school. Parents' support groups, based regionally, but with a national federation, are growing in number, as are self-help groups linked to eye conditions, such as the Albino Fellowship.

> In children, early identification of poor sight enables early provision of specialized help

## Requirements for driving

### Ordinary driving licences

The standard is the ability to read, in good daylight, a number plate with glasses or contact lenses if worn, at 20.5 metres (67 feet). There is no precise Snellen equivalent: a near approximation is 6/9 minus 2 letters. A full binocular visual field is needed—at least 120 degrees within the horizontal and at least 20 degrees width above and below the horizontal, measured by kinetic perimetry to a standard target (see Fig. 12.1). Patients are entitled

**Table 12.4** Visual acuity requirements for professional and vocational driving

*New applicants*
3/60 uncorrected in each eye separately
6/9 corrected in the better eye
6/12 corrected in the worse eye

*Renewing applicants*
3/60 uncorrected in each eye separately
6/12 corrected in the better eye
6/36 corrected in the worse eye

> Driving requirements (ordinary licence):
> • visual acuity, equivalent to Snellen 6/9–2 (number plate at 20.5 m)
> • full visual field within 120° horizontal, 20° vertical above and below fixation

to drive (but not vocationally) with one normally sighted eye but will need a period of adaptation before they feel safe to judge distances.

Diplopia, if insuperable, is a bar to driving; but if it is of 3 months' duration and correctable with a prismatic lens, or avoided by an eye patch, driving is allowed, so long as the prism or patch is worn. Colour vision defects are not a bar to driving. Night blindness precludes driving.

Progressive conditions such as glaucoma, high myopia, cataract and diabetic retinopathy all need to be notified to the DVLC. A licence lasting 1–3 years will then be issued.

### Professional and vocational driving licences
Any pathological field defect, insuperable diplopia or monocular vision is a bar to a vocational licence. This includes Large Goods Vehicle (LGV), Passenger Carrying Vehicle (PCV) (previously HGV and PSV), taxi and car hire licences. Professional driving is defined as being employed to drive.

The requirements for visual acuity are shown in Table 12.4. Glasses or contact lenses can be worn; in which case acuity is described as corrected.

## Occupational requirements
The following employers make variably stringent demands on standards of unaided visual acuity and colour vision in their recruits:
• Royal Navy, Army and Royal Air Force.
• Civil Aviation Authority and Merchant Navy.
• Royal National Lifeboat Institution.
• Rail authorities.
• Police (varies between different forces).
• Fire services.

# Appendix 1 **Formulary for eye care in general practice**

This section details the medications that are most useful to the non-specialist and describes their use and any problems. It is a basic choice—others are described in the relevant chapter of the *British National Formulary*. The preparations most likely to be used are marked by an asterisk.

## Formulations and application

### Patient information leaflets
Leaflets describing the techniques for giving eye medications may be available via some pharmacies, within or outside eye departments. An example is given in Fig. A1.1.

### Drops
These act at the surface of the eye and diffuse into the anterior chamber. Their advantages are speed of action, good vision after use, good cosmetic effect and a reasonably measured dose. Their disadvantages are that they may need to be used frequently, they are not useful for prolonged action at night, and they may sting or irritate the eye surface. Some patients develop allergy to the medication or to preservative in the drop.

The pharmacist will dispense a prescription for drops when written as such or as **guttae** or **gutt**. ('drop' in Latin).

Drops are instilled from a plastic dropper bottle. This is not difficult, but may need initial practice (Fig. A1.2). The patient tips his head back, looking upwards. One hand pulls down the lower eyelid, making a sac. The other (usually right) hand can be steadied on the nose or cheek, holds the bottle tip downwards and squeezes a drop into the sac. Ideally, the bottle tip should be close to, but not touching, the eye surface. Elderly patients, particularly those with poor vision or arthritis, may have difficulty. They should ask the pharmacist if they could be supplied with a special dropper device. Some may need another person to instil drops.

The dose from a single drop is fairly standardized, and only one drop at a time is needed. The total daily dose is determined by the concentration of drop chosen and the frequency of use. If more than one drop arrives by mistake the excess will spill onto the cheek, so it is difficult to overdose. If more than one sort of drop is used at one time the patient should wait until the first has dispersed before applying the next—perhaps about 3 minutes or so. There is no incompatibility problem with eye drops.

After an emergency visit or minor operation the patient will often have the eye padded, but may also be instructed to use drops quite frequently. If so the pad should be removed, but should be replaced as instructed, though it does not have to be changed each time.

In babies and young children it may be difficult to prise the eyes open to give the drop. Rather than struggle, it may be better to lie the child down and put the drop into the inner corner of the closed eye (Fig. A1.3). The child will eventually open the eye, maybe reluctantly, but as long as the child can be persuaded to keep lying down until then, enough of the drop will trickle in.

Drops do drain away from the eye surface into the nose and throat, so they are swallowed. Some drops can have an appreciable systemic effect, particularly if used often. Some taste unpleasant. A few practical points to remember when using eye drops are given in Table A1.1.

### Ointments
These also act at the eye surface, and their medications diffuse into the anterior chamber. Their advantages are a more prolonged action, particu-

# How to use your eye medication

## Drops

- In order to keep the drops clean, do not allow the dropper tip to touch the eye or anything else
- DO NOT allow other people to use your eye drops
- Discard eye drops after 1 month

### Application

1 Sit or lie comfortably with head tilted backwards looking at the ceiling

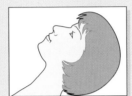

2 Gently pull down the lower lid with one finger to form a sac

3 Holding the eye drops in your hand, bring the dropper close to the eye and squeeze one drop into the sac

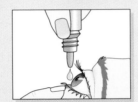

4 Close the eye and blot excess solution with a clean tissue

5 Replace the cap of the eye drops immediately after use

## Ointment

- A small amount of ointment should be squeezed out and discarded immediately before every application to ensure sterility
- Discard eye ointment after 1 month

### Application

1 With head in fairly upright position, gently pull down the lower lid with one finger to form a sac

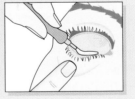

2 Squeeze a 1 cm ribbon of ointment into the sac formed

3 Close the eye and very gently massage with with a tissue to spread the ointment

**Fig. A1.1**  Patient information sheet: applying eye medication.

**Table A1.1**  Practical points about eye drops

Drops sting less when warm — they should be carried in a pocket
Drops should be discarded after 1 month of use
More than one drop will do no harm
A few minutes should be allowed between drops

larly useful at night, and less tendency to stinging with more lubrication. Disadvantages include blurring of vision, which may persist for quite a long time after application, and a sticky appearance which some patients find cosmetically unacceptable. The dose is less accurate than with drops. Ointment is the preparation to choose for eyelid conditions, as it is easier to apply and longer

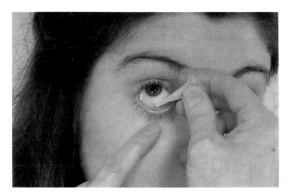

**Fig. A1.2** Method for giving eye drops to the everted lower lid.

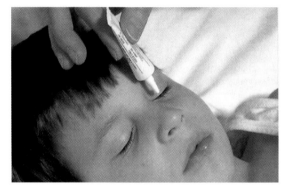

**Fig. A1.3** Giving ointment to the inner corner of the closed eye in a child reluctant to open the eye. (Drops can be given in a similar way with the child lying down.)

lasting. It also softens lid crusts. Ointment that spills into the eye will do no harm, but should be minimized in patients with dry eyes or inflamed lids. Allergy to ointment base is not uncommon.

Ointment is prescribed as such or as **occulenta**, usually abbreviated to **occ**. in hospital departments (Latin for 'ointment').

The technique for giving ointment to the eye itself is similar to that for drops (Fig. A1.1). About 1 cm is the usual dose. If the ointment is stiff at room temperature the tube may be warmed a little before use, in the hand or in warm water. Ointment applied to the eyelids may be rubbed in gently with a cotton-wool bud.

Systemic effects from ointment are not seen in practice, probably because more is absorbed locally and less swallowed.

## Lotions

Patients often ask about lotions for 'bathing' their eyes. Commercial preparations are not recommended because of the risk of transmitting infection. If eyes are crusty, the best lotion is freshly boiled and cooled tapwater. If the eyelids are inflamed, a large pinch of bicarbonate of soda or of salt added to a cupful of this water may be helpful. It should be emphasized that the solution must be freshly prepared and not stored.

## Other formulations

Some preparations are marketed in a viscous base to try and combine the advantages of drops and ointment. In practice, these are poorly tolerated as they also compound the problems.

Occasionally, in a hospital department, drugs may be given by local injection around the eye either subconjunctivally or to the retrobulbar space. Such methods in experienced hands are less hazardous than they sound, and they do not usually upset the patients unduly.

Systemic treatment may be needed for certain infections or for conditions affecting the inner eye, as topical treatment penetrates poorly in the posterior chamber, retina and choroid. In most cases this will be managed in a hospital clinic setting, as the eye response must be monitored carefully.

## Medication in contact lens wearers

It is usually advisable for the patient to stop wearing contact lenses for the duration of a short course of topical treatment. For longer term use, most drops are compatible with rigid lens wear, but not with soft lenses. The soft lens absorbs some of the constituents of drops, and this may be a hazard to the eye or to the lens. One classic novice eye casualty officer's mistake is to give fluorescein to a soft lens wearer without first removing the lens, which turns a brilliant fluorescent green. Although this may be removed by hydrogen peroxide solution or by soaking in several changes of saline for about 1 hour, the patient is usually not amused. Lens wear is not usually successful with ointments, which cause smearing of vision, though they may be tolerated at night if the lenses are removed first. The solutions used for cleaning and disinfecting contact lenses are not available on prescription, but should be bought at a pharmacy and advice about preparations should be given by the lens practitioner who dispensed the lenses.

## Preservatives and minims

Most drop and ointment preparations for eye use are dispensed in quantities suitable for 1 month or less. If used for longer, there is a risk that the preparation itself may become contaminated with organisms, particularly *Pseudomonas*, and patients should be advised not to use time-expired eye medications. All preparations contain preservative to delay this process, except for minims. These are single-dose drop containers prepared without preservative (see Fig. 2.20). They are most useful for diagnostic purposes—dilating drops, topical anaesthetics and fluorescein—but may also be prescribed for patients who are truly intolerant of preservatives. Once opened, they should be discarded after use.

## Side-effects

### Allergic reactions to eye medication

Topical treatments carry the risk of inducing sensitization of the conjunctiva and surrounding skin (see Fig. 5.18). Not all patients will have a history of previous allergy. Some agents carry a high risk, including neomycin preparations and atropine-like dilating drops. The prime symptoms are itching, swelling and redness particularly below the eyes, with characteristic wrinkling and scaling of the skin.

### Systemic effects of absorbed eye medication

These are uncommon. The most common is with topical beta-blockers, e.g. timolol, used for chronic glaucoma, which may cause or worsen asthma or bradycardia. Topical cyclopentolate is used with caution in babies, as there is a slight risk of mild transient encephalopathic symptoms if too much is absorbed. In general, babies have underdeveloped lacrimal drainage, so systemic effects are rare, though chloramphenicol should be used only in short courses.

## Anti-infective preparations

### Topical antibiotics

#### Chloramphenicol*

Eye drops 0.5%, eye ointment 1%. These are a standard first choice for simple conjunctivitis at any age, and for blepharitis, as chloramphenicol has a broad spectrum of activity. There are no contraindications, and it is well tolerated. Worries about an association with aplastic anaemia proved to be unfounded. Allergy is very rare. It is also the choice for prophylactic treatment after corneal abrasion or for a poorly closing eye, as with a facial palsy. The non-proprietary preparations are inexpensive.

Drops given by day and ointment at night is the usual regime. For an acute infection, drops should be given hourly for the first day, then every 3–4 hours for a few days.

Other topical antibacterial agents have little to recommend them against chloramphenicol. Many, particularly neomycin, are prone to cause local allergic reactions.

#### Tetracycline hydrochloride

Ointment five times daily for 4 weeks in addition to systemic treatment (see below) is recommended for proven chlamydial conjunctivitis.

#### Gentamicin sulphate

Drops and ointment are second-line treatment for acute bacterial infections, but should only be necessary for certain unusual conditions, particularly if *Pseudomonas* infection is suspected. The preparations may cause local irritation (see Fig. 5.4). Patients with acute infective conditions that have not responded to chloramphenicol should be referred for hospital assessment rather than delay by changing antimicrobial agent. It may be necessary to culture organisms in such cases.

#### Antibacterial/corticosteroid combinations

These should only be prescribed for certain specific conditions, including marginal ulcers, which should be diagnosed and managed using the slit-lamp.

## Systemic antibiotics

Systemic antimicrobial treatment may be needed in certain conditions. Infection of the internal eye—endophthalmitis—usually follows injury or surgery and requires urgent systemic treatment in a hospital setting. Lid and orbital cellulitis should also be referred promptly to a specialist (see Acute swelling around the eye, pp. 96 and 98).

### Flucloxacillin sodium

Capsules, 250 mg four times daily for 5–7 days, is one possible first-line treatment for infection of an *abcess of a meibomian cyst, cellulitis of the lid in a patient over the age of 3 years*, or acute infection of *the lacrimal sac* (use erythromycin for those hypersensitive to penicillin).

### Tetracyclines

Oral tetracycline hydrochloride, 250 mg four times daily for 2 weeks, or doxycycline hydrochloride, 100 mg daily for 10 days, is recommended for *adult chlamydial conjunctivitis*. Systemic treatment eliminates the organism from all sites, and there is a lower incidence of relapse than after topical eye treatment alone, which should also be given (see above). Babies should be given oral erythromycin, 30 mg/kg daily in two to four divided doses for 3 weeks, combined with topical tetracycline as for adults.

### Amoxycillin

Suspension, 125 mg three times daily for 5 days, is the treatment of first choice for cellulitis of the lid in young patients (under the age of 3 years). The warnings about orbital cellulitis (see Acute swelling around the eye, p. 98) should be heeded.

### Benzylpenicillin

Gonococcal conjunctivitis should be treated systemically with benzylpenicillin and managed in a specialist setting.

### Cephalosporins

Oral cephalosporin or combined co-amoxiclav is first-line treatment for lid cellulitis in those under the age of 7 years. Parenteral cefuroxime or cefotaxime should be used for orbital cellulitis at any age or in lid cellulitis under the age of 7 years.

### Clindamycin

This is the agent of choice for active chorioretinal *Toxoplasma* infections. Its use should be supervised by an experienced ophthalmologist. There is a risk of causing pseudomembranous colitis. Systemic corticosteroids may also be needed.

## Tetanus vaccination

Either primary or booster injections may be given for penetrating eye injuries, particularly those involving an intraocular foreign body, soil or vegetation.

## Antiviral agents

### Acyclovir (aciclovir)*

Ointment is suitable for treatment of herpes simplex corneal infections, applied five times daily. Patients should be under slit-lamp observation. Topical acyclovir may also be needed in patients with zoster ophthalmicus with corneal involvement.

Oral acyclovir is often given to patients with zoster ophthalmicus, but if the cornea is involved topical treatment is also necessary, as oral treatment alone is not as effective.

## Anti-inflammatory preparations

### Corticosteroids

Topical corticosteroids as drops or ointment carry a significant risk of precipitating corneal herpes simplex infection and of raising the intraocular pressure. For this reason the preparations should be used with discretion unless slit-lamp supervision is available. If a course of treatment is prescribed, this should be for a limited period and medication should be tailed off rather than stopped suddenly, to avoid rebound inflammation. Systemic corticosteroids for internal ocular inflammation should be prescribed and monitored by a specialist.

### Hydrocortisone*

Ointment 0.5% or 1% may be useful for acute

worsening of blepharitis or of eyelid allergic reactions, but long-term use should be discouraged. If the lids are sticky, chloramphenicol should be added as a combined preparation. The incidence of side-effects from a short course applied to the eyelids is low.

*Prednisolone\**

Drops 0.5% are the preparation of choice for selected patients with marked episcleritis or allergic conjunctivitis. Treatment is usually started at four times daily and reduced progressively once the condition is controlled. As a rule of thumb, if treatment is needed for longer than 2 weeks, the patient should be referred to hospital. It should be noted that Pred Forte (prednisolone 1%) (Allergan, High Wycombe, UK) is a more potent preparation, equivalent to dexamethasone.

*Betamethasone*

Drops 0.1% are more potent than prednisolone 0.5%. Ointment is convenient for treating with a corticosteroid at night.

*Clobetasone*

Drops 0.1% are of intermediate potency and have less tendency to elevate intraocular pressure.

*Dexamethasone*

Drops 0.1% are the most potent and should be reserved for serious conditions best managed by an expert. Pred Forte (prednisolone 1%) is an alternative high potency preparation.

## Non-steroidal anti-inflammatory preparations

Non-steroidal anti-inflammatory drugs have no place in the management of uveitis or other internal ocular inflammation, though they are useful in some patients with scleritis.

*Flurbiprofen*

Flurbiprofen, 150–200 mg/day in divided doses, may be helpful in patients with scleritis. This is a potentially damaging condition which should be diagnosed and managed by a specialist.

## Anti-allergic preparations

### Antihistamines

These preparations are of limited value in ocular allergic reactions.

*Loratadine*

Loratadine 10 mg once daily can be helpful in hay fever.

*Levocabastine/emedastine*

Levocabastine and emedastine are recently developed topical antihistamines and likely to be much more useful than antazoline in seasonal and allergic conjunctivitis and may have some use in perennial allergic conjunctivitis.

*Antazoline*

Topical antihistamine drops, usually combined with a vasoconstrictor, may be helpful in controlling the symptoms in an acute attack, but have little long-term benefit and there may be rebound symptoms on stopping.

### Sodium cromoglycate\*

Sodium cromoglycate as drops may block mast cell degranulation locally in the conjunctiva. There is no effect on the established symptoms, but treatment is given as a prophylactic. The patient must understand that to be effective the drops must be used regularly and frequently every day, even if symptoms continue at first. Most patients need to start with drops four times a day, trying to reduce towards twice a day if this is effective. A frequent regime causes particular problems when treating schoolchildren. Formulations with a more viscous medium, attempting to reduce the frequency, have been poorly tolerated. It is worth trying a properly maintained course for 1 month in the first instance; the patient can then decide if the improvement in symptoms is worth the trouble of continuing regular medication. Occasionally, patients develop allergy to the preservatives in the preparation and so need preservative-free drops, though these are difficult to obtain.

Nedocromil and lodoxamide are newer mast cell stabilizers and worth trying if sodium cromoglycate is ineffective.

## Medications for the dry eye

### Hypromellose*
Drops are the best first-line measure. Their cost is lower than the standard prescription charge. They may be given as often as the patient finds helpful and contain no active medication, though they do contain preservative. Other formulations of artificial tear substitutes may be better tolerated, and it will be a process of trial and success to find which one the patient likes best.

### Polyvinyl alcohol (Liquifilm Tears)
The manufacturers (Allergan, High Wycombe, UK) have produced a preservative-free drop in unit dose packs of 30 for use by patients allergic to preservatives, in whom they may be worth the extra cost.

### Acetylcysteine
Combined with hypromellose (Ilube, Cusi (UK), Haslemere, UK), 5% drops used three to four times daily may help patients who have adherent mucus.

### Simple eye ointment: ('occ-simplex') or liquid paraffin ointment
Given regularly at night, these may help patients with frequent corneal erosions by acting as a lubricant for the eyelids in sleep. Daytime use of ointment in dry eyes should be avoided if possible, as it may make symptoms worse.

## Drugs acting on the pupil
Contraindications to the use of dilating drops are uncommon. They include acute neurological conditions, patients with an iris clip lens, and precipitation of acute angle closure glaucoma in a small number of susceptible patients with shallow chambers (see Diabetic eye screening, p. 145).

### Tropicamide 1%*
Drops in the form of minims are the choice for dilating the pupil for fundus examination. They act within 10–15 minutes (but may take longer in dark-eyed patients), and the effect lasts for a few hours. Patients should wait and drive only when they feel safe to do so, perhaps after 1–2 hours. They should be warned that reading may be blurred for several hours. Precipitation of acute glaucoma is rare due to the short time of action.

### Cyclopentolate 1%
Drops are useful in anterior uveitis, to dilate the pupil at night and to minimize mydriasis in the day, though they can act for up to 24 hours.

### Atropine 1%
Drops or ointment are useful for prolonged pupil dilatation in severe anterior uveitis or for refraction in children. *The use of atropine should be restricted to the hospital setting and avoided elsewhere.* Allergic eyelid reactions are quite common.

### Phenylephrine 10%
Drops will dilate the pupil weakly and are seldom used alone. Their routine use is also restricted by possible precipitation of arrhythmia or hypertension.

### Pilocarpine
Drops of various strengths constrict the pupil but have *no* effective action in reversing the effect of a dilating drop.

## Diagnostic agents

### Fluorescein*
Fluorescein for staining the tear-film is available as impregnated paper strips which should be moistened with tears or tapwater (see Fig. 2.5). These are easier to use than minims of solution, which tend to deliver too much. The dye shows up defects in the corneal epithelium (see Fig. 2.7).

Fluorescein plus a topical anaesthetic, e.g. minims lignocaine and fluorescein, are used for contact tonometry.

### Topical anaesthetics*
Drops such as minims oxybuprocaine hydrochloride (benoxinate) are useful for examining an eye with a painful corneal lesion, particularly in children, as they may make it possible to open the eye by reducing blepharospasm. *They should never*

*be prescribed for repeat use.* The patient should be warned that the drops sting for a few seconds and then the eye will be comfortable, but that the eye will be painful again as the effect wears off within an hour.

## Drugs to control intraocular pressure

Most of these will be prescribed and monitored by a hospital glaucoma clinic, and practice varies in different clinics. It is useful to know the more common agents prescribed:

• Beta-blockers, e.g. timolol 0.25% drops twice daily, are a common first-line treatment for chronic simple glaucoma. They may exacerbate bronchospasm or bradycardia by systemic absorption.

• Dorzolamide and brinzolamide are topical carbonic acid inhibitors; they are used twice daily as monotherapy or combined with a beta-blocker. Side-effects include a bitter taste and later onset blepharoconjunctivitis.

• Brimonidine is an $\alpha_2$-adrenergic agonist, used twice daily. Side-effects include dry mouth, stinging and allergy.

• Latanoprost is a prostaglandin analogue and is very effective in reducing intraocular pressure. It promotes the outflow of aqueous. It is used once daily, preferably at night. Side-effects are few, but include an increase in iris pigmentation and the growth of longer, thicker eyelashes.

• Miotics, e.g. pilocarpine, are less often used now. They may be of particular value in helping to control an attack of acute angle closure glaucoma. They have no role in trying to reverse the effects of dilating drops.

• Acetazolamide given intravenously has an important first-line use in acute angle closure attacks, though it is best to confirm this diagnosis at the slit-lamp before starting treatment, unless this would mean delay of over an hour. Given orally, it may be useful as an adjunct in the management of short-term and medium-term rises in ocular pressure of less dramatic degree.

# Appendix 2 **List of suppliers and charities**

## Suppliers

Sometimes pharmaceutical companies promote their products by means of torches, cobalt blue filters (for use with fluorescein), neurological pins or pin hole devices.

If you are unable to buy the items you need from a local supplier, the following companies may be able to help. They supply anything from a slit-lamp to a pin hole device.

Clement Clarke International Ltd, Edinburgh Way, Harlow, Essex CM20 2TT (Tel. 01279 414969, Fax 01279 635232, *www.clement-clarke.com*).

Keeler Ltd, Clewer Hill Road, Windsor, Berks SL4 4AA (Tel. 01753 857177, Fax 01753 857817, Email *info@keeler.co.uk*).

Ophthalmoscopes are supplied also by:

Welch Allyn UK Ltd, Aston Abbotts, Bucks HP22 4ND (Tel. 01296 682140, *www.welchallyn.com*).

Instruments for minor operations are supplied by:

John Weiss and Son Ltd, 89 Alston Drive, Bradwell Abbey, Milton Keynes, Bucks MK13 9HF (Tel. 01908 318017, Fax 01908 318708, Email *sales@johnweiss.com*).

## Consumables

Most of these are available through the local pharmacy or the wholesaler with whom the GP may have links. The local hospital CSSD may supply dressing packs and eyepads.

Prescribable items include:
- Therapeutic dilating drops, e.g. cyclopentolate hydrochloride 1% in dropper bottle form.
- Topical anaesthetic drops, ditto.
- Sutures (some).
- Sterile eye pad and bandage.
- Normal saline.
- Skin cleansing agents.
- Dressing packs.

Non-prescribable items must be bought:
- Fluorescein Fluorets.
- Minims, including tropicamide 1% dilating drops.

These are available from:

Chauvin Pharmaceuticals Ltd, Ashton Road, Harold Hill, Romford, Essex RM3 8SL (Tel. 01708 383838, Fax 01708 371316, *www.chauvingroup.com*).

## Charities associated with eyes and sight

Royal National Institute for the Blind (RNIB), 224 Great Portland Street, London W1N 6AA (Tel. 020 7388 1266, *www.rnib.org.uk*).

The Partially Sighted Society, P.O. Box 322, Doncaster, S. Yorks DN1 2XA (Tel. 01302 323132, Fax 01302 368998).

# Appendix 3  **Patient information sheet: applying a pad**

Part of the treatment that the doctor has ordered for you is to have your eye covered by an eye pad for 12/24* hours (* delete as necessary).

It is important that the pad is applied properly so that your eye remains closed underneath it at all times.

This will enable the scratch on the front of your eye to heal more quickly, as the healing process will not be interrupted by continual blinking. It will also make your eye feel more comfortable.

## Method

• First wash your hands. You will have been given two eye pads by the nurse. Fold one of the pads in half, like so (Fig. A3.1).

• Cut four pieces of micropore tape or ordinary sellotape, approximately 10 cm long, and keep to hand. Close your injured eye gently.

• Place the folded pad over the closed eye (the straight edge fits neatly under the eye brow) and secure it with a piece of tape down the centre (Fig. A3.2).

• Place the unfolded pad over the top and keep it in place with a piece of tape down the centre of the pad.

• Apply the other two pieces of tape either side to secure the pad firmly, thus keeping the eye closed underneath (Fig. A3.3).

• Whilst you are wearing an eye pad you will find that your perception of depth and distance will have altered; therefore, it is essential that you *do not*:

    (a) drive;

    (b) operate any machinery;

    (c) climb ladders/scaffolding, for your own safety, and the safety of others.

• Remove the pad 12/24 hours* after application (* delete as necessary).

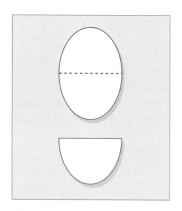

Fig. A3.1

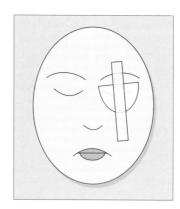

Fig. A3.2

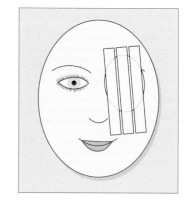

Fig. A3.3

# Appendix 4 **Patient information sheet: blepharitis**

This is an inflammatory condition affecting the margins of the eyelids. The cause is often unknown. Prolonged treatment may be required before it is effective and the condition may recur.

## Signs and symptoms
Red, inflamed eye lids, crusting around the eye lashes with itching and discomfort.

## Treatment
Using bicarbonate of soda, make up a solution with a large pinch of bicarbonate of soda in a small teacup of boiled, cooled water.

## Method
• With a clean cotton-wool bud dipped in the freshly prepared solution, massage the base of the eye lashes to dislodge all crusting. Use at least one bud for each eyelid.
• This treatment should be performed every morning and evening unless otherwise instructed by the doctor.
• Pretreatment with a hot compress may be helpful; using a clean face flannel wrung out in hot tapwater, hold to the eyelids for 1 minute.

# Glossary of terms used in ophthalmology

This section is intended to define terms and explain jargon. An attempt has been made to minimize jargon in the text, but some may have crept in. This list may also be helpful in interpreting information from an optometrist or ophthalmologist.

**accommodation** focus for near, when the ciliary muscle contracts the suspensory fibres to the lens relax and the lens becomes rounder.

**ALT** argon laser trabeculoplasty, in which the argon laser is used to make several small holes in the aqueous drainage area to assist in reducing eye pressure.

**amaurosis** blindness.

**amaurosis fugax** 'fleeting blindness', usually describing transient marked loss of vision in one eye.

**amblyopia** sometimes called 'lazy eye', meaning an eye that has developed reduced vision as a consequence of a fault in early life, e.g. error in focus or squint. In old literature, may mean poor vision from any cause.

**angle** the zone in the recess of the front chamber where aqueous drains.

**anisocoria** inequality of pupil size.

**anterior chamber** the front cavity between the cornea and lens/iris.

**anterior uveitis** inflammation within the front chamber, synonymous with **iritis**.

**aphakia** absence of the lens, usually surgical.

**aqueous** watery fluid filling the front chamber.

**ARMD** age-related macular degeneration.

**astigmatism** uneven focus, usually due to an irregular cornea.

**blepharitis** inflammation of the eyelid margin.

**BR** blind register.

**bulbar** of the eyeball.

**buphthalmos** a form of glaucoma found in childhood when the eye tends to enlarge.

**canthus** inner or outer angle of the eyelids.

**cataract** lens opacity.

**CFS** counting fingers vision—less than 6/60 but better than hand movements.

**chalazion** meibomian cyst.

**ciliary injection** redness of the blood vessels on the eyeball near the margin of the cornea.

**chemosis** swelling due to collection of fluid beneath the conjunctiva.

**colloid bodies** pale lesions within the retina, usually a sign of ageing.

**CSG** chronic simple glaucoma.

**cupping** abnormal enlargement of the central cup in the optic nerve head.

**cycloplegic** agent that dilates the pupil and paralyses accommodation.

**dacryoadenitis** inflammation (usually infective) of the tear gland.

**dacryocystitis** inflammation (usually infective) of the tear sac.

**dendritic** 'branch-like', usually referring to the characteristic pattern of herpes simplex corneal ulceration.

**dioptre** a measure of focusing strength of a lens.

**diplopia** double vision, which may be binocular (only with both eyes open) or monocular (persisting with one eye open).

**disc** optic nerve head visible with the ophthalmoscope.

**drüsen** *see* colloid bodies.

**ectropion** eyelid margin pulled away from the eyeball.

**endophthalmitis** inflammation (usually infection) of the internal eye.

**entropion** eyelid margin turned in towards the eyeball.

**enucleation** removal of the eyeball.

**epiphora** overflowing tears, watering of the eye.

**erosion** spontaneous renewal of a site of previous abrasion or ulceration, usually on the cornea.

**exophthalmos** *see* proptosis.

**exudate** pale shiny retinal lesions related to leakage of plasma and characteristic especially of diabetic retinopathy in which they may be arranged in a circular ('circinate') pattern.

**follicle** pale lump made up of a collection of white cells in the conjunctiva.

**fornix** recess of conjunctiva between the lid and the upper and lower eyeball.

**fovea** small point of fixation and maximum sensitivity in the retina, at the centre of the macula.

**fundus** interior of the back chamber visible with the ophthalmoscope.

**glaucomas** group of conditions in which eye pressure damages nerve fibres within the optic nerve head.

**globe** eyeball.

**guttae** or **gutt.** Latin and its shorthand for drops.

**high myopia** short-sightedness greater than about 10 dioptres.

**HMS** hand movements vision—worse than counting fingers but better than perception of light.

**homonymous** meaning 'same side', refers to the visual field defect characteristic of a disorder behind the optic chiasm.

**hordeolum** stye or inflammation of a lash follicle.

**hypermetropia** far-sightedness or long-sightedness, being able to see more clearly at distance.

**hyphaema** blood in the front chamber which has sedimented at the bottom.

**hypopyon** white cells in the front chamber which have sedimented at the bottom.

**injection** refers to reddening of the eye surface.

**interpalpebral** between the eyelids when the eye is open.

**IOFB** intraocular foreign body.

**IOL** intraocular lens implant.

**IOP** intraocular pressure.

**iridotomy** making a hole in the iris, either surgically or by laser.

**keratitis** inflammation of the cornea.

**kerato** referring to the cornea.

**keratoplasty** corneal graft or refashioning the shape of the cornea, usually for optical purposes.

**KP** keratic precipitates of white cells on the interior surface of the cornea, as in iritis.

**laser** acronym of light amplification by the stimulated emission of radiation.

**LASIK** laser-assisted *in situ* keratomileusis. A technique to refashion the corneal contour for refractive purposes.

**limbus** zone where the cornea meets the conjunctiva, which coincides with the edge of visible iris.

**loupe** small magnifying aid.

**macula** usually refers to the area of retina bounded by the major branch vessels temporal to the optic nerve head. The fovea is at its centre. Sometimes the term is used to refer to the fovea itself.

**media** clear parts of the eye—tears, cornea, aqueous, lens, vitreous.

**metamorphopsia** distortion of central vision, particularly if straight lines look bent.

**miosis** constriction of the pupil.

**monocular** one eye.

**mydriasis** dilatation of the pupil.

**mydriatic** drug that dilates the pupil.

**myopia** short-sightedness or near-sightedness, being able to see more clearly when close (*see* high myopia).

**NPL** no perception of light vision. A completely blind eye, unable to detect a bright light and so worse than 'PL'. There are relatively few causes.

**nystagmus** repetitive to-and-fro movements of the eye in a variety of patterns.

**occulenta** or **occ.** Latin and its shorthand for ointment.

**OD** *oculus dexter* meaning the right eye (RE).

**optometrist** relatively new title for the professional who was formerly titled an ophthalmic optician.

**OS** *oculus sinister* meaning the left eye (LE).

**oscillopsia** sensation that stationary objects are moving.

**orbit** bony cone behind the eyeball.

**pannus** scarring containing blood vessels at the periphery of the cornea.

**papillary** pattern of red lumps suggesting inflammation around small blood vessels in the conjunctiva.

**PC** posterior capsule of the lens. Sometimes post-operative thickening is treated using the argon laser.

**phaco** referring to the lens.

**'phaco'** phaco-emulsification, technique for removing cataract through a small incision.

**PL** perception of light vision. Worse than hand movements but better than no perception of light.

**posterior chamber** back cavity between the lens and retina. If the lens has been removed, this means behind the iris.

**presbyopia** loss of focusing ability for near due to normal ageing of the lens.

**proptosis** protrusion of the eyeball, usually because of pressure behind it in the orbit.

**PS** posterior synechiae, adhesions between the iris and lens that occur in iritis.

**pseudophakia** presence of an artificial lens implant.

**PSR** partially sighted register.

**ptosis** drooping of the upper eyelid.

**punctate** in a pattern of small dots.

**PVD** posterior vitreous detachment, when the vitreous shrinks and pulls away from the retina.

**RAPD** relative afferent pupil defect in which the pupil reacts to bright light in an asymmetrical way. Implies a disorder of the eye or optic nerve on one side.

**red reflex** illumination of the pupil by light reflected from the retina.

**refraction** bending of light rays. Also used for the testing of focusing ability.

**retrobulbar** behind the eyeball.

**rubeosis** formation of abnormal new blood vessels on the iris or in the aqueous drainage angle. May lead to glaucoma.

**scotoma** area of loss of vision within the seeing field, e.g. the blind spot.

**Snellen chart** standard chart for measuring distance vision.

**STFB** subtarsal foreign body.

**strabismus** squint.

**tarsal** referring to the eyelid.

**tarsorrhaphy** stitching together the eyelids, either partially or completely.

**tonometry** measurement of internal eye pressure by externally applied pressure.

**trabeculectomy** operation for glaucoma, to improve drainage of aqueous and lower eye pressure.

**trichiasis** turning in of eyelashes so that they damage the eye surface.

**uvea** literally 'a grape', refers to pigmented tissues, including the iris, ciliary body and choroid, external to the retina.

**uveitis** inflammation of any part of the uvea. Anterior, of the iris and ciliary body (as in iritis or iridocyclitis). Posterior, of the choroid (choroiditis). Pan, of all parts.

**VA** visual acuity. Sometimes recorded separately as RVA (right visual acuity) and LVA (left visual acuity), which may be recorded as just RV and LV. If 'UA' also appears, this refers to 'unaided' vision, without glasses.

**visual acuity** sharpness of vision.

**vitrectomy** removal of the vitreous, replacing with clear fluid.

**vitreous** 'glass-like' jelly filling the back chamber behind the lens.

**vitreous haemorrhage** bleeding into the vitreous jelly, which originates from the retina.

# Index